A Note on the Author

GERMAINE GREER is an Australian academic and journalist, and a major feminist voice of the mid-twentieth century. She gained her PhD from the University of Cambridge in 1967. She is Professor Emerita of English Literature and Comparative Studies at the University of Warwick. Greer's ideas have created controversy ever since *The Female Eunuch* became an international bestseller in 1970. She is the author of many other books including *Sex and Destiny: The Politics of Human Fertility* (1984); *Shakespeare's Wife* (2007); *The Whole Woman* (1999) and *White Beech* (2014).

THE CHANGE

Women, Ageing and the Menopause

GERMAINE GREER

FULLY REVISED AND UPDATED

BLOOMSBURY PUBLISHING

LONDON • OXFORD • NEW YORK • NEW DELHI • SYDNEY

BLOOMSBURY PUBLISHING
Bloomsbury Publishing Plc
50 Bedford Square, London, WC1B 3DP, UK

BLOOMSBURY, BLOOMSBURY PUBLISHING and the Diana logo are trademarks of
Bloomsbury Publishing Plc

First published in Great Britain 1991
Revised edition published 2018
This edition published 2019

Bloomsbury Publishing Plc does not have any control over, or responsibility for, any third-party
websites referred to in this book. All internet addresses given in this book were correct at the time
of going to press. The author and publisher regret any inconvenience caused if addresses have changed
or sites have ceased to exist, but can accept no responsibility for any such changes

A catalogue record for this book is available from the British Library

ISBN: TPB: 978-1-4088-8638-0; PB: 978-1-4088-8637-3; eBook: 978-1-4088-8639-7

2 4 6 8 10 9 7 5 3 1

Typeset by Newgen KnowledgeWorks Pvt. Ltd., Chennai, India
Printed and bound in Great Britain by CPI Group (UK) Ltd, Croydon CR0 4YY

To find out more about our authors and books visit www.bloomsbury.com
and sign up for our newsletters.

For Ann and Julia
(still)

Contents

Acknowledgements

The author and publishers thank the following publishers and literary representatives for permission to quote copyright material.

Elizabeth Bishop: to Farrar, Straus & Giroux, Inc. and Chatto & Windus for the poem 'One Art' from *Poems* (Chatto & Windus, 2011). Reproduced by permission of The Random House Group Ltd. © 2011

Helene Deutsch: to W. W. Norton & Co. for extracts from *Confrontations with Myself: An Epilogue* (1973); to the Institute of Psychoanalysis, London, for extracts from 'The Menopause' published in the *International Journal of Psycho-Analysis*, 65 (1984). Reprinted by permission of Curtis Brown Ltd, © Nigel Nicolson, 1931

Emily Dickinson: Harvard University Press for poems from *The Poems of Emily Dickinson*, edited by Thomas H. Johnson, Cambridge, Mass.: The Belknap Press of Harvard University Press, Copyright © 1951, 1955 by the President and Fellows of Harvard College. Copyright © renewed 1979, 1983 by the President and Fellows of Harvard College. Copyright © 1914, 1918, 1919, 1924, 1929, 1930, 1932, 1935, 1937, 1942 by Martha Dickinson Bianchi. Copyright © 1952, 1957, 1958, 1963, 1965 by Mary L. Hampson

Rosemary Dobson: to Curtis Brown (Aust) for an extract from 'Amy Caroline' from *Collected Poems*, © Rosemary Dobson, 1991

Barbara Evans: to Pan Macmillan for extracts from *Life Change: A Guide to the Menopause, Its Effects and Treatment*, 4th edition (1988). Reproduced with permission of the Licensor through PLSclear

Lillian Hellman: to Hachette Book Group for extracts from *An Unfinished Woman* (Penguin Books, 1973)

Elizabeth Jennings: to Pan Macmillan for the poem 'Let Things Alone' from *Relationships*; to David Higham Associates for the poems 'Growing' and 'Accepted' from *Growing-Points*

Doris Lessing: to Penguin Random House for extracts from *The Summer Before the Dark* (Jonathan Cape, 1973)

Patrick McGrady: to Weidenfeld & Nicolson, Ltd, for extracts from *The Youth Doctors* (Arthur Barker, 1979)

Ann Mankowitz: to Inner City Books, Toronto, for extracts from *Change of Life: A Psychological Study of Dreams and the Menopause* (1984)

Gabriel García Márquez: to Penguin Random House for extracts from *Love in the Time of Cholera* (1989)

Willa Muir: to Enitharmon Press for the poem 'Where is my love, my Dear' from *Laconics, Jingles & Other Verses* (1969)

Iris Murdoch: to Penguin Random House for extracts from *Bruno's Dream* (Vintage, 1987)

Linda Pastan: to W. W. Norton and the Jean V. Naggar Literary Agency for poems from *The Five Stages of Grief* (1978)

Margaret Powell: to David Higham Associates for extracts from *The Treasure Upstairs* (Peter Davies)

Vita Sackville-West: to Penguin Random House for extracts from *All Passion Spent* (L. & V. Woolf, 1931). Reprinted by permission of Curtis Brown Ltd, © Nigel Nicolson, 1931

Stevie Smith: to James MacGibbon for extracts from *The Collected Poems of Stevie Smith* (Penguin Books, 1985)

While every effort has been made to trace copyright holders, this has not been successful in all cases; any omissions brought to our attention will of course be remedied in future editions.

Introduction

The idea of eliminating menopause came not from women but from men who thought that the cessation of ovulation was a premature death, a tragedy. The years of the change are certainly difficult for some of us to traverse, so there have always been women who ask for help from male professionals during the climacteric. The help that was given was, at first, the only treatment doctors had for anything, namely bleeding and purging, accompanied by an array of ineffectual medications, some of which continued to be marketed at high prices for hundreds of years as Dr So-and-so's 'female pills', setting a pattern for the exploitation of the 'little health of ladies' that persists to this day. Next the learned gentlemen tried to reactivate menstruation from another site, by opening issues of blood; from this they proceeded to hysterectomy and castration, in the hope of correcting the mental derangements that were thought to accompany the decline of the catamenia, as the menstrual losses were called. No sooner had electricity been discovered than they began thrusting electrified rods into the uterus; one of the first uses for X-rays was to bombard the ovary with them and so kill it. Marie Curie had not long discovered radium before radium rods were being inserted in the vagina.

There was always another school of thought that held that the climacteric was in truth less stressful than other periods in the travailed female life course. As long as childbirth was unavoidable and dangerous, this was clearly true. Partly because there was a disproportionate number of virgins over the age of fifty, climacteric problems became associated with old maids, adding greatly to the prejudice against them and against menopause. By the mid-nineteenth century, public awareness of a menopausal syndrome was greatly complicating the problems that the middle-aged woman had no option but to face. The irrational certainty that the womb was the real cause of the ageing woman's anger or melancholy effectively obscured the inconvenient possibility that she had genuine grounds for feeling angry or sad. There was no shortage of women who obligingly internalised their own rage and produced a bewildering array of symptoms, many of which responded to hideous invasive procedures that can have had no genuine therapeutic function. Obstacles to negotiation of what is in fact a stressful stage in female life began to pile up, and menopausal distress accumulated around them.

In the guise of immense chivalrous sympathy for women destroyed by the tragedy of menopause, a group of male professionals permitted themselves to give full vent to an irrational fear of old women, which I have called, from the Latin *anus*, meaning old woman, anophobia. These are the men whose names continue to appear on hundreds of learned papers every year, elaborating the possibilities of eliminating menopause and keeping all women both appetising and responsive to male demand from puberty to the grave, driving the dreaded old woman off the face of the earth for ever.

There are positive aspects to being a frightening old woman. Though the old woman is both feared and reviled, she need not take the intolerance of others to heart, for women over fifty already form one of the largest groups in the population structure of the Western world. As long as they like themselves, they will not be an oppressed minority. In order to like themselves they must reject trivialisation by others of who and what they are. A grown woman should not have to masquerade as a girl in order to remain in the land of the living. Capitulation to pressure to do just that has resulted in a gallery of grotesques whose gallant refusals to age are the staple of our gossip magazines. The most spectacular of these was the late Doña María del Rosario Cayetana Fitz-James Stuart y de Silva, 18th Duchess of Alba de Tormes. A series of phantasmagoric cosmetic operations had radically changed her appearance before, in October 2011, aged eighty-five and with a valve installed in her brain in an effort to slow down her mental decline, she made 61-year-old Alfonso Diez her third husband. The wedding was recorded for posterity in photographs of the Duchess dancing a barefoot flamenco at the wedding. Diez, who had signed a prenuptial agreement renouncing any claim to a share in her £2.2 billion fortune, was by her side when she died in November 2014.

There have always been women who ignored the eternal youth bandwagon and agreed to grow up, who negotiated the climacteric with a degree of independence and dignity and changed their lives to give their new adulthood space to function and flower. In a childish world this behaviour is seen as threatening. Nobody knows what to do with a woman who is not perpetually smiling and fawning. Calm, grave, quiet women drive anophobes to desperation. Women who refuse even to try to empower the penis are old bats and old bags, crones, mothers-in-law, castrating women and so forth. Though female culture cannot afford to give such attitudes even token respectability, we could see our way to exploit male panic if we dared. As women are the arbiters of birth, they are also the managers of death, within the womb and out of it. They have the spiritual resources to confront and deal with both, but men are terrified to leave such matters in their hands.

This is one book that seeks neither to trivialise nor to medicalise the menopause. The climacteric is a mysterious time about which sinister myths continue to cling. It is not illuminated by the proliferation of pronouncements defining it by the Masters in Menopause, those male professionals who with the willing assistance of the pharmaceutical multinationals have made a lucrative career out of an experience they will never undergo. It is a continuing aspect of the menopause industry that the women practitioners who allow themselves to become involved seldom corroborate either the evidence for massive derangement of female faculties during the climacteric or the miraculous results of the administration of extracts of mares' urine.

Though there is no public rite of passage for the woman approaching the end of her reproductive years, there is evidence that women devise their own private ways of marking the irrevocability of the change.

The climacteric is a time of stock-taking, of spiritual as well as physical change, and it would be a pity to be unconscious of it. Certainly many women do not seek medical help for climacteric distress, but this has more to do with their attitude to doctors and their coping style than with the extent to which they experience symptoms. It is probable, however, that menopausal symptoms are becoming objectively more serious as a result of pre-menopausal medical intervention, especially sterilisation and hysterectomy, and of the pressure to keep young, fit and beautiful if you want to be loved, and of addiction and of environmental poisons. There is a proportion of women who suffer unbearable symptoms during the climacteric but the unluckiest ones are the ones who undergo destructive procedures, sometimes a series of destructive procedures, to eliminate disorders that time and patience would have dealt with unaided.

In most medical literature addressed to women there is a tendency to exaggerate the extent to which women have brought their difficulties upon themselves. Arguments based upon the assumption that women are in control of their own lives and get the menopause they deserve simply absolve the practitioner of any obligation or responsibility. Many women only realise during the climacteric how little of what has happened to them in their lives has actually been in their interest. Women discovering for the first time that they are actually poor, dependent, insecure and lonely don't need to be burdened with a weight of guilt as well. They do need, on the other hand, to take the control of their own lives that is now available by default. To be unwanted is also to be free.

The fifth climacteric is the time when a woman plans the rest of her life; if she has not the financial resources, the education or the energy, it is not too late to acquire them. If she approaches this challenge in apologetic mode, haunted by guilt or by fears of psychological inadequacy, she cannot make the decisions upon which her future happiness depends. She must reject any argument that holds that she has brought her present distress upon herself. On the other hand, if she persists in imagining that control of her life is exercised from outside herself, she will not achieve well-being. She will go down into darkness as a complaining, querulous, naughty, old, girl.

Whatever her temporary discomforts, the menopausal woman has eventually to confront the problem of ageing. Again medical science can give her very little help. Ageing is the most idiosyncratic of all human processes and predictions cannot be made about any individual's ageing career. Still, the wise woman can decide to age no faster than she absolutely must. This may involve her in drastic alterations of lifestyle and complete reordering of priorities. Some of the crutches she has been using will have to be kicked away. Bad habits will have to be given up. The role of menopause in her ageing is not easy to evaluate;

some women produce significant amounts of oestrogen after cessation of ovulation, others do not. Replacement oestrogen may protect against the effects of ageing on the cardiovascular system and the skeleton, or it may not.

The enormous proliferation of menopause literature belies the utter lack of understanding of what is really going on. No one knows why ovulation ceases or even when it ceases, or what symptoms are caused by it and not by ageing, or even whether younger menopauses are more easily lived through than older ones. Nothing about menopause can be predicted, no risk factors can be isolated, no preventive measures suggested. Every year adds new symptoms to climacteric syndrome and every year takes some off. We have lost involutional melancholy and gained autogenic dysregulation. At all levels and in all therapies placebo response is high, sometimes dominant. All experimental results are compromised by the multiplicity of symptoms and by the self-limiting nature of the phenomenon.

Officially the medical establishment has one treatment for the climacteric, and that is hormone replacement therapy (HRT); in fact this is a multiplicity of regimes using a multiplicity of products in various combinations and strengths. No single individual can find her way around the whole gamut, and patients certainly will not be given the option. Selection of patients suitable for treatment is governed by the subjective impressions of the practitioner, and selection of the treatment regimen is a matter of serendipity. Investigations of counter-indications ignore important and common ailments such as varicose veins and give far too much attention to the risk of cancer. Opposing oestrogen with progestogens probably undoes its most important protective effect. The administration of oestrogen by the oral route makes no sense at all. Apart from these considerations, HRT is a valuable contribution to the pharmaceutical armamentarium, particularly for the multinationals who have patented the oestrogen preparations.

Traditionally women have not made a great fuss about menopause. When older women were in charge of the birthplace they witnessed frequent agony and death among the childbearing women, and had reason to congratulate themselves on having survived. They medicated themselves when necessary with simple preparations of plant material according to the season. There is no agreement in this vast pharmacopoeia because it is entirely reliant upon microclimates and cannot be duplicated in different circumstances. When male professionals took over medical practice they too developed nostrums of their own, but the principle of useless standardisation was early set. The least destructive doctors prescribed a cooling diet for their female patients, or adding a little wine to their regimen to keep their spirits up, and recommended a change of air, a long stay in one of the many spas where the middle-aged woman could not only take the waters but rest or walk, fast or diet, and recover from the multiplicity of childbed accidents she was likely to have undergone. Recourse to spas, which was part of traditional medical practice since the Iron Age, fades into hydrotherapy and alternative medicine, which offers an array of treatments for climacteric distress, most of which have the advantage of being relatively non-invasive and harmless.

No matter how good or effective the treatment of physical symptoms at the climacteric may be, there are some aspects of being a fifty-year-old woman that cannot be cured and must be endured. Sooner or later the middle-aged woman becomes aware of a change in the attitude of other people towards her. She can no longer trade on her appearance, something she has done unconsciously all her life. There is no defined role for her in modern society; before she can devise one for herself she experiences a period in free fall, which brings with it panic. Her physical symptoms may be such that she is always tired and cannot summon up the energy to haul herself through to the next phase. There are two aspects of her emotional condition at this time; one I have called misery, which has no useful function and should be avoided, and the other grief, which is wholesome, though painful, and must be recognised. The misery of the middle-aged woman is a grey and hopeless thing, born of having nothing to live for, of disappointment and resentment at having been gypped by consumer society, and surviving merely to be the butt of its unthinking scorn. Grief at the death of the womb is, in Iris Murdoch's phrase, an 'august and terrible pain' unlike anything a woman can have experienced before, but she comes through it stronger, calmer, aware that death having brushed her with its wing has retreated to its accustomed place, and all will be well.

Most books about women and ageing devote a significant proportion of their pages to the discussion of sexual activity, regardless of whether the middle-aged reader has the prospect of sexual activity or not. Rather than reassuring the sexually inactive woman that she will become neither mad nor ill as a result of her failure to exercise her genitals, such books address themselves to the wife who is losing interest, encouraging her to use medications and any other resources she can find to fan her waning flame. Rather less is said about what she might do to stimulate her partner's flagging interest, or what she might do to repel his/her advances if they were unwelcome. If the sexuality of older women were allowed to define itself, it is possible that we would discover that older women are not overwhelmed with desire for even older men or women. There may be something more to be said for the bar on the Piccola Marina where love came to Mrs Wentworth-Brewster than has hitherto been admitted. The secret lusts of old ladies are not the important point here, however; what is important is to debunk the reverence that hushes the voices of all other writers on this topic, who present sexual congress with one's spouse as a duty from the altar to the grave, rather like cleaning one's teeth and keeping one's bowels open. It is a variant on this author's often-quoted if misunderstood position that 'no sex is better than bad sex'.

There are of course women in history who have inspired love in middle age and kept it till death intervened, without the aid of cosmetic surgery or oestrogen replacement. The stories of Diane de Poitiers and Madame de Maintenon, both of whom in middle age won and kept the love of a king of France who might have had as concubine any of the most beautiful women in the country, are encouraging, if only because they imply that there is more to a woman than two taut breasts and ankles that she can cross behind her head. Neither of these grandes dames would have looked good in shorts. The hardy perennials of our own time are less encouraging, because their charms depend upon expensive imitations of the girlish charm of much younger women. They must take up hours every day preparing the imitation body that is all their stock-in-trade. In 2008, when she was sixty-one, Cher told her audience at the Grammy awards, 'In my job becoming old and becoming extinct are one and the same thing.' At the premiere of her film *Burlesque* in 2010 she was seen to be wearing facelift tape just beneath her jawline. Times change; beautiful women are now unashamed to tell their fans that their nubile bosoms are fake but many would be ashamed, on the other hand, to admit that they were on HRT.

This book suggests other role models for the ageing woman, role models who are not simply glittering threads, some bones, some silastic and hanks of hand-knotted bought hair. If the world has dubbed you crone, you might as well be one. There is no point in growing old unless you can be a witch, and accumulate spiritual power in place of the political and economic power that has been denied you as a woman. Witches are descended from the sibyls and female saints; their lineage is noble and no woman need be ashamed to call herself a witch. This does not mean that she has to dress up and babble meaningless formulae in cellars and crypts. The wild white witches live outdoors and hobnob with creatures as wild as themselves.

The object of facing up squarely to the fact of the climacteric is to acquire serenity and power. If women on the youthful side of the climacteric could glimpse what this state of peaceful potency might be, the difficulty of the transition would be lessened. It is the nature of the case that life beyond the menopause is as invisible to the woman who has yet to struggle through the change, as the top of any mountain would be to someone in the valley below. Calm and poise do not simply happen to the post-menopausal woman; she has to fight for them. When the fight is over her altered state might look to a younger woman rather like exhaustion, when in reality it is anything but. The dependent woman is obliged to believe that only her turmoil of passion, fear, rage, expectancy and disappointment is living, and that when she is no longer tormented by it she will be as dead as a spent match. The difference between her clamorous feelings and the feelings of the silent, apparently withdrawn older woman is the difference between what someone tossing upon the surface can experience compared with someone who has plunged so deep that she has felt death in her throat. The older woman's love is not love of herself, nor of herself mirrored in a lover's eyes, nor is it corrupted by need. It is a feeling of tenderness so still and deep and warm that it gilds every grass blade and blesses every fly. It includes the ones who have a claim on it, and a great deal else besides. I wouldn't have missed it for the world.

I

The Undescribed Experience

The experience of menopause is and will remain undescribed, because menopause is a non-event. It doesn't happen on a day or in a place. It is not announced, or applauded or deplored. It is not the last menstruation, which is by definition pre-menopausal, not to mention that you can't know that a menstruation is your last until months have passed. And that was before hormone replacement therapy, which may mean that a woman can go on having monthly bleeds as long as she chooses, maybe for the rest of her life (Rees & Barlow). In mid-2016 60-year-old Kris Jenner's daughters were calling her 'Miss Menopause'; viewers of *Keeping up with the Kardashians* might have seen tampons popping out of her purse. Commentators chattered away about her much younger boyfriend's desire for children as if they were a realistic prospect. Though information about menopause abounds, nearly all of it is unverifiable, and most of it is wrong.

A few months after my fiftieth birthday, on a bright spring morning, my friend Julia and I were sitting in a pavement café in Beaubourg. Around the corner we could buy wonderful things to eat with the dew of the country still on them, wild mushrooms and bitter salads, and armfuls of cornflowers to look at while we ate them. Our coffee had been delicious and the croissants light and buttery.

'I won't live like that,' said Julia. Her eyes were fixed on a little grey lady with a plastic shopping basket apologetically threading her way through the gaudy prostitutes and lounging boys on the pavement opposite. 'I won't live in some bedsit with a plate and a knife and a fork and creep out to the market each day for a slice of cheese and a baguette.

I won't become grey and invisible. I think what happened to my mother, those years of not knowing where or who she was. I'm not taking that road. I've thought about it. It won't be an unconsidered decision. I don't see the point of the next twenty, thirty years. To get so's your own body makes you sick, no matter how hard you struggle to keep your looks, and keep fit. I can't see the point of battling against it, when you know the outcome can only be defeat. It's so unfair.'

Julia's anxiety, with its telescoping of the next thirty years into a single grim tomorrow, is typical of the climacterium. We had both sailed through our forties with very little awareness of growing older. We had each buried a parent; she had shed a husband, but we had each remained at the centre of the life we had built. Suddenly something was slipping away so fast that we had not had time quite to register what it might be. All we knew was that it was irreplaceable. The way ahead seemed dark. Somewhere along the line optimism seemed to have perished. Neither of us could identify this feeling of apprehensive melancholy.

Julia nodded towards a table where two grey-haired men were being listened to by two sleek, expensive and very much younger women: 'Those men are our age, probably older than we are. It's bloody unfair. Those men can have their pick of women of any age. They can go on for years, and here we are, finished. They wouldn't even look at us.'

The unkind sunlight showed every sag, every pucker, every bluish shadow, every mole, every freckle in our fifty-year-old faces. When we beckoned to the waiter he seemed not to see us, and when he had taken our order he seemed to forget it and we had been obliged to remind him.

'Now what do I do?' Julia asked. 'Am I supposed to haunt the singles bars and try to pick up younger men? Am I supposed to descend lower and lower into squalor because I won't live without love? Or am I supposed to just work, and come home and eat and watch telly and go to bed day after day, until I get too old to work? Am I supposed to become that?' Her eyes followed the anonymous lady delicately picking her way home, the end of her baguette poking out of the plastic shopping basket. 'Just thinking about it fills me with terror. I lie awake at night, worrying. What will become of me?'

I would have rattled off some names of other fifty-year-old women who had overcome the climacteric and been reborn into a different kind of life, but they were not names that sprang readily to mind. I needed role models for a woman learning to shift the focus of her attention away from her body ego towards her soul, but for the life of me then and there I couldn't bring to mind a single one. The journey inwards towards wisdom and serenity is as long, if not longer, than the headlong rush of our social and sexual career, but there are no signposts to show the way. If there are leaders beckoning, most of us have no idea who they might be.

In fact Julia did find love. She married, worked until she retired, and in her late seventies lives in the midst of her family, at peace with herself and them.

Though the literature on menopause is vast, until recently very little of it had been written by women. When women have tried to bring menopause into the story, as Virginia Woolf did in earlier versions of *Mrs Dalloway*, references to menstruation and menopause were edited out. Until recently, nearly all of the millions of words written about menopause had been written by men for the eyes of other men; thousands of middle-aged women trooped meekly through the pages of hundreds of studies assessing their health, their well-being, their status, their needs, their opportunities, and their problems. Before 2000 we heard hardly one word in their own voices; now online blogs and chat rooms resound to a chorus of female protest and complaint, most of it ill-informed and misguided. Health professionals find no difficulty in ignoring all of it.

The following examples of online anguish were chosen at random in October 2016: 'I have a cabinet full of supplements that don't relieve my symptoms. Broke down and finally am taking a very low dose of an antidepressant. I can't be sitting at work crying every day, I need to be able to function.' Another goes like this: 'The constant tearfulness is hard for me and then the sudden rage of wanting to run over people in the grocery store with my cart LOL … I just finished a 24 hour straight hot flash, which made me miserable, which in turn made anyone around me miserable!' And yet another is almost incoherent:

When I look back, mine started with severe dizziness, dry eyes,
Most of the time I just used to feel (as I used to put [it], I am not
firing on all 4 cylinders – haha after about 6 months the anxiety
kicked in and boy has it gotten worse, plus bouts of feeling like

down a dark hole and I just want to get back to me, it's almost
as if I am on a different wave length, a lot of the symptoms seem
to come in phases, I just can't understand why this anxiety one is
staying so long, I am at the edge at the moment x.

Some women are eager to share their newly discovered miracle
cure: 'I've started taking a magnesium tablet daily, I'm on hrt patches
but breakthrough bleeding and terrible hot flashes night and day were
just getting me down, I've been referred to a menopause clinic, whatever
that is lol! But read about magnesium, seriously, what a difference,
maybe a couple of night sweats and a couple of sweaty day moments,
my hubby is so happy, I've actually been out with him today and not
had any sweats at all, worth a try ladies, xx'. (The only way to find out if
you need added magnesium is to try one of the commercial preparations
and see if you feel better. Actual deficiency cannot be tested for but is
very common.)

The contradictoriness of information about menopause is not the
fault of the women whose responses are so unpredictable but stems from
the lack of understanding by health professionals of the complexity of
the endocrine processes ongoing in the human female. Blood tests,
urine tests, saliva tests are of little use in determining what reproductive
hormones are circulating in any particular case, and even when details
of the picogram to millilitre level have been established, they can't be
shown to have any relation to the formation of symptoms. A survey
of 3,275 women by Nuffield Health in October 2014 found that 'just
over a third (38 per cent) of women sought help from a GP. However, a
quarter of those who visited a GP said the possibility of the symptoms
being menopause related failed to come up.'

The names that cropped up most often in discussions of menopause
in the Seventies and Eighties are still cropping up. They are the names
of the men I call the Masters in Menopause (by analogy with masters in
lunacy and masters in bankruptcy). The Grand Master in Menopause is
Wulf H. Utian, who discovered menopause in 1967. His own account
reveals how the discovery of a remedy inspired his search for a disease to
treat with it: 'In 1967 I happened to be in West Berlin and was invited to
visit a major international pharmaceutical firm. A new female hormone
was mentioned and thereby started my interest in the subject.' (Utian,
1978, p. 9)

Utian then set up the first menopause clinic in the world, at Groote Schuur; its name was later changed to the Femininity Clinic and then, as the notion caught on that menopause could be 'eliminated', it was renamed the Mature Woman Clinic. In 1976 Utian moved on, from Cape Town to the Mount Sinai Medical Center in Ohio, and founded the International Menopause Society. In 1989 he set up the North American Menopause Society, with himself as director, a position he held until 2009. Utian, who served as the medical editor of *Maturitas* from 1983 to 1993, and Honorary Founding Editor of *Menopause* (1994–2010), and editor of *Menopause Management* between 1987 and 2009, still is the Grand Master in Menopause. His view of menopause is undeniably bleak; he sees it as the result of an evolutionary lag in the development of the endocrine system of the human female that did not keep pace with the increase in life expectancy. He believes menopause to be a potential endocrinopathy with potential destructive consequences involving, as well as womb and ovaries, bone, the cardiovascular system, brain, skin and sensory organs.

The multinational pharmaceutical company that had its head office in Berlin in 1967 was Schering AG, manufacturers and distributors of a formidable array of steroidal preparations for the dosing of women under the names Anovlar, Controvlar, Cycloprogynova, Eugynon, Gynovlar, Logynon, Microgynon, Minovlar, Neogest, Norgeston, Noristerat, Primolut N, Progynova and Proluton. The new hormone in 1967 was oestradiol valerate, marketed as Progynova and with a progestogen as Cycloprogynova. Oestradiol valerate is described variously as a 'naturally occurring oestrogen' 'chemically and biologically identical to human oestradiol' and a synthetic ester, specifically the 17-pentanoyl ester, of the natural oestrogen, 17β-estradiol. It is now marketed under many brand names, Schering's patents having expired. In common with other plant-derived steroids, it is marketed these days as a 'bio-identical' hormone.

While Wulf Utian was preparing the ground for Schering, the multinational Akzo group was limbering up for its own onslaught on the replacement steroid market. In 1969 Akzo endowed the magniloquently titled International Health Foundation with headquarters in Geneva and 600,000 Swiss francs a year to spend on furthering 'the health of mankind by identifying and contributing to the solution of human physical, mental and social problems through programmes of research and education and by providing information in medical and all related sciences'. The immediate beneficiary was their wholly owned subsidiary Organon International BV, manufacturers of ethinyloestradiol in tablet form and as implants, and of Ovestin vaginal cream. The International Health Foundation seems to have come into existence to publish three studies on menopause; its director-general was the Dutch Master in Menopause Pieter van Keep, MD, second only to Wulf Utian in generating learned articles, all based at first on the same Akzo-funded studies. In 2007 Akzo, by then AkzoNobel, sold Organon to Schering's American subsidiary Schering Plough for 8 billion euros.

The ultimate aim of such developments was to get government funding to spread the gospel of HRT into every hovel on the planet, and, despite the catastrophe of the suspension of the Women's Health Initiative and the Million Women Study, Big Pharma still hasn't stopped trying. The arithmetic is simple. Post-menopausal health problems, notably osteoporosis, tie up expensive hospital facilities for hundreds of thousands of woman-hours a year and they will tie up hundreds of thousands more, as life expectancy improves around the globe. Educating women to accept HRT makes sense. Let it not be thought that I am implying that Schering and Organon, Utian and Van Keep were motivated by any but the highest motives.

The official view of the International Menopause Society is that menopause is a social construct, that illness is not the only response, that women need to know what a normal menopause is, whether their own is abnormal, and what doctors can do about alleviating their symptoms, that the approach to menopause is polarised between dismissing the menopausal woman and telling her to get on with it, and treating menopause itself as a deficiency disease, and finally that 'new lifestyles' that stress youth, fitness and active sexuality are leading to a new consciousness of the ageing body. Now that menopause has achieved a high profile, other professional bodies have held, are holding and will hold further conferences on menopause management. The pharmaceutical multinationals would be only too happy to finance international junkets all over the world in order to publicise their products so that they can be administered to women on a daily basis for billions of woman-years. Given the freebies and the junkets in the Seventies and Eighties, we were not surprised to find Third World professionals joining in the discussion and gleefully contemplating the scope for marketing steroids to a huge new population of post-menopausal peasant labourers. That was before 2001, before the Women's Health Initiative, before the flight from HRT.

Menopause is a dream specialty for the mediocre medic. Dealing with it requires no surgical or diagnostic skill. It is not itself a life-threatening condition, so a patient's death can always be blamed on something or somebody else. There is no scope for malpractice suits. Patients must return again and again for a battery of tests and check-ups, all of which earn money for the medic. In the Nineties ladies in the provinces held bring-and-buy sales to finance the setting up of menopause clinics – that is, outlets for the distribution of replacement hormones – working without reward, as women always have done, for the further enrichment of some of the richest institutions in the world. In the summer of 1988 the Amarant Trust was officially promulgated as a UK charity, its function to 'usher in a new lease of life for mature women', by increasing the pressure on doctors to prescribe and on women to accept HRT. In the Trust's first newsletter (March 1988), which was a four-page advertisement that made misleading claims for the proven effects of HRT, women were told that they could pay a monthly levy to support the good work.

> Women who work can now give to the Amarant Trust directly,
> through their pay packets. With your permission your employer
> can send us up to £10 a month from which he will deduct about £7
> from your pay packet; the rest is made up by saving the tax. But if
> you wish to give less, 'give as you earn' is still a good way to support
> the Amarant Trust because the government gives us back the tax
> you would otherwise have paid.

A small announcement at the bottom of the back page imparted the interesting information that the costs of producing the newsletter had been defrayed by 'an educational grant from [Swiss pharmaceutical company] Ciba-Geigy plc, and Novo Laboratories'. The merger of Ciba and Sandoz in 1996 would form Novartis, which would become the second-biggest pharmaceutical company in the world. As an embittered observer once remarked, women are the perfect guinea pigs; in the case of HRT they not only fed themselves and kept their cages clean, paid for the medications both through taxes and directly, administered the drugs themselves, and recruited further experimental subjects, they were also willing to subsidise the promotion of the products out of their own slender funds. The history of the medication of women in the climacterium is peopled with patients who have said, 'Thank you, doctor, I feel so much better,' whether they have been irradiated, electrocauterised, electroconvulsed, dosed with animal extracts, hysterectomised, dunked in cold water or given placebo.

In the ten years to 1978 Wulf Utian 'authored' or 'co-authored' twenty-six publications on the menopause. He had virtually commandeered the field of research into the usefulness of replacement hormones, which is characterised by poorly designed studies reflecting an unacceptable degree of bias. In 1984 clinical psychologist John Gerald Greene, who had been working at Dr David Hart's Menopause Clinic at Stobhill Hospital in Glasgow – the first menopause clinic in Europe – attempted to 'construct a cohesive sociopsychological model of the climacteric' using the existing 'substantial body of empiric research'. Though he paid tribute to Utian's grasp of the biology of menopause, he was obliged to point out that there is no evidence of the deficiency disease that Utian and his cohorts assume to be the cause of climacteric distress, that no one knows how to disentangle the climacteric itself from ageing, and that in properly designed double-blind cross-over trials, the placebo effect is so great as to weaken or even to invalidate the claims made for the medication of choice. Although he made no direct attack on Utian, and a practitioner in the menopause industry would have been be ill-advised to do so, he did manage to imply that Utian's enthusiasm for the 'mental tonic' effect of HRT was not justified by his own scientific research (Greene, 1984). The effect of Greene's rigorous review of the literature on climacteric 'syndrome' is greatly to weaken our certainty that there is such a thing, let alone whether there is a cure for it.

One of the basic tenets of feminism is that women must define their own experience. The climacteric needs to be rescued from the fog of prejudice that surrounds it. The menopausal woman is the prisoner of a stereotype and will not be rescued from it until she has begun to tell her own story. Besides, anxiety about menopause can only complicate the event itself. Negative attitudes to menopause result in menopause being blamed for events and situations that have nothing to do with it. When retail guru Mary Portas was sixteen, and her father away on a business trip, her 52-year-old mother became ill; doctors said it was 'the change'. The children struggled to get someone to believe that their mother was really ill, but to no avail. She slipped into a coma and died a week later. What had been dismissed as menopause was in fact meningitis.

Interestingly, women themselves seldom admit to having negative attitudes towards menopause. In 1980 a review of the available evidence reported that 'women consider menopause as requiring little readjustment when compared with other life events … it appeared also that menopause is not viewed with trepidation by younger women, nor remembered as a stressful period of change by the elderly. In fact negative stereotypes of the menopause are less prevalent among women than among men. The climacteric is viewed by men as a major life change.' (Asso, p.113)

Certainly the campaign to eliminate menopause has been initiated and is run by men. Since menopause became big business there has been a vast explosion of propaganda disseminating male views of menopause. The fact that male researchers remain attached to a view of menopause as catastrophe despite the necessary conclusions from their own research indicates an emotional loading that they themselves are unable to let go. The authors of the 1975 International Health Foundation survey make repeated references to 'menopausal crisis' and even conclude that 'for many women the menopause is a period of disorientation, physical problems and psychological imbalance' (IHF, 1975, p. 49) even though their own evidence proves that ageing is far more problematic. Such skewing of the argument represents something more than researcher bias.

Women who have graduated in a scientific discipline at a university have had to adapt in a very obvious way to the demands of a masculinist discipline, but even so they tend to resist the irrational certainties of the Masters in Menopause. Men see menopause as the cancellation of the only important female functions, namely attracting, stimulating, gratifying and nurturing men and/or children and, given that they believe that carrying out these functions constitutes women's happiness, it makes sense that they should seek to keep women unchanged. Women who have not internalised this view will not fear the cessation of ovulation like the plague.

The Masters in Menopause bask in the certainty that they are motivated not by greed or the lust for power, but by the purest chivalry. They offer replacement oestrogen not for their own convenience, but to relieve the anguish of good women. What is at work here has been described by psychoanalyst Karen Horney as the profound desire men have to put women down (Horney, 56–7); it is a need to show that women cannot manage their own lives without the aid of men, a delusion that women themselves have gone some way to foster. The post-menopausal woman is not allowed to have no further need of men. She is not permitted to transcend her biology once for all. She is defined as suffering from a deficiency disease, and men will once again demonstrate their superiority by supplying the remedy for her defect. Some of the inquiries into menopause demonstrate this mechanism more clearly than others, by including, for example, the question whether or not women become more 'self-centred' at menopause. (If only they did!)

Until the twenty-first century women remained relatively silent on the matter. When female researchers test the male hypotheses about menopause, they tend to find them unsubstantiated; when they assess the performance and rationale of hormone replacement therapy, they remain sceptical. The woman who rejects the male construction of menopause and turns to other women will find it difficult even to broach the subject. Women are not given spontaneously to describing their own menopause experiences; women writers, memoirists, *bellettristes*, diarists, novelists, poets, rarely so much as hint at menopause as an event. In the vast majority of cases women do not see the climacteric as a factor in their development. It seems unlikely that what we are up against is lack of awareness or lack of insight, and only slightly more likely that we are contemplating the more sinister phenomenon of denial. If the denial is simply denial of a male construction of a female event, it is only proper; if it is denial of the event itself, it is neurotic. If acceptance of HRT is the behavioural expression of that kind of denial it cannot be justified.

If fifty-year-old women were visible in our culture we would know that every climacteric is different; it is only our ignorance that implies that all menopausal women are enduring the same trials and responding in the same way. What happens during what one nineteenth-century gynaecologist called 'this interesting process of the human uterus' summarises a woman's life and career and provides the impetus for the rest of her life. It is a time of taking stock and making decisions; as such it is stressful. The stress may be complicated by physical symptoms or not.

Since I have been fascinated by fifty-year-old women I have turned to biography after biography, memoir after memoir, seeking out the moment of change, the turning of the corner, the beginning of the third age, but have found very little. This is partly, but only partly, because many of my heroines did not make it to fifty. Some, like Mary Wollstonecraft and Charlotte Brontë, died in childbed or of the consequences of miscarriage or giving birth, others of infectious disease. The ones who survived to menopause choose not to discuss the matter in literature, even in the most densely encoded fashion. To appear in print is to expose oneself in mixed company. The cessation of the menses is no more likely to be discussed in literature than any other female bodily function. Even so, the utter invisibility of middle-aged women in English literary culture is baffling. The years of the climacteric are, even for the most vociferous of women, silent years, and this phenomenon adds not a little to our anxiety regarding them.

As I have become accustomed to this reticence, I have learned to interpret the signs not only of the climacteric itself, but of the lunatic procedures menopausal women were subjected to by doctors. We read, for example, that in 1818 Maria Edgeworth was severely depressed and suffered 'alarming weakness' of her eyes. Both are usually explained as a result of family troubles and the worry of serious illness among the Irish peasantry, but they may mean more to us when we realise that in 1818 Maria Edgeworth was fifty-one. She gave up reading, writing and needlework for two years, and recovered. Disturbances of vision are sometimes reported in the climacteric; the person who was alarmed was probably her doctor who, if he was anything like his male contemporaries, almost certainly overinterpreted the symptom. Edgeworth's depression cannot have been materially assisted by the enforced inactivity he prescribed. Sixteen years later she was hale enough to tour Connemara, and then began, at the age of seventy, to learn Spanish. Jane Austen sent her a copy of *Emma*; 150 barrels of flour were sent to her from Boston to help with her relief work during the Irish famine, and when the porters would accept no pay, she knitted each one a comforter. She was very lively right up until the age of eighty-two, when she died peacefully in the arms of her dearest friend, her father's fourth wife, Frances Anne Beaufort.

In fiction, whether written by men or by women, middle-aged women are virtually invisible. All our heroines are young. Even women writers who are themselves fifty or over write about young women. Barbara Cartland, who was ninety-nine when she died in 2000, wrote 723 novels, but I doubt that any of them has a heroine over twenty-five. Older women themselves suffer from youthism, and contribute to the prejudice against themselves; they endure the never-ending jibes against menopausal women, against mothers-in-law, against crones in general, without a word of protest. Even the Women's Liberation movement has consistently identified with young, sexually active women, and treated the older woman as one of her oppressors. Virginia Tiger, discussing Doris Lessing's novel about the rebirth of a woman in the climacterium, *The Summer Before the Dark*, feels that she has to ask: 'Was Summer's emotional austerity, its insistence that women must develop an impersonal sense of self, evidence that Lessing is now alienated from the authentic feminist perspective?' (Tiger, p. 81)

In fact *The Summer Before the Dark* is not simply about the old theme of the discovery of self, but Tiger did not recognise its exact description of an utterly and solely female experience, possibly because she had not confronted it herself and nothing in the literature has prepared her for it. The 83 per cent of the British population who are not women over fifty are uninterested in women who are over fifty primarily because they are not interested in women. History is replete with the documentation of women who heroically or uproariously or problematically served men; their stories end when the relationship with their man ends. History records Lady Christian Acland, for example, for her valiant exploits at her husband's side in the Canadian campaign, but after his death in 1778, when she was only twenty-five, she disappears from the record though she lived until 1815.

It is unlikely, if we read *Emma* by Jane Austen, that we even remember Miss Bates. Emma is rude to Miss Bates, whom she finds so 'silly – so satisfied – so smiling – so prosing – so undistinguished and unfastidious …' Mr Weston describes her as 'a standing lesson in how to be happy' (p. 255), though 'her youth had passed without distinction, and her middle of life was devoted to the care of an ailing mother, and the endeavour to make a small income go as far as possible.' Mr Knightley is severe with Emma for humiliating this poor lady; his reasons for condemning her thoughtlessness, that Miss Bates 'is poor; she has sunk from the comforts she was born to; and if she live to old age must probably sink more'

(p. 375) must have struck dread into the hearts of Austen's unmarried female readers.

All our heroines are young. The implications of this statement are serious. If women themselves are not interested in mature women, if even mature women are not interested in mature women, we are faced with a vast and insidious problem. Women over fifty make up one of the biggest groups in Britain, being 17 per cent of the population. Any view of such a group as marginal must be based upon an inaccurate notion of who or what the typical Briton is. Mary Wollstonecraft (who died at the age of thirty-eight) wrote crossly in 1792 of a 'sprightly male writer' (whose name she had forgotten) who asked what business women over forty had in the world. We can afford to dismiss the sprightly writer, for we neither know him nor care for him, but what if we share his ignorance? What if we, the horde of women of fifty, cannot see what business we have in the world? Most of us are no longer sought as lovers, as wives, as mothers, or even as workers, unless there is a conspicuous dearth in our profession, and then only until we are in our sixties. We are supposed to mind our own business; if we are to do this we need to find business of our own.

Elizabeth Gaskell wrote *Cranford* when she had just turned forty. The novel was a wild success. Everybody loved the dotty ladies of Cranford, and especially dear old Miss Matty, with her tremulous motion of head and hands and well-worn furrows in her cheeks, Miss Matty who says, 'I had very pretty hair my dear, and not a bad mouth,' and who also says (a thunderclap this), 'Martha, I'm not yet fifty-two.' She is already getting dithery and sometimes wears one cap on top of another. A hundred pages later Miss Matty cannot walk very fast; she has a touch of rheumatism and her eyes are failing. In case we should console ourselves with the thought that old people get younger with every generation that passes and fifty-year-olds are younger and spryer now than they were then, we are brought up short by Miss Matty saying, 'We are principally ladies now I know, but we are not so old as ladies used to be when I was a girl' (p. 76).

None of these ladies knew the word 'menopause', though the educated among them did know the more correct expression 'climacteric', taken from the Greek word *klimacter*, meaning 'critical period'. The notion of the climacteric is as old as medicine itself; Aristotle noticed that women cannot bear children after the age of fifty, but until very recently only the truly irreverent, like the poet Byron, would dream of making an explicit reference to 'that leap-year, whose leap in female dates, strikes Time all of a heap' (*Don Juan*, XIV, 52). Byron dares even to refer to the climacteric of Catherine the Great (X, 47). He is unusual among poets in that he was genuinely interested in women as people and aware of the fundamental gravity of the woman question:

> But as to women, who can penetrate
> The real sufferings of their she-condition?
> Man's very sympathy with their estate
> Has much of selfishness and more suspicion. (XIV, 24)

The general public did not begin to discuss the climacteric until after it had been captured by the medical profession and defined as a syndrome, by which time it was too late to render it respectable. The medical notion of 'menopause' was the brainchild of C. P. L. de Gardanne, who described a syndrome he called 'la Ménéspausie' in *Avis aux Femmes qui entrent dans l'Age Critique*, published in 1816. 'Menopause' was not defined until 1899, in an article on 'Epochal Insanities' contributed by Dr Clouston to *A System of Medicine by Many Writers* (Allbutt, viii, p. 302) under the heading 'Climacteric Insanity'. By describing a set of symptoms, and identifying it as a syndrome with a dramatic name, the medical establishment was empowered to treat the 'critical phase', de Gardanne's *'âge critique'*, as a complaint in which their intervention was to be sought, rather than as an important process in female development with which women themselves would have to deal.

Menopause is the invisible Rubicon that a woman cannot know she is crossing until she has crossed it. Insistence on an inappropriate idea of a kind of invisible leap leads to some utterly mystifying data on 'age at menopause'. Women are asked, some many years later, when they 'went through menopause'. It would make more sense to ask them when they had their last bleed, which might with reason be dated to a month and a year. The last bleed itself is not the menopause, though some websites will say otherwise.

The climacteric is actually composed of three periods, two that exist and the one that does not; the first is the peri-menopause, the time leading up to the last bleed and the bleed itself, the second is the menopause proper, the bleed that does not come, and the third is the post-menopause. The whole process occupies the fifth climacter of a woman's life, the fifth of her seven ages. Her first age is infancy and childhood, her second adolescence and nubility, her third wifehood, her fourth motherhood, and her fifth the end of mothering and the beginning of grandmotherhood. Generally speaking, we can assume the climacteric to begin at about age forty-five and end at about fifty-five. Most women will traverse the difficult transition from reproductive animal to reflective animal between those years, which we could call middle age. Almost half a modern woman's life lies beyond the transition, yet nothing in her education or her conditioning has prepared her for this new role.

Though women's life expectancy at the beginning of the twentieth century was no more than forty-eight years, most of the women who died did so when they were infants or during their childbearing; the female population has always included a visible proportion of old crones. Women who survived to menopause might live on indefinitely, in ever worsening health. A disproportionate number of them would have been spinsters, who did not run the risks of childbirth, so that the old maid was a more familiar and therefore less cherished figure than the old matron. In the literary culture of the élite, impatience with the symptoms of menopause thus blended with casual ridicule of marginalised, dependent, unattractive old women. From the turn of the century, when the word 'menopause' began to figure in medical literature, the notion that the climacteric was a time of mental and physical derangement became one of the things that everybody knew. There seemed no need to investigate it.

The prejudice was international. The fortunes of an obscure Danish writer called Karin Michaëlis were transformed when, in 1904, she published a novel called *The Dangerous Age* which swept German-speaking Europe, then France, then the English-speaking world (see also p. 93, below). Every character in it was obsessed by the idea of a dangerous age, although none had any clear idea of when it might arrive or what form it might take.

Books on the menopause addressed to women were rare before the 1970s. The worst of them began with diagrams of the female reproductive organs, as if women had not ever since their schooldays had to consider their bodies as permanently in the lithotomy position, thighs apart, labia held asunder, jabbed with long lines with labels on the end – 'Glands of Bartholin', 'Vaginal Introitus'. (Never 'Clitoris'.) Even at menopause woman is to most medical writers nothing but a reproductive machine on stilts. The laborious description of the machinery that is now obsolete drags on and on; there will be another diagram of the lower half of a female sliced down the middle to show her reproductive organs, more labels – 'Germinal Epithelium', 'Tunica albuginea' – and another sliced along the midline to show how the womb fits in with her bladder and bowels, and another of the breast. The women reading these books are acutely aware of themselves as reproductive animals who can reproduce no longer, and are panicked to think that they are coming to the end of their useful life. What they need is a new perspective on themselves as people, to be able to feel that they are at least as important as hearts and minds as they were as wombs. They open a book called *The Menopause*, and find themselves again confronting the same old diagrams that their doctor has been drawing on the office blotter ever since they can remember. They are forced to chart the involution of the womb stage by painful stage, a peculiar palliative for grief.

When I complained to another middle-aged woman that there are no novels written about middle-aged women, she said at once, 'Oh, that's because nothing happens to us.' How can this be, I thought, our hearts break, our lives are overwhelmed, spectres of pain and fear loom at every turn, and this is 'nothing happens'? If there is a belief that nothing happens to middle-aged women, it is only because middle-aged women do not talk about what does happen to them.

Take the case of Kathleen Sutcliffe, for example. Nobody in her family could remember if it was actually on her fiftieth birthday that her husband rang her at work to tell her (probably untruthfully) that he'd be working late.

'Who's that?' she asked.

'Who d'you think it is?' her husband asked. She'd never actually heard his voice on the phone before and he was tickled that she couldn't recognise it. Her reply floored him.

'Oh, is it Albert?' she said.

It had never occurred to John Sutcliffe that the woman who served him his meal before he went off on the night shift might have an admirer. When he got engaged to her in 1941, her big brown eyes and masses of black curls had all the boys running after her, but those days were long gone. Like a good Catholic girl Kathleen got pregnant on her honeymoon. After she'd borne seven kids (and buried one) she had no time to go to Mass, especially as her husband was too busy with his sporting and theatrical activities to give her a hand. She'd become a motherly homebody who moved her old mum into the house in 1952 and looked after her till she died in 1964. After that Kathleen went out cleaning every week-night and on Saturday and Sunday morning so that her kids could have decent clothes. Her husband spent a good deal of his money on himself, his entertainments and his other women, but Kathleen didn't seem to mind. Even when her husband groped her sons' girlfriends Kathleen turned a blind eye. She was famous on the estate where they lived for her warm heart and her sweet manner. Her third son used to say, 'She were a right honest sort of person, me mother. Right gullible. You could tell her owt an' she'd believe you without wanting to delve … she'd stick up for you, me mother …' Kathleen's one indulgence was that every other Thursday she went to the hairdresser.

So who was Albert? Albert was a policeman who lived two streets away. His wife worked long hours and Albert sometimes had time on his hands. When Kathleen was walking her son's terrier by the canal he'd be walking his. They'd got to talking, to like talking to each other, and then to need to talk to each other. They made love rarely, in his house, when his wife was out at work, and in his car. He'd telephone her sometimes when she was at work; her husband never did.

'Is it Albert?' she said, because I dare say she so much wanted it, needed it to be Albert. 'Oh, Albert, when can I see you again?' Cruelly her husband decided to pretend that he was indeed Albert. As Albert he rang her several times and finally persuaded her to spend the night with him at a local hotel. He told her to bring something fetching to change into and had the bitter satisfaction of finding in their bedroom a pretty new nightgown in a Marks & Spencer bag. He commanded three of their older children to meet him at the hotel at the appointed time. Two of them turned up, and were the more mystified to see their mother pacing nervously up and down on the pavement outside. Their father let her pace for a minute or two and then went out, grabbed her arm and marched her in to face her kids. One of them remembered that 'she didn't remonstrate with him, or cry, or do anything dramatic;

she seemed numb; and all the blood had drained from her.' I cannot tell you what she felt when he leaned over, and took her handbag and pulled out the new nightgown.

Kathleen tried to get her husband to believe that the relationship with Albert was innocent, but the evidence of the nightgown damned her. He threatened to go to Albert's house and confront him and his wife, so Kathleen confessed. Albert was summoned to their house and ordered never to see Kathleen again. The lovers disobeyed and met once more, but Kathleen's husband caught them. This time he threatened to denounce Albert to his superior officers in the police force. Albert had his pension to consider. He gave Kathleen up.

Her husband thought he probably ought to show her a bit more affection, so when he was watching television he would reach for her hand or put his arm around her shoulders. At such moments, according to her daughter, Kathleen seemed 'dead embarrassed'. She was not well; she was putting on weight, and kept having pain around her heart and difficulty in breathing. She had every possible test but nothing organic seemed to be wrong. She had to give up her Boxing Days when she had all the old people from her own and her husband's family to dinner. She had to give up work. The council moved her to a more convenient flat; the priest began to bring her fortnightly communion. If her eldest son was driving past in his lorry he would always drop in to see her and would never leave her until he had coaxed her to smile. He reckoned that the scene in the hotel and its aftermath had broken her heart; it was as if she was slowly dying before his eyes. She died in November 1978, less than ten years after she lost Albert, and three years before the world came to know her loving firstborn son as the Yorkshire Ripper.

This is just one reality behind the 'nothing' that is thought to happen to middle-aged women. Most people who read Gordon Burn's book about the Ripper, *Somebody's Husband, Somebody's Son*, will not be reading it for the story of Kathleen, but for the gruesome story of Peter Sutcliffe and his wife Sonia. All credit must go to Burn for rooting out Kathleen's story as we have it, but he and his readers should be aware that they do not have the flesh of it. What did Albert mean to Kathleen? What did their physical lovemaking mean to her? Was she so apathetic when her husband humiliated her because the worst pain was simply that Albert was not there and she wanted him so much? Or was the worst grief that Albert didn't have the gumption to take her away from her overbearing, unfaithful, neglectful husband for good? Or was it guilt and contrition that menopausal lust had undone a lifetime of fidelity to her role of Catholic wife and mother? Did she will herself to death? The story of Kathleen Sutcliffe could, like any great myth, be written a thousand different ways, if only we could place a middle-aged charlady at the centre of our mind-stage. This is one change that needs to happen if middle-aged women are to succeed in regaining their balance and living the rest of their lives in an unapologetic fashion.

In 1973 Doris Lessing published *The Summer Before the Dark*. The novel's heroine, Kate Brown, 'is faced for the first time in twenty years with the prospect of being alone, because her husband, a successful neurologist, is going to work for some months in an American hospital. Urged by him to take a job, she embarks on a summer of exploration, freedom and self-discovery, during which she rejects the stereotypes of femininity which like her conventional clothes, do not fit her any more ...' Because Doris Lessing is an important writer, rather than a 'women's novelist', *The Summer Before the Dark* was reviewed by men, mostly respectfully but not enthusiastically. Lessing had already become interested in Sufism and had begun writing non-realistic stories; she had returned to realistic narration to describe the important processes that unfold in a woman at the time of the climacteric.

> We are what we learn.
> It often takes a long and painful time.
>   Unfortunately, there was no doubt, either, that a lot of time, a lot of pain, went into learning very little ...
> She was really feeling that? Yes, she was.
> Because she was depressed? Was she depressed? Probably. (p. 10)

The cancelling of the heroine's role as consort and mother is dramatised in Lessing's book by her husband's suggestion that they let their big house while he is away and the children are about their own affairs. Lessing carefully pares away the usual assumptions about 45-year-old women; this one is well-dressed and well-preserved, but 'she did not walk inside, like the fine, almost unseeable envelope of a candle flame, that emanation of attractiveness ...' (p. 39) She changes her image, in order to send a stronger signal, and it works; she attracts a younger man and goes to Spain with him. Lessing coins an unforgettable image

of unnatural life to encapsulate Kate's uneasiness about the role she is
playing:

> She dreamed as soon as she went to sleep. She was sitting in a
> cinema. She was looking at a film she had seen before ... of the poor
> turtle who, on the island in the Pacific that had been atom-bombed,
> has lost its sense of direction and instead of returning to the sea after
> it has laid its eggs, as nature ordinarily directed, is setting its course
> inwards into a waterless land where it will die. (p. 71)

Once at home she had taken in a stray cat:

> The family had treated Kate like an invalid and the cat a medicine.
> 'Just the thing for the menopause,' she had heard Tim say to
> Eileen.
> She had not started the menopause, but it would have been
> no use saying so: it had been useful, apparently, for the family's
> mythology to have a mother in the menopause ... oh, that had
> been an awful spring, to follow a bad winter. She had feared she was
> really crazy, she spent so much of her time angry. (p. 99)

Part of the difficulty with *The Summer Before the Dark* is that the
climacteric is never identified as a factor and may not be intended to be
understood as a cause of Kate's spiritual malaise. In fact her sensations,
that a cold wind is blowing on her, that the stuffing is running out of
her, that she is being flayed alive, are all typical of the climacteric. The
affair fizzles out; Kate is feverishly ill for some weeks and comes out of it
all bones, with her hair grizzled and frizzy, as if the weeks of illness had
devastated her as much as the years of the climacteric. Shabby, scrawny
and grey, Kate finds that she is invisible. Lessing's writing of this change
is classic.

> It seemed a long time before the food came. Kate sat on, invisible,
> apparently, to the waitress and to the other customers: the place
> was filling now. She was shaking with impatient hunger, the need
> to cry. The feeling that no one could see her made her want to
> shout: 'Look, I'm here, can't you see me?' She was not far off that
> state that in a small child is called a tantrum. (p. 166)

Kate discovers that by concealing the evidence of age she can become visible again. Eventually, after a good deal of turmoil, she decides that she will accept her new condition.

Lessing's novel is an important text in the self-definition of late twentieth-century woman. However, it inspired few emulators. Rachel Billington's novel *A Woman's Age* is more typical of the mainstream in that it deals with anything but the topic named in the title. As soon as Violet, the heroine of the first part, is widowed and she decides to go into politics, the novelist switches her attentions to her nubile daughter. Violet makes only summary appearances for the last 200 pages.

If older women look about them for role-models they may see politicians like Golda Meir, Sirimavo Bandaranaike, Indira Gandhi, Gro Harlem Brundtland, Aung San Suu Kyi, Khaleda Zia, Sheikh Hasina, Hillary Clinton, Helen Clark, Angela Merkel, Theresa May, Julia Gillard, all of whom came to power in midlife, but it is difficult to see how we can profit by their example. They demonstrate that there is no responsibility too great for a fifty-year-old woman to assume, but their careers can hardly be imitated by the mass of women. One thing is obvious, they did not begin their acquisition of political power at fifty. By fifty the long years of committee work and party service were bearing fruit. These women had a compensation for the losses of middle age, a compensation for which they had in a sense bartered the years of their youth. Most fifty-year-old women are simply mocked by such examples. Mrs Thatcher's career gives us no clue how to deal with the loss of parents, with the growing away of children, with the increasing infirmities of age. We were told that she used hormone replacement, but didn't know whether to be encouraged or disheartened by the result, especially once she was tossed out by her male colleagues and condemned to silence. We could see that Mrs Thatcher's image was tailored by professionals; she illustrated a standard of middle-agedness to which most of us cannot aspire, partly because we were not so canny as to marry a millionaire in the first place. Instead we sit on the bus looking at the faded faces of the other women using off-peak transport and we wonder how old they are. 'Is she older or younger than I?' we ask ourselves. 'Am I ageing better or worse than she?'

There may be positive sides to lack of interest in oneself, but there is nothing positive about having a 'low self-image'. If mature women simply forget themselves, that is one thing, but if they actually dislike or even despise themselves, we can expect all kinds of evils to ensue as a consequence. Despite the advances in recognising women's rights, women, even educated sophisticated women, prefer not to admit their age, and even lie about it. The Wikipedia entry for ITV newscaster Sue Jameson does not supply her birth date. This would seem to imply that being old, for a woman, is somehow shameful. Simone de Beauvoir said that when she admitted at the end of *Force of Circumstance* to being on the threshold of old age, people were shocked and annoyed with her. 'You're not old,' people say to fifty-year-old women. 'Fifty is young.' In 2004 the *Guardian* announced that fifty was the new thirty 'so drop the Zimmer frame jokes'. Once upon a time, age had traditional transitions. 'Now, if fifty is the new thirty, then sixty-five is probably where the midlife crisis has gone.' Part of what makes such nonsense nonsense is that the sloganisers cannot tell the difference between midlife and old age, which is even greater than the gulf between adulthood and middle age.

Every twenty-year-old knows that fifty is old. Abbie Hoffman used to say in the Sixties, 'Never trust anyone over thirty.' He himself was close to thirty then; it was not thirty but fifty that did him in. This book is not about the anxieties of ageing men and will not devote any of its limited space to the 'male menopause'. The purpose of this book is to demonstrate that women are at least as interesting as men, and that ageing women are at least as interesting as younger women. The climacteric and women's experiences during it and their strategies for managing it are fascinating. It is not a stage to hasten through, let alone obscure or deny. On these years depends the rest of your life, a life which may be as long as the life you have already lived.

2

No Rite of Passage

In her book *Change of Life*, Jungian psychotherapist Ann Mankowitz quotes a menopausal woman as saying: 'Sometimes I feel I am twelve years old, sometimes seventy … I feel uncertain how to behave, how to relate to people, especially men. How do I seem to them? I just don't know … I've never felt like this before' (p. 43). The problem is not a new one. In 1820, the fifty-year-old Marquise de La Tour du Pin began her memoirs: 'My thoughts ramble. I am not methodical. My memory is already much dimmed … At heart I still feel so young that it is only by looking in the mirror that I am able to convince myself I am no longer twenty years of age' (Harcourt, p. 13). The Marquise's is a typically menopausal state of mind; her acquisition of a notebook and inscribing the first page of her autobiography was a DIY ritual to mark the otherwise unmarked transition from the two functions that according to Rousseau justified a woman's life, those of spouse and mother, to something new and undefined. The male theoreticians of the Marquise's epoch held that it was a woman's duty to please; in embarking upon her memoirs the Marquise was taking a long, invisible step. After a lifetime of pleasing others, she was about to please herself. In fact, for many years, she didn't find time to continue the memoirs; it was the beginning, the inditing of her title page that was her rite of passage.

If the Marquise had not chosen to mark the change herself she might have found herself in the muddle that afflicts most women at some stage during the climacteric. 'What are we supposed to wear?' my friend

Vivian asked me one day. 'I find it so difficult to choose clothes. How do we dress our age? Everything is either pastel crimplene safari suits or tat for the teens and twenties. There isn't anything that is just grown-up and elegant. Half the things I bring home the girls pinch, and tell me that I'm too old for them.' A. S. Byatt lamented in the *Independent Magazine* (16 June 1990, p. 18):

> Clothes manufacturers are waking up to the fact that over 50 per cent of women are over size 16, but they are still hooked on the idea that the waistless want to flaunt themselves as though they were nubile children … I want to look quietly elegant … . I've got the money, not the teenagers. Where are the designers?

Designers there are but, unless a woman's shoulders are broader than her hips, she cannot wear their clothes. Designers seldom allow their designs to be made up in sizes over twelve. Still less are they prepared to tailor them to fit. Dressmakers have gone extinct. Nowadays women over fifty who have no intention of putting themselves through the ordeal of the fitting room have to rely on website outlets. Though the middle-aged woman has the money to pay for quality, what can be found for sale online is cheap and mass-produced, nearly all of it in Asian sweatshops.

It is not simply a matter of designers. There has always been pressure upon the middle-aged woman to make herself inconspicuous. Kitty, Duchess of Queensberry, scandalised everyone in 1771 when at the age of seventy she wore a pink lutestring gown at a wedding. The narrator of *Cranford* refused to allow Miss Matty the turban she longed for but pressured her to content herself with 'a neat, middle-aged cap'. In this case it is a younger woman who constrains the older to forgo bright colours and exciting clothes. As Simone de Beauvoir observed in *The Prime of Life*, first published in 1962 when she was fifty-four, 'Young women have an acute sense of what should and should not be done when one is no longer young. "I don't understand," they say, "how a woman of forty can bleach her hair; how she can make an exhibition of herself in a bikini; how she can flirt with men."' (p. 291)

There is, as we all know, no possibility that the glow of youth could be outshone by the savoir-faire of the middle-aged woman, but the young themselves are unaware of their bloom, and deeply insecure about their attractiveness. The middle-aged woman for her part is confused; she knows from her own perception that nothing is so macabre or ridiculous as mutton dressed as lamb, but how is mutton supposed to dress? No fifty-year-old woman actually wants to compete with her daughters for attention, or that they should compete with her, but more and more in our society such competition is forced upon us. There is no accepted style for the older woman; no way of saying through dress and demeanour, 'I am my age. Respect it.'

At no time in our history have the generations been pitted against each other as they are now, when households contain only parents and children and no representatives of intervening age groups, no young aunts and uncles, no older cousins, and very few brothers and sisters. The interaction is all parent–child and child–parent, so that the group as perceived by both polarises into their generation and our generation, them and us. Yet outwardly, in dress and manner, there is no distinction. Parents cannot disentangle themselves from their children's affairs or vice versa, nor can they insist on any degree of formality or respect in their relationship with their children. Women who are now fifty called their parents 'mother' and 'father', or names to the same effect, but they often prefer that their own children call them by their Christian names, as if to set aside their own seniority.

There is no point at which a middle-aged woman can make plain her opting out of certain kinds of social interaction. She has a duty to go on 'being attractive' no matter how fed up she is with the whole business. She is not allowed to say, 'Now I shall let myself go'; letting herself go is a capital offence against the sexist system. Yet if a woman never lets herself go, how will she ever know how far she might have got? If she never takes off her high-heeled shoes, how will she ever know how far she could walk or how fast she could run? The middle-aged women who begin to train for marathons will never run as far or as fast as they might have in their teens and twenties, but the women who study to develop their souls can find their full spiritual and intellectual range on the other side of fifty. Developing the muscles of the soul demands no competitive spirit, no killer instinct, although it may erect pain barriers that the spiritual athlete must crash through.

The fifty-year-old woman has no option but to register the great change that is taking place within her, but at the same time she may well feel the need to keep this upheaval secret. The shame that she felt at the beginning of her periods is as nothing compared to the long-drawn-out embarrassment occasioned by their gradual stop–go ending; no woman would step into a shop or an office or a party and announce in ringing tones that she expected special consideration because she was struggling through menopause. She would not wear a badge that said 'Beware menopausal mood swings'. In the UK Nuffield Health (in 2014) and the Chief Medical Officer (in 2016) have both suggested that employers make efforts to extend special consideration to their menopausal employees; this resulted in a declaration by one section of the police force that they would raise the issue with women they thought might be going through menopause, a suggestion that raised a shudder with women everywhere. Questionnaires about menopausal status will do nothing to help women through their 'dodging time'. A rite of passage would surround the middle-aged woman with solemnity while preserving her privacy. Best of all would be the conferral of superior status on women as they enter midlife but there is no prospect of any such thing.

The social invisibility of the menopause serves no useful purpose. In 1973 a researcher reported:

> I was surprised to find that those most interested in the subject were young people, of both sexes, who had been affected by their mothers' menopause. One young man told me that his mother's 'change' came when he was fourteen, and she did indeed change toward him – from an affectionate and indulgent parent to a moody and rejecting one. Unable to understand what was happening, he felt confused, miserable, guilty. Naturally he felt that the whole subject needed to be brought out into the open. (Mankowitz, p. 11)

An alarm bell rings when one reads this kind of thing. There is here no suggestion that the young man may have behaved in such a way as to provoke his mother's rejection, though fourteen-year-olds often do. The possibility that the teenager might have been too demanding is not considered. If the climacteric is thought to be one more pathological manifestation, it becomes one more reason why women should not be taken seriously. In the same way that the completely negative construction put on the menstrual cycle acts against women's interest, the identification of menopause as the sole cause of changes in women's attitudes strips those attitudes of respectability. What would fulfil the purpose of warning off self-obsessed spouses and children at a time when the woman is preoccupied with an upheaval within herself, without caricaturing the woman as sick and deranged, would be a rite of passage.

To make matters worse there has been a concerted attempt to blur the boundaries of menopause by extending the peri-menopause way back into a woman's thirties and forties. More recently women readers of tabloid newspapers have been informed that if they are muddling and forgetful, they are victims of the 'pink fog'. Sue Carpenter asks herself in the *Daily Mail*, 'Could my mental fuzziness really be due to the menopause – or even the peri-menopause (the bit before, which can start as early as your late 30s)?' In view of the fact that when she penned this in 2012 Carpenter was fifty-six, the answer to both questions would seem to be 'no'. Extending the peri-menopause backwards by ten years is easily accompanied by the suggestion that women should start taking replacement oestrogen long before their last period.

The pink fog notion seems to have been born of a misinterpretation of a small 2013 study by Miriam Weber, which concluded that 'women in the first year of post-menopause performed significantly worse than women in the late reproductive and late menopausal transition stages on measures of verbal learning, verbal memory and motor function. They also performed significantly worse than women in the late menopausal transition stage on attention/working memory tasks.' The study was rigorous but the sample was small. In fact 'pink fog' was an expression borrowed from cross-dressers to describe the feminine feeling they get when sitting at the vanity doing their hair, 'body smooth and silky … painted fingers and toes … smell of perfume in the air … Jewelry and heels on … legs crossed … taut garter straps … sheer nirvana' (crossdressers.com). Another version uses the expression to refer to the period of euphoria experienced by the cross-dresser who has come out to his female partner. Pink Fog is also the title of a transgender cartoon series.

It is Christiane Northrup who believes that the peri-menopause, in the words of her acolyte Oprah Winfrey, 'can start as early as 35 (yes, 35) and can last anywhere from 5 to 13 years'. In 2009 Oprah believed that the peri-menopause could last from two to eight years. In fact she has been preaching the gospel of peri-menopause since 2002, when she put women who had experienced peri-menopausal symptoms for the first time aged thirty-one, thirty-seven and thirty-eight on her show. To extend the concept of menopause to cover thirteen years is to make the notion of a transition even more difficult to grasp. The experience is by now almost completely amorphous. What reduces it to mere wraithdom is the acceptance of replacement steroids that perpetuate the cycle and keep the elderly woman experiencing regular monthly bleeds. Add to that the number of women who undergo hysterectomy and oophorectomy and therefore have a surgically induced menopause, and the picture becomes even more cloudy.

We cannot be surprised that the menopause keeps appearing and disappearing like the Cheshire Cat. According to Mankowitz, 'the menopause was and is virtually a non-event in all societies'. Mankowitz explains the function of a rite of passage as 'to give significance to a crucial change in the life of the individual, to give one the support of society during this change and to attempt by means of the ritual to bring down the blessing of the gods at this time of danger both to the individual and to society' (p. 20). Historically, few women lived long enough to ensure that society evolved a ritual to mark the cessation of the menses. More important however may be the fact that menopause involves no one but the individual woman; her birth and her death are both celebrated by others; her arrival at puberty, her marriage and her childbearing all involve the exercise of her most important social function and the rituals to celebrate them all dramatise the fact. The menopause signals the woman's withdrawal from this social context and perhaps that is why it is ignored.

In a culture where women are obliged to maximise their reproductive opportunities, that is, to become pregnant as often as ever they can, menopause is masked by the last pregnancy. Many human societies have suffered such high rates of child mortality from infectious disease, as well as miscarriage and stillbirth, that their women were pregnant or lactating throughout their reproductive life. In such societies amenorrhoea is the normal condition and menstruation a relative rarity. The last menstruation is likely to occur before the last pregnancy, at a time not obviously connected with the cessation of ovarian function. In such an instance the woman only slowly realises, when she does not fall pregnant when she weans her last baby, that her childbearing years are over. Lactational amenorrhoea merges indistinguishably with the amenorrhoea of menopause. So many pregnancies, so much labour and lactation, together with the struggle to produce food and keep the growing children healthy, make hard work. Provided she has enough surviving children, the ageing wife is not likely to regret the fact that she will not have to endure another pregnancy. On the other hand she may not be keen to advertise it either, for a wife's menopause can provide a reason for a husband's taking a second, younger wife (Beyene).

In their three-volume study of woman, published in Leipzig in 1885 and in an English translation in 1935 as *Woman: an Historical, Gynaecological and Anthropological Compendium*, anthropologists Hermann Heinrich Ploss and Max and Paul Bartels list hundreds of female rituals associated with birth, puberty, marriage and childbearing. Older women merit a single, brief, dismissive chapter. This seems both obvious and explicable, yet, though there is no public celebration of the beginning of the last third of a woman's life, it is not quite true to say that no rites of passage are celebrated at all. Though the male hierarchy may be unaware of women's rites of passage, and therefore the lore of the elders contains no recognition of them, women themselves may have their own ways of signalling their new status, and their acceptance of it, which have escaped the attention of anthropologists.

At age fifty Barbara Hannah Grufferman ran the New York marathon, something she never thought she would do. Having succeeded at that she decided to become a full-time writer. Now she exhorts women 'Run a marathon, Change your Life'. Fifty- to fifty-four year old women constitute about 2 per cent of marathon runners, completing the course in about five hours. When Sharon Largent ran the Philadelphia marathon in 2012 she decided that the experience taught her 'to believe in life again', which is pretty much what rites of passage are meant to do for you.

In 1998 California artist Sue Ellen Cooper bought two red hats, one for herself and another for a friend about to turn fifty-five. She was inspired by the famous Jenny Joseph poem 'When I am an old woman'; the hat signified a move towards female solidarity and fun. The idea caught on and the Red Hat Society, 'an international society of women that connects, supports and encourages women in their pursuit of fun, friendship, freedom, fulfilment and fitness while supporting members in the quest to get the most out of life', was born. In April 2004 Cooper published *The Red Hat Society: Friendship and Fun after Fifty*, and a year later *The Red Hat Society's Laugh Lines: Stories of Inspiration and Hattitude*. By 2011 there were local chapters of the society in Argentina, Australia, Austria, Canada, Ecuador, England, Finland, Germany, Greece, Guam, Ireland, Italy, Japan, Luxemburg, Mexico, Namibia, The Netherlands, New Zealand, Norway, Panama, Peru, Scotland, South Africa, Sweden, Taiwan, Trinidad and Tobago, and Wales.

In 2001 members of the Red Hat Society flocked to see *Menopause the Musical*, book and lyrics by Jeanie Linders, when it opened in a small theatre in Orlando, Florida. The cast consisted of four women, 'Power Woman', 'Iowa Housewife', 'Earth Mother' and 'Soap Star', shopping for lingerie in Bloomingdale's department store. They sang twenty-five songs adapted from hit songs of the baby boomer era, with new lyrics dealing with hot flashes, nocturnal sweats, chocolate cravings, loss of memory and sexual predicaments. The show was an instant success; productions were staged all over the US where it is now permanently housed at Harrah's in Las Vegas. In February 2017 the show began touring provincial theatres in the UK, but given the reaction to a trial run in Ireland in 2016 its reception was not likely to be ecstatic. Readers may make their own assessment from the numerous videos available online.

In Jenny Joseph's famous poem the old woman signals her change of life by wearing purple as Australian feminist Dale Spender has always done and members of the Red Hat Society do on high days and holidays. More often women choose to emblematise an invisible, inner alteration by changing the way they do their hair. In 1924, when Harriet Shaw Weaver, James Joyce's patroness, mentor and champion, was forty-eight, her photograph was taken by Man Ray. This famous portrait shows her in pure and severe profile and, for the only time in her life, with shingled hair. Usually she wore her abundant dark hair in a heavy chignon; few of her old friends can have recognised her in Ray's photograph. Her family objected. Miss Weaver grew her hair long again and wore it in whorls over her ears, as befitted the maiden aunt impeccable who cared for all her ageing and ailing relatives, but for a year, whether in mourning or renunciation or rebellion, 'Aunt Hat' or 'Josephine' (as she called herself) was shorn. The drastic alteration in her appearance externalised an important alteration in her Gestalt, but Miss Weaver did not explain it and people did not wonder for too long what had 'come over' her.

In Doris Lessing's novel *The Summer Before the Dark*, Kate Brown marks the change within her by deciding that she will never again have her hair coloured and shaped.

> Her experiences of the last months – her discoveries, her self-definition, what she hoped were now strengths – were concentrated here: that she would walk into her home with her hair undressed, with her hair tied straight back for utility; rough and streaky, and the widening grey band showing like a statement of intent. It was as if the rest of her, body, feet, even face, which was ageing but amenable, belonged to everyone else. But her hair – no! No one was going to lay hands on that. (p. 237)

It would appear, from the reference to a 'widening grey band', that until this moment Kate had been dyeing her hair. In the 1950s fewer than 15 per cent of American women dyed their hair. In a Procter & Gamble survey of 2005, 65 per cent of women admitted to colouring their hair in the previous year, which could be thought to indicate that twenty-first-century women find it harder to reconcile themselves to going grey than their mothers did.

When Anne Kreamer was forty-six she decided to stop colouring her hair; the decision was so transformative that she decided to write a book about it. The result was *Going Gray: How to Embrace Your Authentic Self with Grace and Style*, published in 2007. Now Kreamer says, 'Nothing's really changed since I wrote the book. I'm still generally the only woman in the room with white or grey hair, but it's always a positive experience, whether at work or in my personal life' (*Guardian*, 25/4/16). The promotion of what has become a veritable avalanche of books exhorting women to embrace the change and stop colouring their hair can strike a repellent note. The dust-jacket of Maggie Rose Crane's *Amazing Grays: A Woman's Guide to Making the Next 50 the Best 50 *Regardless of your hair color* promises a 'uniquely refreshing and candid look at midlife for those unwilling to become feeble old women with boobs in their laps, dreams on the shelf, and Memory Lane their only destination'.

Ellen Lee, who went grey long before menopause, in a guest blog she wrote for timegoesby.net, explains her rationale for refraining from colouring her hair because it 'is just another example of age-denial; that with enough collagen, botox, nips and tucks, and hair colouring, we can keep age at bay and look thirty- to forty-something indefinitely.' She goes on:

> To me, this only adds to the problem of invisibility for elders. It's
> bad enough that our youth-obsessed society doesn't want to see
> elders – except in stereotyped cute, crotchety or forgetful, dim-wit
> roles – we elders are making ourselves invisible by trying to look
> like something other than what we are. If we can't be comfortable
> in our own skins, then we're contributing to the ageism that views
> growing older as a negative.

She concludes rather tartly 'The grey-haired have become invisible and it's our own fault.'

In 'The War over going gray' that appeared in *Time* magazine for 31 August 2007 Anne Kreamer interprets this kind of thinking as signalling 'a contentious new baby-boomer argument over gray hair that is as mutually judgmental as the mommy wars between working and stay-at-home mothers was in the 1980s and '90s.' These have not eventuated; rather most women in the public eye still colour their hair; even Gloria Steinem still colours her hair. Children are now growing up to believe that as women grow older their hair turns blond.

The most insidious aspect of the commercial promotion of hair-colouring is the suggestion that grey hair is not the 'real you' and that by bleaching or colouring her hair a woman becomes her 'real self'. The postmodern beauty industry has adopted as dogma the nonsensical notion that artificial colour expresses a deeper truth about who one is. According to Clairol's in-house director of colour and style, Marcy Cona, hair-dye helps 'each woman create an authentic connection between how she feels internally versus how she looks externally'. Some such notion might make sense if you were dyeing your hair green or purple, but brown?

If we look about we can see signs of more dignified celebrations of the change of life. Because these rituals do not involve the priestly caste of men and do not enhance getting and spending activities they are often unpopular, and are even seen as subversive, backward or superstitious.

In traditional Mediterranean societies women of a certain age begin to wear black. When a parent dies, an event which usually occurs at about the same time as menopause, a daughter will don black and never again wear any other colour. This custom is regarded by younger people as morbid behaviour, and is nowadays strenuously discouraged. The women in black are those who register bereavement and carry out the duties of mourning by regular visits to the graves of dead relatives. These practices too are nowadays discouraged. Very few people would agree that the women's quiet activity among the gravestones has any value; they do not see it as part of a contemplative phase in human development, or as a way of conferring form and dignity upon the serendipitousness of life. There may have been no time to mourn the child who died while its brothers and sisters needed all their mother's attention; those children gone their ways, the ageing mother may bring each day the best flowers from her garden to the small grave. Passers-by can click their tongues. The woman herself does not expect them to understand. Her behaviour is proper to her at her time of life, and that thought suffices her.

In countries where these practices are still alive, the cemeteries are not dreary places. In the small town in the Ticino where my mother's ancestors are buried, the cemetery is clean, neat and alight with flowers. On the Feast of All Souls the older women will bring their grandchildren to the cemetery and tell them the story of each relative who is buried there, and pray with them for the repose of those souls. In modern progressive societies graves are untended, unmarked or defaced. Cemeteries are bleak and empty. Most people no longer know, let alone inhabit, the places where their ancestors are buried. We do not value continuity, nor do we value the contemplative life. This indifference creates the meaninglessness and marginality of middle age; it is the cold wind that the fifty-year-old woman feels upon her skin.

The woman who chooses to wear black and live in perpetual *lutto* is eschewing the life of spouse and embracing the role of grandmother. Usually she binds up her hair as well, and covers her head with a shawl or *fazzoletto*. These are all signs that she is not to be flirted with or addressed familiarly by men, although she should walk slowly in the street and even choose to sit down on a park bench without being molested. She is to be treated with respect. Her black liberates her by allowing her to remain invisible, as a kind of secular nun, who is allowed to indulge in her own thoughts.

In Sicily in 1985 I decided to dress in black as an expression of my mourning for my father. At first men displayed no awareness of my unavailable status and still ogled and came sneaking up behind me as I wandered through the temples at Segesta and Selinunte. It was only when I put up my long hair and covered my head that my mourning was respected. I found the new freedom from men's attentions exhilarating rather than depressing. There was also tremendous liberation in not having to think what to wear. Black goes with black. One has only to think of textures, of the part of one's clothing that matters to oneself.

When the Mediterranean woman takes all her outer clothing and throws it in a copper full of boiling black dye, she is enacting a rite of passage. She is renouncing one kind of life and taking on another. She may weep bitterly for the end of her young womanhood, and she may look to the years ahead with foreboding, but she has also the consolation of fulfilling a prescribed procedure. There will be privileges attached to her new status; she will be allowed to rest more, to spend more time sitting at her house door talking with other women, or praying in church, and even to go away for weeks at a time, on her own, on pilgrimages, so seeing the outside world through her own eyes for the first time.

To the young all these activities are utterly unattractive; they can see no point or pleasure in reflection. They neither know nor care about the spiritual landscape that opens out before older people. Consumer culture denies that such a landscape exists. In the free-market economy the frugality and simplicity of old age is anathema. Yet to many troubled souls the calm austerity of old age is a goal to be striven for 'in life's cool evening'. Poets since classical times have celebrated an ideal stage of tranquil thoughtfulness to round off a busy life. The woman of fifty has even more reason to long for that time; after menopause, when she may be permitted to give up being someone's daughter, someone's lover, someone's wife and someone's mother, she may also be allowed to turn into herself. In 1933, when she was forty-seven, the poet H. D. embarked on analysis with Freud, because, she said, in her *Tribute to Freud*:

There was something that was beating in my brain; I do not say my
heart. My brain. I wanted it to be let out. I wanted to free myself of
repetitive thoughts and experiences. (pp. 16–17)

As analysis proceeded she felt herself struggling against an oceanic
swell of unexamined life that threatened to engulf her:

I must not lose grip, I must not lose the end of the picture and
so miss the meaning of the whole, so painfully perceived. I must
hold on here or the picture will blur over and the sequence be lost.
(p. 80)

Changing into yourself doesn't mean becoming obsessed by
yourself, although doubtless there are those who will think the idea no
more than another indulgence of the 'me generation'. It means rather
that you don't continue living your life mainly through responses
to the needs of those in your own household and workplace. You
no longer suppress your own curiosities, and your own insights and
opinions, in order to let other people express theirs. Your mind and
heart, which have always been full of concern for others and interest
in the pursuits of others, may now begin to develop spaces where your
own creativity might begin to extend its range, feel its strength, make
its contribution on a wider stage, a different stage. This need not be a
public stage; the threshold where you stand may open upon a region
of the mind, or of the soul. You may be seeking not to express, but to
understand.

There are many books written now for ageing women which argue
that there need be no change, that the middle-aged woman can continue
being what she always was, an attractive and responsive lover, a dutiful
wife, an efficient employee. These books never consider the possibility
that a woman could actually be tired of being all these things, or that
she might be conscious of having led an unexamined life. Such books
assume that what the middle-aged woman is afraid of, that there is
no point in a woman's life if she is not functioning as lover, wife and
employee, is actually true. You are not reading one of those books.
This book argues instead that women are whole people with a right to
exist and a contribution to make in and as themselves. Moreover, the
climacteric is real; it is a fundamental change, which, like the other

fundamental changes in women's lives, needs mental preparation and profound acceptance if it is not to be experienced as unbearable.

Though I have no intention of minimising the impact of menopause or falsely presenting it as avoidable, I do not argue as Ploss and Bartels do, in the few words that they can be bothered to spare for the ageing woman in volume 3 of *Woman*:

> The climacteric is an indication for woman that the period of her vigour is beginning to disappear forever. With more or less rapid steps but steps which admit of no return, woman now proceeds towards old age. (p. 351)

This 'scientific opinion' is stunning in its banality. Every day that passes takes us closer to our death 'with more or less rapid steps'; as we do not know whether the process will take a day or fifty years, the knowledge cannot avail us much. The clock cannot be turned back for anyone of either sex. In explanation of their premature consignment of the fifty-year-old woman sooner or later to the tomb, Ploss and Bartels quote the utterly absurd observation attributed to the 'father of modern pathology' Rudolf Virchow: 'Woman is a pair of ovaries with a human being attached; whereas man is a human being furnished with a pair of testes' (p. 351). Those men whose interest in women is mostly dictated by the testes do not consider women as human beings but as objects of their sexual attention. For the likes of Virchow post-menopausal women, being unattractive to them, might as well be dead. For women who justify their existence by the amount of male attention they can command, the truth of Virchow's argument is self-evident, but women with more pride than libido do not see their emancipation from the duty of sexual attraction as death-in-life.

Menopause is a change but if that change removes us from attentions of the Virchows of the world, it must be a liberation. It would be easier to grasp this if the ageing woman could point to, as well as all the losses that accompany the climacteric, some gains – gains in seniority, privilege, rank, respect, or privacy. Such gains need to be institutionalised by an outward sign, a change in the form of address, in the style of dress, in the attitude of others. The climacteric is signalled by none of these. Part of the difficulty that women face in dealing with the last great change in lives which have gone through so many fundamental changes already is that the change from mother to grandmother has no outward sign – indeed, women who are being buffeted by this tempestuous passage are supposed to pretend that it isn't happening at all. This is the kind of contradiction that has teased and tormented women all their lives.

There was a time when the beginning of menstruation was marked by the lengthening of skirts and the putting up of hair, which did not necessarily coincide with the biological event, but was an acknowledgement that it had happened, that the girl had become a woman or, as they say in Italy, *si era fatta signorina*. All societies place new restrictions on the fecundable female, but usually there are privileges to accompany them which are thought to compensate in some measure. The 'grown-up' girl can wear scent, make-up and high heels, and pretty underwear, and can stay up late. Glamour is her compensation for the squalor of menstruation. A similar strategy might help us to deal with the upheaval of the climacteric.

Though 'civilised' cultures have given up marking the first great upheaval in women's lives, namely the menarche, the onset of the menses, it is still a huge alteration; the boyish little girl watches herself turning into a womanish individual. Though she might not necessarily groan under puppy fat and pimples, she is aware that her body looks different and smells different, and behaves in a new and not exactly pleasant way. One of the first skills young women have to develop is that of dealing with menstruation in mixed company without anybody guessing what they are about, slipping into the lavatory with a sanitary napkin up a sleeve, washing stained underwear on the sly in co-ed digs. It is arguable that young women would find menstruation less problematic if they did not have to behave as if they were ashamed of it. Seclusion of menstruating women in traditional societies wouldn't have endured in practice for so many centuries if it didn't have a positive aspect. The little girl who retires with the menstruating women has conspicuously grown up; she is admitted to women-only conversations, the like of which she has never experienced before, and she is allowed a time of rest from her hitherto incessant duty of waiting on the family. She does not cook, but is fed, washes only her own clothes, and rests.

The almost entirely negative feelings of women in the developed world towards menstruation are as nothing compared to the embarrassment of the climacteric. The women who are most blasée about menstruating, not caring a whit who knows it, are likely to be the most anxious to conceal the fact that their ovarian function is on the blink. A very intelligent fifty-year-old woman told me once that she had slipped and broken her ankle coming out of a chain-store pharmacy. 'Serves me right,' she said, 'I was so proud to be seen buying tampons at my age! Out I swept and boom! down I went!' I couldn't help wondering if the cashier noticed the age of the woman buying the tampons or if she thought that she was probably buying them for someone else or if she gave a damn. I also wondered if the ankle snapped because bone loss was already taking place; the monthly bleeding of which she was so proud could have been anovulatory, breakthrough bleeding and not menstruation at all.

In the developed world more is made of retirement from paid employment than of menopause. Getting your pensioner's bus pass is a far more significant indicator of changed status than anything we have to mark death of parents, adulthood of children and cessation of ovulation. The state and the employer have constituted themselves the arbiters of lifespan events and they issue the markers. A bereaved mother in our society may not wear her dead relative's picture on her bosom, but she must show her bus pass and her pension book to any of the many strangers who have a right to see them. We have tacitly allowed visceral events like birth and bereavement to fade from public recognition, and some of the evidence seems to show that we are therefore finding them harder to deal with. If the woman who accepts hormonal replacement of the kind that causes breakthrough bleeding imagines that she is holding her menopause at bay she may be complicating the transition and adding to her psychic load in a way that may prove ultimately destructive. We would have a better idea of whether or not this does happen if we had any clear idea of the ideal shape of human life. If neither religion nor psychology nor anthropology nor sociology can offer such a thing, we can only improvise, staggering from expedient to expedient and evasion to evasion.

Odd and disturbing as it may seem, the demand for hysterectomy could be thought to reflect a desire on the part of some, indeed many, women for a definitive rite of passage. In 1981, at the third international congress on the menopause held under the auspices of the International Menopause Society, gynaecologists Barbara Ehret and Louise Dennerstein contributed a paper on 'Psychosocial, Emotional and Medical Sequelae of Hysterectomy'. Ehret described her experiences with 3,000 women treated at her institute at Bad Salzuflen in West Germany. In the course of the discussion she asked:

> What is it that makes such a large number of women allow the prophylactic removal of a healthy organ in the sexual sphere? ... It is very difficult to find an answer to this question. Actively courageous decisions rarely form the basis for consent to an operation. On the contrary, the decision is often influenced by passive, partly autoaggressive tendencies. These women view themselves and are viewed by others as sexual objects; they behave in many aspects of life as passive objects and are considered to be physically and psychically inferior. The removal of the uterus from such a woman is comparable to removing the tearducts from a crying person. (Van Keep et al., 1982, pp. 78–9)

In 40 per cent of Ehret's cases the grounds for hysterectomy were insufficient, being moderate prolapse, ovarian cysts and small fibroids; what was more, the 87 per cent who suffered post-hysterectomy abdominal pain, disturbed sexuality and depression had complained of these symptoms before the operation.

Marcelle Pick, obstetric/gynaecological nurse practitioner, writing on the American website Women to Women feels obliged to begin an entry on hysterectomy with a general comment:

> Every year, more than 600,000 women undergo a hysterectomy. Despite the fact that some progressive doctors claim that up to 90% of hysterectomies are unnecessary, more conservative estimates put that number between 20–30%. Either way, that is a lot of women that may be having unnecessary hysterectomies.

Hysterectomy used to be the most frequently performed surgical procedure in the United States, where in 1988 30 per cent of women aged between forty-five and forty-nine had had their wombs removed (Riphagen et al., 1988); the rate remains high, with a third of American women hysterectomised by age sixty, but it has been overtaken by caesarean section. The incidence drops by about 1 per cent every decade, but even so 20 per cent of women in the developed world will have parted company with their wombs by the age of fifty-five. For every five hysterectomies performed in the US only two are performed in England and only one in Sweden. These contrasts cannot be justified by differences in the health status of the women in the three countries or by the greed of practitioners in America. Extirpation of the uterus is considered justified not only by surgeons but also by women for relatively minor uterine dysfunction. In 2002 a British study led by Michael Maresh of St Mary's Hospital for Women and Children in Manchester found that of 37,298 hysterectomies performed in one year, 46 per cent were carried out for heavy bleeding, which could have been dealt with by endometrial ablation (Maresh et al.).

Women themselves seem to share the view expressed in 1969 by R. L. Wright (quoted in the *Lancet*, 26 September 1987, p. 789):

> After the last planned pregnancy the uterus becomes a useless,
> bleeding, symptom-producing, potentially cancer-bearing organ
> and therefore should be removed.

The discussion run by British website Mumsnet in answer to the question 'Can I request a hysterectomy?' revealed that many of the respondents had insisted upon hysterectomy. A 27-year-old announced that she was soon to undergo the procedure that she had in her own words 'to push for'. Another respondent begged, 'Just be sure that the womb is the source of your problems' – the difficulty is that the woman she was addressing already was sure – quite sure.

The usual justification for hysterectomy in women approaching menopause is that the operation cures flooding: as long ago as 1987, an editorial in the *Lancet* (15 August, p. 376) summarised the fringe benefits of hysterectomy as 'greater reliability at work, availability at all times for sexual intercourse, saving on sanitary protection, freedom from pregnancy and freedom from uterine cancer'.

At the same time that the *Lancet* was defining the blisses of womblessness, psychologists who were discovering that women who reported depression after hysterectomy had very often reported depression before hysterectomy (Gath et al., 1982) began to consider the possibility that the womb had been blamed for problems that had nothing to do with it, by both patients and doctors. It was realised that a significant proportion of the women of all ages whose healthy wombs were removed for pelvic pain were possibly suffering from a 'somatisation disorder' which caused them to convert stresses and unease of non-corporeal origin into symptoms that demanded self-mutilating treatment.

By and large surgeons are loath to entertain the suspicion that they are being exploited in a mutilation ritual, and they have so far been quite willing to perform the operation despite their awareness that uterine bleeding is a notoriously idiopathic phenomenon. Indeed, they have accepted 'anxiety' about the uterus and its potential for developing cancer as sufficient justification for the procedure. In an article on menopause in *Harper's and Queen*, John Studd was reported as saying that in twenty years

> A lot of women will elect to have a hysterectomy when their
> families are complete at forty or forty-five ... That operation will
> remove their ovaries, cervix and endometrium, the three major
> sites of gynaecological cancer. They will then start taking Hormone
> Replacement Therapy and continue it indefinitely.

Evidently Studd then believed that the progressive women of the future would undergo devastating major surgery, to mutilate themselves in order to acquire synthetic sexuality, courtesy of the pharmaceutical multinationals. That was rather more than twenty years ago and Studd's vision has not come to pass. In 2012 the number of hysterectomies performed in the UK fell from 57,669 to 44,634, which signifies a change of heart.

About half of all hysterectomies are carried out because of the presence in the uterus of what women call fibroids and health professionals myomas or leiomyomas. These are overgrowths of smooth muscle. Fibroids are common in women in their forties. Quite large fibroids can be quite asymptomatic; others will cause some pain and increased blood loss at menstruation. Fibroids usually shrink and disappear with the involution of the uterus after the cessation of ovarian function. Hysterectomy is a major operation and has a number of common and serious after-effects; of the 37,298 cases reviewed by Maresh's team in 2002, 14 women died within six weeks of the surgery, 30 suffered complications and 130 needed further treatment.

Clearly, hysterectomy is not an appropriate treatment for disorders that are milder and less dangerous than the effects of the procedure itself. Both eagerness to undergo hysterectomy and the evangelism of hysterectomised women are irrational. To some extent both are the result of abuse of their authority by professionals, but there is also an element of women's own urge to mutilate themselves and in particular to inflict wounds upon the abdomen. It is curious that hysterectomy should be trivialised and presented as routine while mastectomy is dramatised and regarded as a catastrophe. The visible mutilation (a comparatively minor operation) is dreaded in the same irrational proportion as the massive internal mutilation is courted.

No woman traverses the climacteric without experiencing vivid awareness of a change; if the adult can only live out the blueprint provided by pre-verbal experience, as in traditional Freudian views of human development, there can be little optimism about this change. Nowadays even in psychoanalysis Freudian determinism has had to give way before developmental accounts of the human career.

Lifespan theories were for a time very fashionable, but there is no unanimity in them. In 1950, Erik Erikson defined 'Eight Stages of Man'. Daniel Levinson elaborated this idea into a staircase model, which shows how the successful negotiation of each phase allows progress to the next, but this model was challenged by sociologists who argued that changes are not triggered by chronology or biology, but by the timing of crucial life events and the individual's response to them. The two schools of thought have agreed to differ. It is difficult to relate this view of the human career to women, whose lives encompass so many changes. The growing up of children, the death of parents and the cessation of menstruation are upheaving for women regardless of social class; some of the evidence goes to show that lower-middle-class or blue-collar women are more aware of the change than more privileged women (e.g. Van Keep and Kellerhals, 1974; Severne, 1979; Greene and Cooke, 1980; Polit and Larocco, 1980; Campagnoli et al., 1981). One might also have thought that most women's work, being dead-end, offers little opportunity for alternative patterns of development.

If the theorists can disagree on the fundamental question of whether or not human life proceeds through passages, we clearly cannot expect the revival of rites of passage. The theorists do not consider the importance of cultural stereotyping and projection of appropriate models, for their research is predicated on questionnaires of individuals. However, they do raise an important question, which is whether or not menopause has been overemphasised and has become a scapegoat for other more disorienting changes in occupation and social role experienced by women in midlife. Margaret Gullette has argued that menopause has been socially constructed as a 'magic marker of decline'.

Fortunately, a book like this one does not need to enter into the questions of definition and discipline that must be addressed by social scientists; it is the woman's awareness of a fundamental change that is the important factor, whether it occurs with menopause, or divorce, or widowhood, or the departure or sexual activity or marriage of her children. The change may come early or late; it may be sudden and catastrophic, or it may be slow and long-drawn-out, or it may be jerky, or it may be divided into strands some of which go fast and are sudden, and others that are slow and inexorable. One thing is certain; it will come and it will keep on coming.

The women of the Newfoundland fishing village studied by Dona Lee Davis between October 1977 and December 1978 saw the female lifespan as 'characterized by a series of seven-year-cycles' (p. 79). Davis had a good deal of difficulty in eliciting from these women, toughened by a hard climate and harder work, any subjective account of their own symptoms at menopause. They often described themselves and other women as 'on their changes', whether referring to the processes of pregnancy, birth, lactation and weaning, or the menstrual cycle, or the menopause. They placed a high value on courage and coping in relative silence, although they had a complicated rhetoric of 'nerves'. If asked about the subjective symptoms they attempted to compare or contrast them with the symptoms of others, in preference to making avowals on their own behalf. They did not give themselves the kind of enthralled introspective attention that could give the researcher answers to her questionnaire. As far as they were concerned, a woman who could not cope with her changes was unlikely to be able to cope with anything else; to admit to having symptoms was to complain and to complain was to admit being unable to cope. Davis was obliged to conclude that the standard questionnaires on menopausal symptoms were useless in the circumstances. She had to let the women express their concept of their own situation using their own vocabulary, which invited no comparison or translation into the language of hot flushing, irritability, joint pains, insomnia and so forth.

Modern concepts of four ages or eight ages or no ages seem to me to have no greater validity and a good deal less cultural importance than the seven-year stages of the Newfoundland women's lifespan theory which, like Shakespeare's, uses Hippocrates' division of human life into seven ages, each divided by a critical passage or climacteric. Mostly the seven ages thus defined are 'ages of man'. Women's lives are constructed of changes so vivid that they might well be called metamorphoses; often these changes, from child to woman to lover to wife to mother to grandmother, are signalled by contrasting body states from skinny to curvaceous or pregnant or obese and back again. The underlying biological changes are mostly to be hidden or denied. Only the change from single woman to married woman, which paradoxically may involve no fundamental change of lifestyle or biological status, has an outward, ceremonial sign, exaggerated even, in the change of the woman's name. The fifth climacteric signals the end of all the disruptions and remodellings involved in defloration, conception, pregnancy, childbirth and lactation; it is the change that ends changes. It is the beginning of the long gradual change from body into soul.

My definition of the seven ages of woman does not correspond with Shakespeare's ages of man in all respects. Women's seven ages begin with the first critical phase or climacteric, which is birth and infancy; the second stormy passage is adolescence, the third defloration, the fourth childbirth, and the fifth, menopause. Between them lie the relative calms of childhood, maidenhood, wifehood, and motherhood. The fifth is exceeded in significance only by the grand climacteric of dying. The climacteric is not a rite of passage, but the passage itself. The menopause, being a non-event, the period that does not come, cannot be turned into a ritual. Nevertheless if we look about us we can find examples of female recognition of a change. Josephine Baker began adopting children, when? When she was fifty. When did Helene Deutsch leave Vienna? When she was fifty, with half her life still to live, for she died at the age of ninety-seven. Few women devise as drastic a ceremonial as Helen Thayer who, at fifty-two, 'skied to the magnetic North Pole with her dog. She pulled a 160-pound sled for twenty-seven days and 345 miles, surviving seven polar bear confrontations, three blizzards, near starvation and several days of blindness'. Thayer courted annihilation, and several times must have thought she had found it; she emerged reborn.

If women are to celebrate the fifth climacteric by claiming special privileges, they will have to award them to themselves. If we consider the behaviour of fifty-year-old women, we may discover that in fact they do. Among the traces of vanished rites of passage we may include the new attitude of older women to jewellery; sometimes this is precipitated by the inheriting of a mother's jewellery, and the rationalisation is that it would be a pity to break up the pieces. Gems have a significance of their own; they are emblems of unchanging beauty and spiritual power; the ageing woman who wears a diamond necklace on a picnic is pleasing herself. The middle-aged woman may declare a taste for her own tipple, and for the first time a bottle of her own appears on the drinks tray. She may become interested in betting on horses or playing bingo. She might even decide to change her house for a smaller one, or for a house in the country, or for a house that demands less housework and more gardening. She might even decide, after years of putting up with him for the children's sake, to divorce her husband. Whatever she decides, the younger generation will click its collective tongue. The younger generation is not used to her deciding anything, and has never doubted that the pinnacle of her happiness has been achieved waiting on it hand and foot.

Other women content themselves with subtler changes in their image at a psychological stage that seems to them appropriate. Lots of middle-aged women begin to leave off make-up which long-sighted eyes cannot see to apply very well. They don't shop for clothes with the same indefatigability as younger women, and they want the clothes they buy to last longer. With the gradual erosion of their narcissism, many women become more adventurous in their conversation; they begin to make their own jokes instead of laughing at the jokes of others, and to express their own opinions in the face of the most assured derision. In *La Fin de Chéri* Colette lets us see Léa de Lonval after this change has taken place. The voluptuous *femme d'un certain âge* enveloped in cunningly chosen draperies has become a massive, sexless figure like a jolly old man with a shock of white hair and a vulgar manner, who believes that the solution to all human ills can be found in good food. This figure is regarded by Colette without enthusiasm; she is not interested in how Léa became like this, or why, but we are. Colette herself did not follow the same route; she never stopped making herself up and wearing scent, and never allowed her husband to see her before she was presentable. To the last, we are told, she retained her 'femininity'. If femininity is real, it should amount to more than a streak of kohl and a squirt of scent.

Colette, like many other women, feared the virilisation that accompanies old age. In *Chéri*, published in 1920 when she was forty-seven, she invented a gallery of grotesque older women who represent her middle-aged heroine's future: the Baronne de Berche, whom age is virilising to a terrifying extent, so that bushes of hair burst forth from her ears and nostrils and flourish on her lip, or the ancient Lili, with her giggling ways, her round face made up like a doll on top of a neck like a belly, who threatens to marry the adolescent Prince Ceste. Léa is to avoid following in the footsteps of Lili by undergoing the ordeal of giving Chéri up to be married to a woman of his own generation, as the much younger Marschallin does in *Der Rosenkavalier*.

For Léa femininity is a matter of iron self-discipline; she allows no scenes, permits herself no reproaches, never in fact raises her voice. She would never leave off her corset, no matter how it pinched – '*Nue si on veut, mais jamais depoitraillée*' – if her legs are swollen, she wears her little blue boots to hide it. She knows she needs white near her face, and very pale pink for her underwear and her *déshabilles*, if the slackening of her muscles and the loosening of her skin are not to become unattractively apparent, but she tells herself too that as soon as Chéri is married and happily disposed of, she will no longer have to exercise such vigilance. Colette's contempt for old age and fear of it is evident in many small touches:

> Sitting with her cheek resting on her hand, she penetrated in a
> dream into her imminent old age, imagined her days each exactly
> like the other, saw herself with Chéri's mother, kept alive for a
> long time by a lively rivalry which shortened the hours, and the
> degrading carelessness which induces mature women first to leave
> off their corsets, then dyeing their hair, and at last fine lingerie. She
> tasted in anticipation the rascally pleasures of the aged which are
> nothing but secret mourning, murderous wishes, and lively hopes
> springing eternal for catastrophes that spare no one, and no part of
> the world ... (p. 103)

Colette was obese; she would have been surprised to hear that women nowadays consider obesity a much greater crime against femininity than wearing cotton underwear. 'Feminine' women these days prefer to maintain their flesh in a self-supporting condition.

Colette also suffered from arthritis, almost certainly complicated by osteoporosis, aggravated by a lifestyle that had always been sedentary. Her version of femininity is theatrical, a set of assumed behaviours and an appropriate costume. Older women can afford to agree that femininity is a charade, a matter of coloured hair, écru lace and whalebones, the kind of slap and tat that transvestites are in love with, and no more. What women in the climacteric are afraid of losing is not femininity, which can always be faked and probably is always fake, but femaleness. The people who read Colette now are unaware of her dyed hair, her fine lingerie, and her corsets. They are also unaware of her contempt for age. What remains vivid and unforgettable across page after page is Colette's femaleness, which is not a matter of a rag, a bone and a hank of hair.

After centuries of conditioning of the female into the condition of perpetual girlishness called femininity, we cannot remember what femaleness is. Though feminists have been arguing for years that there is a self-defining female energy, and a female libido that is not expressed merely in response to demands by the male, and a female way of being and of experiencing the world, we are still not close to recognising it. Yet every mother who has held a girl child in her arms has known that she was different from a boy child and that she would approach the reality around her in a different way. The onset and retreat of her reproductive years cannot alter that. She is female and she will die female, and though many centuries should pass, archaeologists would identify her skeleton as the remains of a female creature.

What actually happens to the ageing woman during the climacteric is that men lose interest in manipulating her femaleness; they no longer sniff around her. They do not bother to intimidate her by whistles and catcalls as she passes the building site. They no longer communicate their confidence that she exists for them by assessing her physical charms or acknowledging them. The kerb-crawling stops. In 1973 Doris Lessing told an interviewer in *Harper's Magazine*:

> ... you only begin to discover the difference between what you really are, your real self, and your appearance, when you get a bit older ... A whole dimension of life suddenly slides away and you realize that what in fact you've been using to get attention has been what you look like ... It's a biological thing. It's totally and

absolutely impersonal. It really is a most salutary and fascinating
thing to go through, shedding it all. Growing old is really
extraordinarily interesting. (Tiger, 1986)

The change hurts. Like a person newly released from leg-irons,
the freed woman staggers at first. Though her excessive visibility was
anguish, her present invisibility is disorienting. She had not realised
how much she depended upon her physical presence, at shop counters,
at the garage, on the bus. For the first time in her life she finds that
she has to raise her voice or wait endlessly while other people push
in front of her. She doesn't remember how bitterly she resented being
hunted and harried through the world as a desirable female, doesn't
remember having to take in the most spectacular monuments while
walking briskly and keeping her eyes trained purposefully ahead, to
avoid being accosted by the men who prowled on either side, doesn't
remember being groped in cathedrals and frightened out of cinemas.
She learns to avoid the heavy swing doors that are no longer held open
for her, and to avoid places where her new invisibility means that she
will be trampled and jostled.

The woman who retains the viewpoint of the young, to whom
older people are not only invisible but uninteresting, will manage this
transition badly. Yet if there is no objective correlative outside herself
by which a woman may take her bearings, no marker buoys for the
channel, the most intelligent and sensitive woman can find herself
drifting at the mercy of destructive currents.

Simone de Beauvoir struggled for years with her contempt for her
own age group. As a result, though she had every resource that any
human being could have, intelligence, prestige, work worth doing that
health and opportunity allowed her to continue, and an impressive circle
of friends and acquaintances, she aged ungracefully and ungratefully.
Every day she told herself, 'I am not what I was', and wasted precious
time in bitter regret. Though she was spared for longevity, and an old
age unbedevilled by poverty or disease, she felt no gratitude, no sense of
her good fortune whatsoever. Many happier people have died younger
and unwillingly left a life they loved, but Simone de Beauvoir felt she
owed them nothing, certainly not to be happy.

Women will have to devise their own rite of passage, a celebration of
what could be regarded as the restoration of a woman to herself. The

passionate, idealistic, energetic young individual who existed before menstruation can come on earth again if we let her. In a symposium on 'The timing of psychosocial changes in women's lives', Californian researcher Emily Hancock 'took as a given that women themselves are the experts in understanding their own lives and that they need to take the description and analysis of their own experiences into their own hands' (Reinke et al., p. 275). For her doctorate at Harvard she interviewed twenty middle-aged women (1989). She discovered that most of them had a well-articulated sense of self in childhood that is lost in adolescence in the process that feminists call conditioning when girls learn feminine behaviour, and become less assertive, smaller and weaker than boys.

> Only when women confronted what life had laid at their feet
> and began to question where they themselves stood in the
> configuration of their lives, did they become aware that they had
> pictured themselves happily embedded in enduring relationships.
> With these images shattered, they began to realize that investing
> in relationships without articulating a sense of self could not
> ensure against change, damage, or loss. Women who could forge
> a new framework for living in which the self became the subject
> of experience and the object of care credited their maturity to this
> process.

The tone of Hancock's prose suggests a fair degree of researcher bias. We wonder whether the women she was studying would have used the same words to describe their experience, but even so, the case is persuasive.

> A woman who could respond to the disintegration of old
> assumptions by threading her way back to childhood and catching
> hold of a girl she could draw strength from and rely on matured.
> Women who had no such childhood self to retrieve succumbed to
> defeat. (p. 278)

It is the women who find themselves turning back into themselves during the peri-menopause who will experience what Margaret Mead called 'post-menopausal zest'.

Before she herself had traversed the climacteric, Helene Deutsch took a dim view of the post-menopause years as a retreat from genitality to immaturity. In her old age, her view changed:

> The biological destiny of old age varies from one individual to another. Like all the developmental periods of life, it depends greatly on the events of adolescence. To our stereotyped way of thinking, the process of growing up is identical with the conquest of the stormy forces of adolescence. Yet I feel that my *Sturm und Drang* period, which continued long into my years of maturity, is still alive within me and refuses to come to an end … I find that there are still ecstasies and loves within me, and that these feelings are rooted in my adolescence. They may be reaction formations against the threat of death, but at the same time they represent the generous impulses of the most energetic period of my life. (Deutsch, 1973, pp. 215–16)

We might develop better strategies for the management of the difficult transition if we think of what we are doing not as denial of the change or postponement of the change, but as acceleration of the change, the change back into the self you were before you became a tool of your sexual and reproductive destiny. You were strong then, and well, and happy, until adolescence turned you into something more problematical, and you shall be well and strong and happy again.

3

The Lucky Ones

If turning fifty gave us the keys to the city, if turning fifty entitled us to first place in the queue, if turning fifty gave us the right to sit down, the physical discomforts of the climacteric would be a small price to pay. In 1988 Dr Barbara Evans, in the preface to the fourth edition of her book *Life Change*, told us:

> Women from countries where age is venerated suffer less
> physically than other women at the change of life, or menopause.
> Unfortunately, ours is not one of those societies. (p. 11)

What was true then is still true. Even in the twenty-first century there are societies surviving on the planet where the principle of seniority is generally respected and where the seniority of the older woman is not negated by the fact of her sex, but none of them is a society in which any of us would want to live or in which any of us could live if we wanted to. We don't actually know whether venerated women 'suffer less physically' at menopause, because no systematic study of their subjectively perceived well-being has ever been undertaken. Against the spectrum of toil and pain which is the life of a Third World woman, the distress of the climacteric could hardly be said to bulk large.

It is true that in hundreds of thousands of village communities in Asia and Africa older women find themselves at the centre of social organisation, but every one of those societies is under extreme stress. With every year that passes more and more of those communities succumb to the pressures of urbanisation and modernisation. In any case it should be clearly understood that, though the extended households of traditional Asia represented something for which most people might aim, they were never the majority of households in any settlement. Poverty, conflict, changes in the system of land tenure, famine, migration, illness and death could all frustrate the family building process and often did. The success of the extended family involved not only success in bearing the required number of male children and bringing them up to competent adulthood but also complex social strategies, together with skilful management of the household capital and of the intrapersonal relationships that guaranteed the quality of life, plus a modicum of sheer good luck. The bigger the family the better it weathered upheavals, because the loss of one senior male did not leave the family rudderless or fragmented. In societies dominated by such families there is not the traditional gulf between public and domestic life that guarantees the subjection of women. The contribution of the senior female to the extended family is second in importance only to the role of the patriarch, and in some cases not even to that.

Mohammed Jamil Hanifi, writing about Afghan society in 1988, described the extended family as 'practically the only organized economic unit in Afghan rural society, sharing production and consumption ... The Afghan extended family is also the primary social unit. Individuals are identified primarily by the family to which they belong. Enculturation and socialization take place primarily within the household; children learn the roles that they will perform as children, adolescents and adults ... the extended families are the base social units through which individuals interact with the larger socio-cultural environment' (Hanifi, pp. 50–51). In such families a single woman is not given total responsibility for the socialisation of her children, which is the duty of her whole family, nor are children taken out of the home to be indoctrinated in child ghettos by a horde of underpaid professionals. In all such families women are subject to men, but the fact of segregation means that in terms of daily interaction the women are not at the mercy of the men. They cannot be terrorised or beaten, for example, unless the other women in the family agree to it. Or as Antje Olowali put it, in describing the culture of the matriarchal Kuna people of Panama, 'Due to the absence of privacy there is no domestic violence.' Husbands are usually not permitted unlimited access to the bodies of their wives, who often sleep alongside their children. Though the relationship of consort is important, and women often have a vivid and hilarious imagery of their own for matters sexual, it is not the only or even the primary relationship. There is no public display of affection between spouses.

> A man must never show affection for his wife in front of anyone else, and it is assumed that there are few common grounds for conversation between an Afghan husband and wife. The relationship is confined to economic cooperation and sexual intimacy. Such a relationship does not preclude affection, but the only permitted public manifestations of it are economic cooperation and the procreation of children. (Hanifi, p. 52)

For the Asian woman in a traditional family the affection of her mother-in-law and her sister-wives, and of their children, and even of her younger brothers-in-law, may well be more important to the quality of her everyday life than her husband's degree of partiality to her. In Western society, by contrast, it is assumed that an ideal sexual relationship should outweigh all other relationships. This notion in itself increases the load of anxiety on the menopausal woman who feels her interest in sex declining. No other role within her personal relationships is open to her, her mothering function having withered away to that of short-order cook and bottle-washer for a family that more and more nowadays cannot be bothered even to eat together. The Western woman has no option but to regard possible loss of sexual interest as tantamount to utter uselessness. The ageing woman in the Afghan household moves closer and closer to the centre of activity at the same stage in her life that the Western woman finds herself pushed to the margins.

> Much household activity is outside the concern of husbands and this guarantees a wife autonomy to manage these affairs. The wife, like all women, accepts her overall inferiority as part of the Afghan social order, but her immersion in her own affairs greatly mitigates this sense of inferiority. Beneath the outward submissiveness is a realization and understanding of the indispensability of her own household activities. (Hanifi, p. 52)

Those activities are not merely cooking and cleaning. The Afghan, like any other traditional south Asian household, produces its own foodstuffs or buys them in bulk, unpackaged and unprocessed. The amounts needed have to be carefully calculated; the quality of the food must be controlled and maintained. The senior wife is responsible for controlling the release of supplies stored in the household. Mistakes in her calculations, or in buying goods of inferior quality, can be catastrophic. A shortfall before the next harvest or rot or infestation in the storage bins can mean having to acquire further supplies when the price is high. The successful economic management of such a household is at least as demanding as the successful management of a small restaurant. As the wife ages and ascends in the seniority scale, more and more of this responsibility with its accompanying power falls to her. If she is incompetent the whole family suffers and may break up.

Malika Grasshoff describes 'the central position of women in the life of the Berbers of Northern-Africa exemplified by the Kabyles ...' 'the woman is the foundation of the house and the family, but her role as woman and mother is only completely fulfilled when she becomes a grandmother.' The role of the senior woman in traditional society can be illustrated not only from village societies in the Asian subcontinent, but also in Niger, Yunnan, Ontario, Surinam, Vietnam, Micronesia and New Mexico. 'It is normal in most parts of the world, where women have low status when they are young for the power and status of women to increase over the life course' (Wilson, G., p. 24).

Consideration of the role of the older woman in the extended family has given rise to the belief that the cessation of ovulation long before death has been selected for in the human female, so essential is the role of the post-menopausal woman to the survival of her family. The hypothesis voiced by Cambridge sociobiologist Donald Parry that 'the menopause is nature's original contraceptive that freed women for leadership in the extended family and in the broad community' has by now become orthodoxy. Discussions of the evolutionary origin of menopause make regular appearances in journals such as *Climacteric* and *Menopause*, broached in some cases by animal-behaviour experts like Mirkka Lahdenperä and Andy Russell, who lock horns with such Masters in Menopause as David Sturdee and Alastair MacLennan (Pollycove et al.). Entertaining as such *jeux d'esprit* may be, they offer little in the way of practical advice.

A new explanation of the phenomenon of menopause, which is unknown in other terrestrial species except for two kinds of whales, has recently been put forward by evolutionary biologist Rama Singh of McMaster University in Canada. He reckons that what causes the premature end of fertility in the human female is the human male's predilection for younger females (Morton et al.). His theory is that, rather than the menopause preventing older women from continuing to reproduce, it is lack of reproduction that resulted in the evolution of the menopause. 'How do you evolve infertility?' he asks. 'It is contrary to the whole notion of natural selection. Natural selection selects for fertility, for reproduction – not for stopping it. This theory says if women were reproducing all along, and there were no preference against older women, women would be reproducing, like men, for their whole lives.' Another evolutionary biologist, Dr Maxwell Burton-Chellew, of Oxford University, rejects Singh's hypothesis, which is in truth rather lame, pointing to the evolution of worker bees, all of them sterile females, and questioning whether it might not be that men choose younger mates because older ones are less fertile, thus putting the horse back before the cart.

The happy ending envisaged by Parry and his successors is not only no longer available to women facing the challenges of consumer society, it was only ever available to a minority of women. The life career of a woman in the traditional family in preliterate society is both difficult and dangerous; as a young bride she comes into the house of strangers where she is last in the pecking order and has to wait upon everyone else. Her status changes noticeably with the bearing of her first male child, but in all things she is subject not only to her husband but also her husband's mother and has to study to please her. As her sons approach adulthood, the wife's prospect of becoming mistress in her own household draws nearer and nearer. She may initiate the splitting off of her nuclear family from the household of her husband's parents, for example if her husband is a younger son or if she is at a disadvantage in relation to another of the wives, so that she can begin to build up a household of her own to which her own sons will bring wives in their turn. She may on the other hand find herself assuming command of the other women and children as her mother-in-law becomes too frail to do so, or dies. At all points in this development she is required to adjust, and the adjustments are often so difficult that she becomes ill. In pre-capitalist or pre-literate societies pregnancy and childbirth themselves are dangerous; survival is anything but assured. The woman who finally makes it and finds herself assuming authority over new daughters-in-law and running the large household must usually have done so during the climacterium, but we would be surprised to find any significant amount of evidence relating to its discomforts on the part of women who have everything to congratulate themselves upon in having reached it.

The importance of climacteric distress grows as the lives of younger women become more liveable. As most women no longer have to endure the bitter grief of infant death, or dread each childbirth as a time of danger, or spend most of their reproductive years pregnant or lactating, all the negative aspects of the years of fertility have faded from recall. We have only the relatively minor inconveniences of practising contraception and regular menstruation to mar 'the best years of our lives'. As most of our dealings with traditional families have involved us in concerted attempts to control their high fertility, we have always addressed ourselves to the reproducing women, and have always assumed that their mothers-in-law were tyrannical, unsexed figures who treated their daughters-in-law like breeding machines. Because we encountered stress and unhappiness among young wives we assumed that the husband's mother was by definition a hated, repressive figure. If in fact she is, the extended household will soon fission.

The successful mother-in-law rules the extended family by love. Her wisdom, based upon her experience, should protect and guide the economic activity of the whole group to the perceived advantage of all its members. In a well-run extended household life should be perceptibly easier than in separate nuclear families. If there is less work for individuals because it is done collectively, if there is more food because it is more efficiently produced or economically bought, stored and prepared, if children are safer and happier, there can be small motivation for splitting up. If on the other hand a younger wife feels herself persecuted or put upon, she will stop at nothing until she can escape into a home of her own, even if it is a rented hovel or a slum on the outskirts of a city. The woman who wins the love of her daughters-in-law and extends her household by keeping all her sons and their wives and children with her is vividly aware of her success and good fortune, even if she is not to be spared the heavier household tasks, not to be offered the choicest morsels at each meal or allowed to spend all her time playing with the babies and young children, or allowed to smoke tobacco and drink with the male elders.

In the 1920s the American anthropologist and missionary William Wiser studied life in Karimpur, a village near Agra. This is his account of the role played by one grandmother:

> Balram's wife is now undisputed mistress of the household …
> Because of her age and greying hair she moves about the
> neighbourhood with her face only partially covered. She enjoys
> diversions as much as does Balram. Once when a special fair was
> held at the temple near Mainpuri, six miles from here, she wanted
> to go. They do not own an oxcart nor did she have the bus fare.
> So she went and returned on foot, delighted with all that she had
> seen and heard, and, except for tired feet, not much the worse
> for wear …
>
> She spends most of her time sitting in her own courtyard where
> she can watch all the comings and goings in the lane … She is old
> enough to be free of most restrictions, so when one of the sons of
> Prakash's family comes into the courtyard and younger *bahus* cover
> their faces, Balram's wife carries on in her high-pitched voice with
> whatever tale she is relating … Jiha and the *bahus* enjoy her. She
> is not fussy, nor is she easily offended, and seems able to create
> laughter at all times. Circulating gossip – amusing gossip – is her
> chief contribution … (Wiser, pp. 81–3)

This situation had not changed much when a new generation of anthropologists spent time in south Asia in the Seventies. What could be observed in societies organised upon such lines was a female hierarchy existing alongside the male power structure, with its own sphere of influence and considerable bargaining power. Liesa Stamm described the lives of the women of Ksar-Hellal in the Tunisian Sahel as 'an expectable series of age roles in which they establish skills and personal relationships in the family and household through which they exert influence and control' (Stamm, p. 26). Marriages were arranged, usually by negotiations with neighbouring families initiated and conducted until the final stages by the older women. For many women the most painful aspect of the system was their separation first from their own mothers, and then from their daughters. The painfulness of this separation from the mother, considered to be the source of love, was eased by the allowing of long visits by daughters to their mothers' homes. It was common for wives to return to their mothers' houses for their first and subsequent confinements, and to remain there for weeks and sometimes months after the child is born. With the birth of sons and the cementing of the relationship within the new family the woman gradually acquired influence in this new sphere, but she never forgot her strong attachment to her own mother.

> It is in her role as mother of adult children that a woman has the opportunity to exert the greatest degree of social power ... adult children more frequently turn to their mothers for advice and support ... with increasing age ... women in Ksar-Hellal continue to represent a source of affection, assistance and advice for their adult children, and thereby maintain their role of influence within the family. Rather than losing the main orientation of her female role in her older years a woman in Ksar-Hellal extends her influence into the households of her married children. (Stamm, pp. 28–9)

The fact that the Ksar-Hellal used to love and honour old ladies is not going to popularise their lifestyle in our own countries, nor did it materially aid its survival in Tunisia. As Pat Caplan observed in South India *c*.1980 these matrifocal values can survive transplantation to the cities.

> Many women become grandparents in their early forties and this adds a new dimension to their domestic roles. Daughters come home for their confinement, and stay for long periods. If they live in Madras, they visit very frequently ... Most women welcome and accept eagerly their role as grandmothers and if they have grandchildren living with them they devote a great deal of time and attention to them ... the position of a wife is one of subordination, that of a mother is much more powerful. (pp. 58–9)

Ken David, working at much the same time as Stamm and Caplan amongst the Tamils of Jaffna in northern Sri Lanka, observed much the same phenomena:

... the middle-aged woman can wield great influence over her family. She retains the auspiciousness of the married state and is less fettered by the social reticence expected of a young bride. She is in the optimal position to influence decisions of significance in her family, especially in the crucial matters of marital alliances for her sons and daughters. (David, 1980, p. 99)

Few women living in modern society would regard the supremacy of mothers-in-law as a desirable phenomenon. Clearly, too, such a system was and continues to be very hard on childless wives. The lucky women for whom the climacterium is associated with positive gains in prestige, freedom, leisure, authority and influence are a minority; they have always been outnumbered by the women who have not yet made it or did not make it. The sufferings of widows in such societies can be terrible: Indian widows are not usually permitted to remarry and often stripped of their possessions and forced into perpetual mourning and seclusion. In the Seventies in Iran, where men marry women much younger than themselves, 23 per cent of women aged between forty-five and fifty-four were already widowed; among women aged fifty-five to sixty-four the proportion rises to 48 per cent (Rudolph-Touba, pp. 233–4). In most Asian communities such women are entirely at the mercy of their relatives. The lucky mother-in-law must keep not only herself and her sons alive long enough for her to come into her own, but her husband as well. Where the middle-aged woman with a husband is powerful and auspicious, the middle-aged widow is an outcast.

In modern nuclear families there is only one relationship of intimacy and importance and that is the relationship between spouses. If that doesn't work the family must be jettisoned, the feelings of the children being of relatively little account.

Some of the limited studies that have been done seem to indicate that women who have rewarding work to do deal best with menopause; it seems fairly obvious that women with work they enjoy doing will ignore symptoms, if they form them, for as long as they can, so that they can continue effectively with the work they love and will refute any suggestion that the effects of the climacteric may disqualify them from doing it. Though the menopause itself may have no positive aspect, there are positive reinforcements for making light of it.

The women who have satisfying, well-paid work to do are another lucky minority. Many of the studies of their attitudes can hardly be applied to the condition of minority women or working-class women, many of whom have endured the hardships of the life of a junior female only to find when they themselves become senior that the rewards have been cancelled. Nowadays fifty-year-old women who respected their mothers and nursed their grandmothers find themselves without honour and left to the care of strangers. They have been caught in the transition from one kind of system, a system identified perhaps with the self-help networks of the working class or the ghetto, to another generally considered better, more progressive. At worst the woman who grew up in a house with her Gran and her mother and her aunts and did her bit to help out for them will eventually find herself imprisoned in a house she cannot afford to heat, that she is too frightened to leave because old women are easy pickings for the muggers on the streets outside. For a woman in such a situation every marker of advancing age brings real dread. Symptom formation for her is part of a strategy of survival, for only if she is sick will someone look after her.

The loneliness and vulnerability of old women is the ultimate achievement of a centuries-long campaign in the Western world to destroy the power of the mother. She has relinquished her sway not to the sire of her children but to the patriarchal bureaucratic state of which each authoritarian family is a microcosm. In order to maintain his authority in our tiny households a husband must continually assert the primacy of his needs over the demands of the children. The mother in such a family must play the consort before all else; she can expect no fulfilment in her mother role. Indeed, she may be required to give the care of her children into the hands of menials and professionals, in order to concentrate all of her attention on her functions as her husband's sexual partner and the principal indicator of his wealth and social standing. Though twenty-first century wives do not have armies of servants to care for their children, they are obliged to commit the children to nursery school, to school, to camp, to bed in their own rooms before daddy gets home, and even to the tender mercies of the babysitter. The woman who works outside as well as inside the home has even more difficulty in giving in to the demands of the love affair with her babies. As Estelle Leontief put it in her poem 'Painting in Pompeii':

We shut the album on the mother
who's always crying,
always wild
with unrequited love.

(Luria and Tiger, p. 144)

In terms of the individual woman's life, the attack upon her mother-right was mounted as soon as her children were conceived, when professionals took over the management of her pregnancy and the birth. The mother's body was denied her children, who slept apart from her. They were driven about in carts and carriers instead of carried in her arms or on her back, and for some generations at least were even denied the breast. It is not up to a mother to socialise her child or to teach it the family's way of doing things. These functions having been taken over and carried out inefficiently by the state, the mother is denied the honours of maternity.

All that remains to the mother in modern consumer society is the role of scapegoat; psychoanalysis uses huge amounts of money and time to persuade analysands to foist their problems on to the absent mother, who has no opportunity to utter a word in her own defence. Hostility to the mother in our societies is an index of mental health. Mothers whose hearts yearn for their children are told that they have overidentified with their mothering role, that they were possessive or overprotective. Mothers are forced to learn to dissimulate their vulnerability, to harden their hearts, and this often before their children are at all able to cope alone. Whether immature, confused or even disturbed, at eighteen years old our children are no longer our business, though they have no compunction in using us whenever they wish to exploit our vulnerability to them. In societies where this is not the case, where a mother's love and nearness are considered among the sweetest sweets of existence, seeing one's daughters become mothers is a joyous experience.

Organising relationships so that mothers accumulate prestige, power and autonomy as they grow older requires matrilocality, which simply means that the mother is within physical reach of her grown-up children, who are not being moved about at the behest of an employer. Equally essential perhaps is a degree of social stability which allows the development of patterns of interaction and accretion of experience that can only remain relevant in the absence of rapid technological or economic change. In traditional societies, the ageing mother has mothering functions to perform in the families of her grown-up children, caring for the birthing woman, mothering the older children when their mother is involved with a newborn, disciplining and socialising them according to the family's system of values. In such families there is not a single scapegoat mother, but a succession of big mothers and little mothers, some of whom are male.

We can see some such mechanisms surviving in some working-class communities in Britain, or in black communities in the United States.

> The patterns of black female role behaviour rarely result in
> depression in middle age. Often the 'grannie' or 'auntie' lives with
> the family and cares for the children while the children's mother
> works; thus the older woman suffers no maternal role loss. (Bart
> and Grossman, p. 215)

The mother-centred household is associated with stagnation, with high fertility and with poverty, all indices of backwardness. Most people in the industrialised world see such systems as situations to escape from, rather than to aim for. Aiming to build an extended family in Western society would be futile in any case, for one cannot live in such a system without intensive training from birth. The nuclear family has difficulty lasting until its children are grown up, and could only in the most exceptional circumstances turn into a larger and more durable social unit. Having to live with one's in-laws is regarded principally as a penalty for improvidence. Though many couples have to do it, none of them is proud of the fact and nearly all of them experience the situation as all but unbearable. Living with the in-laws is regarded as sufficient explanation for marital break-up.

With every year that passes, the role of the grandmother is further weakened so that there is in it for most women absolutely nothing to be looked forward to. Older women must look for satisfaction where men do, in their relations with their employer, which will end with a crunch at retirement age. Studies of the well-being of women in their middle years are few on the ground. A 1984 study followed the trend in finding that the principal determinant of women's perception of the two factors studied, 'mastery' and 'pleasure', was employment status; the higher the prestige of the job they held, the higher their well-being rating.

The findings of this study cast doubt on the utility of the constructs often cited as critical for understanding the psychological well-being of women in the middle years. The major correlate of the sense of mastery was employment status, a construct rarely given serious consideration either in theory or in clinical practice, as central to psychological well-being. Occupational prestige, even more neglected as a 'woman's issue', is also an important determinant of well-being. (Barnett and Baruch, 1978, p. 109)

The greatest subjective awareness of pleasure was in the combination of married state (husband present) plus high-prestige employment (cf. Nathanson, 1980). Menstrual status, subjectively assessed as pre-menopausal, menopausal and post-menopausal, was irrelevant. When asked if they would have lived their lives differently the unmarried women said they would not have married, and the childless did not regret their childlessness. The 'empty nest' was of no importance. The results are less surprising when we learn that the sample was composed only of white women living in a small town in the Boston metropolitan area. Less privileged inhabitants of our world might find little to admire in their system of values. Later studies, which are more likely to address themselves to the age group without distinction of gender, tend to conclude that middle age is much more stressful now than it was thirty years ago.

Though most of us would shudder at the thought of being coopted to the zenana or the harem in the interests of a happy post-menopause, we might feel more attraction to the Tiwi way of organising sexual relationships, at least as it was practised in the 1950s when Jane Goodale was collecting data for her book *Tiwi Wives*. The older Tiwi woman has many consolations for the stopping of intercourse, for 'as a woman approaches menopause, her power and prestige directly increase' (p. 227). Not only does she have a position of particular authority with regard to her son-in-law, she may also be a first wife, who 'can sit all day in a camp and send the other wives out hunting' and instruct the other wives in the manner of rearing their children, for she is the 'supreme mother' of all the co-wives' children. Moreover, 'Old women are ... treated with a great deal of respect by their sons. They are not only looked after and cared for but their advice is sought and frequently taken' (p. 227).

We can only wonder how much less women might suffer at menopause if they were to acquire power, prestige and responsibility instead of losing all three. We can barely imagine a world in which fifty-year-old women are routinely asked to advise their adult sons, and that advice is taken, or where grandchildren are reared according to grandmothers' ideas of child management. Already, when Jane Goodale was working with the Tiwi in 1954, the system had begun to break down; widows were not remarrying, officialdom was treating husbands as heads of families and ignoring female authority, and young women were demanding modern monogamous marriage.

African women writers are aware that the power and influence of matriliny are being corroded by the effects of modernisation and its attendant social disruption. With the mechanisation of agriculture women are being driven off the land while their families are menaced by the iniquity of outwork and migration to urban centres. In a short story called 'New Life at Kyerefaso', Efua Sutherland fashions a new myth for dispossessed women in which the matriarch is served and honoured by the new men and enriched by their technology.

> 'See!' rang the cry of the Asafo leader. 'See how the best in all
> the land stands. See how she stands waiting, our Queen Mother.
> Waiting to wash the dust from our brow in the coolness of her
> peaceful stream. Spread skins of the gentle sheep in her way, gently.
> Spread the yield of the land before her. Spread the craft of your
> hands before her, gently gently.
>
> Lightly, lightly walks our Queen Mother, for she is peace.'
> (Sutherland, pp. 22–3)

This tranquil, majestic figure does not exist. Western mythology furnishes many examples of groups of female types that may be no more real. One is the group of women who go mad and commit suicide both at and because of menopause; the other is the group of women who blithely traverse the climacteric years with never a moment of panic or a hot flush. Just how many such women there might be and who they might be is impossible to discover. Everyone who has considered the problem has targeted a different group and questioned them about different sets of symptoms. Some questionnaires muddle up symptoms of ageing with symptoms thought to be caused by cessation of ovarian function, and others make an equally misguided attempt to separate them. Some try to question well women, others women reporting to clinics, others all women between the ages of forty-five and fifty-four, and others the female population of all ages. Questioners discovered that women who had never complained of a symptom would nevertheless admit to suffering from it if questioned. They were not so quick to figure out that, if they asked about symptoms that they associated with menopause, the woman who admitted to experiencing them might have suffered from them for most of her life. The questionnaires were specifically designed to circumvent the women's own definition of menopausal experience; the women were seldom offered the opportunity to distinguish between chronic problems and new ones that they connected with menopause. It was as if the researchers were defining the experience and then challenging the women to admit to it. It is conceivable, for example, that the successful matriarch or prime minister when questioned about climacteric symptoms could admit to having symptoms of considerable severity and because of the design of the questionnaire, or the terms of the interview, would not have the opportunity to add that severe or not, they were unimportant. Given women's tendency to underrate their symptoms on one hand and the common prejudice that they overrate them on the other, the outcome of investigations of apparently symptomless women at menopause is completely inconclusive.

Researchers sought to prove one or other of two hypotheses, one that menopause is insignificant, the other that it is catastrophic. American historian Lois Banner summarised the 'no pathology' school of thought of the turn of the century as follows:

In 1880 A. Arnold, Professor of Clinical Medicine and of the Diseases of the Nervous System in the College of Physicians and Surgeons in Baltimore, contended that all the recent studies of menopause reported no pathology associated with it. In 1897 Andrew Currier called the negative view of menopause a 'hoary' tradition with no basis in fact. In 1900 Dr Mary Dixon Jones writing in the Medical Record angrily called the notion of menopause as a 'dangerous period' 'a libel on the natural formation of one half of the human race'. In 1902, writing in the *Transactions*

of the Tennessee State Medical Association, M. C. McGannon wrote
with regard to menopause that 'it is in no sense a critical period'.
(Banner, p. 6)

In her note to this passage Lois Banner quotes nine more authorities,
all of whom argue that there is no pathology connected with menopause,
and balances them against the medical propaganda of 'climacteric
insanity' and 'involutional melancholy'. Despite the sturdiness of the
opposition, however, belief that the climacteric is a problem phase
remained unshaken.

Thinking about menopause, then, is rather like thinking about the
menstrual cycle: the schools of thought are two. One holds that nothing
of any significance is taking place, and the other that the stress and
strain of what is taking place are so acute that sensible behaviour is not
to be expected. Both kinds of arguments conceal crude misogyny. The
'nothing happening' school reserves the right to despise women who are
encountering difficulties, and the '*Sturm und Drang*' school allows itself
to treat femaleness as a pathological condition.

Mary Margaret Anderson, writing at the behest of the Medical and
Nursing Editor at Faber & Faber in 1983, recommended the positive
approach:

> It is important that women should keep the menopause in
> perspective, and remember that it has been estimated that only
> one-third of menopausal women will experience symptoms of any
> degree of importance to them … so strongly does the author feel
> about this point that *no apology will be offered in the next chapter for
> reiteration of the fact that the topic discussed may never be experienced
> by the individual woman.* (pp. 35–6)

The next chapter discussed 'Menopausal symptoms and signs', and
again at the top of the list Anderson placed in capitals the word 'none'.
And at the end of the chapter she reiterated, if rather chillingly:

> There may be many symptoms and signs associated with the
> menopause but, especially in the well-balanced, educated,
> contented woman who finds her family, sexual and professional life
> fulfilling, *there may be no symptoms whatever.* (p. 58)

Researchers at King's College Hospital Medical School, who included John Studd, British Master in Menopause and founder of one of the first British menopause clinics, put the case rather differently:

Far from being a welcome relief from fertility, these years may be a time of great stress and are currently regarded as being more than a mere manifestation of the normal ageing process, but as a chronic endocrinopathy associated with varied symptomatic and degenerative changes which may be greatly affected by the patient's socio-cultural background. The symptoms are severe enough in 25 per cent of women for specific replacement therapy to be considered. Fifty per cent of women have minimal symptoms which last for up to a year and the remainder seem to be untouched by any characteristic climacteric problems. (Studd et al., 1977, p. 3)

Studd's method of arriving at these figures is nowhere explained. It seems unlikely that only a quarter of the women attending the King's College clinic in the Seventies and Eighties would be offered hormone replacement therapy, but it is difficult to see what other statistical basis Studd has available to him. The clinic population is already atypical in that it is attending a clinic at all. As G. E. Herman noticed in the principal students' handbook *Diseases of Women: A Clinical Guide*, 'Women will not keep under medical care for what they know to be a natural process' (Herman, 1898, p. 585). Studd's division of the female population passing through the climacteric into a quarter who feel symptoms grave enough to require treatment, a quarter who have 'minimal' symptoms, and a half who are 'untouched' is possibly completely arbitrary.

As the people who are pushing oestrogen replacement are peddling a remedy, they have to encourage people to feel the illness. Sir John Peel, surgeon-gynaecologist to the Queen from 1961 to 1973, wrote an introduction to Wendy Cooper's *No Change*, a polemic intended to persuade women to demand hormone replacement therapy, in 1987 and described menopause in terms that make us wonder how every woman traversing it does not capsize:

The changes that affect both the body and the mind at and after the menopause are immensely complicated. Not only are there

hormonal changes, but also emotional, social and family changes,
and no one really knows why in fact some women, albeit the
minority, pass through their fifties and sixties with little physical or
emotional disturbance. (Cooper, 1987, p. 7)

What Sir John, Fellow of the Royal College of Physicians, Fellow
of the Royal College of Surgeons, meant by 'immensely complicated'
changes is simply that he and his distinguished colleagues did not
understand them. They are capable of understanding much more
complicated phenomena, but the endocrinology of femaleness has never
commanded sufficient attention or sufficient funding to make a tenth
of the advances made in, for example, sports medicine. In the hierarchy
of medical specialties, gynaecology has always been among the least
prestigious. As the famous medical epidemiologist Archie Cochrane
once said, gynaecologists have the lowest IQ of any group of doctors.

Raewyn Mackenzie, who set up the first menopause clinics at the
Auckland branch of the Family Planning Association in 1981, would not
agree with Anderson that the women who traverse this tricky period
without noticing anything amiss may be as many as two women out
of three:

Some women, and usually those whose hormonal systems have
slowed gradually, find that they have few problems at menopause.
But others of us experience sudden drops and then accompanying
bursts of hormones, and our bodies may act in a confused and
deprived way until the transition back to a non-fertile state
is achieved. According to surveys about 80 per cent of us will
experience some symptoms ... (Mackenzie, 1985, p. 18)

Mackenzie was using data from a United States National Health
Survey made between 1960 and 1962 in which 16 per cent of
respondents said that they had 'experienced no symptoms at all'. There
is clearly a difference between this percentage and the 60 per cent of
Anderson's English patients who experienced no symptoms 'of any
importance to them'. Anderson's two-thirds probably did not realise
with complete equanimity that their periods had stopped, throw away
their unused sanitary napkins and face the future with optimism and
confidence, glad, if anything, that the worries of contraception and the

inconvenience of 'the curse' have both gone away, but they did not recognise their difficulties as symptoms requiring treatment. Again the situation parallels the conflicting attitudes to menstruation described by Doreen Asso in *The Real Menstrual Cycle*:

It appears that two broad approaches among relatively 'aware' women can be discerned. Some will feel that, because they are being controlled by biological processes, they are helpless to remedy the situation. Others will use their knowledge to attribute adverse responses to the cycle, and will compensate for its effects ... As regards the 'unaware' women, there are also two broad groups. Firstly, those who do experience and report biologically-based variations which they do not relate specifically to the menstrual cycle. Secondly, there are those, apparently a small minority, who state that they do not experience any significant changes. There is some evidence ... that this group do in fact experience changes of the same magnitude as the women who do report changes. (p. 175)

Indeed, some of Asso's evidence seems to show that women who do not attribute their problems to the menstrual cycle find them harder to deal with than the ones who do. Her conclusion is at least as true for the climacteric as it is for the cycle:

All women have to incorporate and adjust to the changes as best they can, with very little information or support, and some have preferred to see them as an unremarkable matter of course rather than to appear awkward, self-important, neurotic and so forth. We have seen, for example, that in general some individuals label their internal sensations as important, and some do not. The point of interest is that profound changes take place in the cycle in all women, including those who do not report them. (p. 176)

Applying Asso's observation of the menstrual cycle to the climacteric, then, we can agree that the climacteric is a difficult period for every woman; the real difference between the 'lucky' and the 'unlucky' is that some women experience their difficulties as medical problems and others do not. A 1980 study by gerontologists Eileen Fairhurst and Roger Lightup found that the climacteric symptoms experienced by women who did not call upon their doctors were much the same and of the same severity as the symptoms of the ones who did.

When women managed their own bodies, delivered their own children and medicated themselves, the difficulties they encountered in managing their reproductive processes were dealt with within the female community. Women were shy of sharing such matters with strange young men, and such shyness still discourages many older women from seeking treatment for trivial but sometimes humiliating and painful ailments. Women's shyness colludes with men's lack of interest in older women to produce our present ignorance about the avoidability and otherwise of climacteric distress. This is not a tendency that anyone would wish to encourage, but the medicalisation of menopause is equally undesirable.

There is much to be said in support of Anderson's attempt to stress the possibility and even likelihood of a symptom-free transition from fertility back to infertility, for anxiety about symptoms can well produce them, but pretending that most women find traversing the climacteric easy is equally counterproductive. Women who find menopause difficult are the more likely, in the presence of a mythology that says it is usually easy, to believe that they are part of an unlucky minority and in need of treatment. As every menopause is different, doctors can hardly be blamed for refusing to tell women what to expect, but it should also be understood that symptoms become more manageable if we have an explanation for them. One of the problems that appear in menopause literature is 'fear of serious disease' or 'worry about health'; the woman whose joints are paining her might fear, for example, that she is rapidly developing a chronic arthritis. To learn that severe and inexplicable joint pain can be connected with menopause is consoling rather than otherwise.

In 2014 *Menopause Review* aka *Prezglad Menopauzalny* published an article called 'Epidemiology of the symptoms of menopause: an intercontinental review' by researchers from the University of Lublin in Poland. This attempted to boil down the conclusions of sixty-four of the most important studies published between 2000 and 2014 from Africa, both Americas, Australia and Eurasia. The researchers, led by Professor Marta-Teresa Makara-Studzinska, summarised their conclusions as:

> The prevalence of menopausal symptoms in African women is disconcertingly high. Women from South America complain

about occurrence of depressive, sexual dysfunctions and discomfort associated with muscle pain and joint aches. Symptoms most reported by women in the United States are pains associated with muscles and joints. Women in Australia suffer mainly due to vasomotor symptoms and sexual dysfunction, while in the group of women surveyed in Asia there is observed an alarming increase in the proportion of women reporting depressive disorders. In Europe there was a much greater incidence of sleep disorders and depressive disorders.

The usefulness of these conclusions is put in question by another observation about the quality of the material they were using, here rendered verbatim:

It was very difficulty to find a comparable number of available studies in each continent, often with a small population of women surveyed. Available studies were characterized by a variety of research protocols and use of different research tools, which created difficulty in defining and grouping of symptoms. The average age of occurrence of the first symptoms of menopause is different for women from different regions of the world; therefore in this paper the data concern women of a wide age range, between 40 and 64 years.

Nevertheless the review concludes that women 'all over the world suffer from ailments characteristic for the menopausal period regardless of ethnic origin, skin color, and socio-demographic factors', a conclusion hardly justified by the softness of the evidence.

The truth seems to be that the fifth climacteric is hard for every woman, but some are able to deal with it unaided, and others are not. To differences in the kinds and degrees of difficulties encountered must be added the woman's greater or lesser tendency to self-reliance and/or the degree of her acceptance of pain and misery and/or her perception of how much others, and particularly younger women, are suffering. Once women are actually being questioned about their symptoms in the climacteric and they have agreed to talk about them, it is very difficult to assess how much subjective importance those symptoms have. If the questioners have already decided what symptoms constitute the climacteric syndrome, and asked about these, we can no longer tell if the woman herself relates them to the climacteric. Headaches are a case in point. Headaches are listed among climacteric symptoms; menopausal women have admitted to having headaches; subsequent researches have tended to show that women who are headachy at menopause have reported headaches at other times, and sometimes more often. It would of course be very strange if a woman who responded to stress by developing a headache did not have headaches at menopause. It would also be odd if these women thought that the headaches they had during menopause were menopausal headaches. On the other hand, many women do not know that joint pains, pins and needles and crawling skin are more often experienced at menopause and may be expressions of vasomotor disturbance.

Many women have discovered, moreover, that complaining does not always make things better. The reactions of others, whether members of the family or health professionals, can make us regret that we ever allowed a groan to pass our lips, for many of us find that we are better able to cope with our own distress than anyone else. Nobody wants to be fussed over at menopause, nor does any woman want to invite callous indifference. Rather than add other people's reactions to her problems she may well decide to button her lip and tough it out.

The increasing tendency of younger women to show an interest in menopause and to begin to ask for information about it is due in part to their growing awareness of their bodies and their understanding of the importance of being in good shape to handle whatever might be demanded of them. They exercised for efficient childbirth and they expect to be able to prepare for the stress of the climacteric. The current concern may be summed up as: 'The climacteric is a period of exceptional somatic stress and we need to be fit to deal with it, but what kind of fit should we be?' What they encounter when they begin to ask for information about the management of their post-reproductive career is utter befuddlement. Women who have achieved their reproductive aims go on menstruating notwithstanding. This may be a good thing but equally it may not. Modern women menstruate more than any other women in history, and some of the evidence seems to indicate that the repetition of dozens of episodes of frustrated ovulation does constitute a stress upon the female body.

Women who have been pregnant for more of their lives tend to cease menstruating later; perhaps by imitating pregnancy and resting the ovaries, as it were, for more of a woman's reproductive career we could delay the final cessation of ovulation. It would be interesting to know for certain if the women who encounter menopause as simply the non-appearance of the menses after their last childbirth develop symptoms or not. The scanty evidence we have seems to indicate that they do not. Alternatively, menopausal symptoms in such cases may be masked by the stresses of late childbirth and lactation, exacerbated by the exhaustion caused by the unremitting demands of manual work and a large family. Climacteric distress may be noticeable only to women who are well enough to feel it. This, however, does not constitute a ground for ignoring it in the women who do feel it.

The woman who asks for information because she doesn't want to make heavy weather of her climacteric will find little understanding of the nature of her request. One thing she is likely to be told is that she will probably have the same kind of menopause as her mother did. This could be encouraging or deeply depressing, depending upon the mother in the particular case. The likelihood is that a daughter's reproductive career has been so different from her mother's that the small degree of probability represented by heredity is counteracted by factors such as their differing marital status, ages at childbearing, different number of children borne, whether they lactated or not, used contraception, smoked, were obese, worked outside the home. Your mother's menopause may give an indication of what yours will be like, but only if all other things are equal, which they are unlikely to be.

While British doctors tend to discourage a younger woman from trying to prepare for menopause and even to withhold helpful information, some had no sooner observed what they took to be beneficial effects of hormone replacement on the health of women post-menopause than they began prescribing replacement hormones for women who were still menstruating regularly, as part of a strategy for deferring the ageing process. This is the dippy and dangerous side of menopause medicine, the side that peddles eternal youth. Most women are too sensible to toy with any such notion. It is the more reprehensible then that to the woman who accepts the fact of transition and simply wishes to handle it wisely, the medical profession can say nothing helpful.

Should we wish to be younger at menopause to cope with menopausal stress or is it better to delay it? Should we lose weight or try to put it on? Should we exercise or rest? Can we take a little more wine than usual, or is this more likely to burn up our oestrogen supply? Should we eat more, differently, less? Should we give up red meat, cheese, chocolate? What is it that the women who experience 'no symptoms at all' are doing right? What has Barbara Metcalfe been doing wrong? This is part of her description of her menopausal symptoms in an article in the *Daily Mail* for 12 June 2013:

> There really is nothing like a hot flush. If you've never had one, you may think it's just like going red with embarrassment. But it's so much worse. It starts from within – like molten lava – and slowly takes you over. It stops me mid-task and I am overwhelmed by the heat. It makes my ears ring and I feel sick and forget what I am doing or what I am saying.
>
> Sometimes the side-effects are so debilitating and distressing that it's tempting not to leave home …
>
> To get out of bed in the morning is a relief from the night sweats, but then begins a day marred by terrible tiredness, hot flushes and confusion. I constantly write lists so I don't forget things. On bad days I feel as if I'm losing my mind, just clinging on to reality …

If our medical practice followed the rules of common sense (or motor mechanics) we might know enough about well women to understand what was not working for Barbara. We should by now have identified the mechanism that enables two-thirds or 20 per cent or 16 per cent or indeed any women to feel no unmanageable physical symptoms during the climacteric. If one woman on earth can get through the climacteric without missing a beat, then all women should be able to. Many of the women who suffer symptoms during menopause want to know if 'there is anything wrong' with them. They are told either that their suffering is not the symptom of an illness, but normal and to be borne, or that it is the symptom of a deficiency disease for which they should be treated. What they are not told is why some women do not suffer during this natural process, from which we may infer that though the process be normal suffering is not an intrinsic part of it, or why some women have developed a deficiency and others have not.

While preserving due scepticism about the existence of a group of women who are absolutely 'symptom-free' at menopause, we must not forget that the existence of a proportion of 'lucky ones' provides the justification for the view that menopause is a natural process and not a disease entity.

4

The Unlucky Ones

'I will now show you,' Emil Kraepelin, founder of modern psychiatry, used to say in his lectures at the university of Munich, 'a widow, aged fifty-four, who has made very serious efforts to take her own life'.

> This patient has no insane history. She married at the age of thirty, and has four healthy children. She says that her husband died two years ago, and since then she has slept badly. Being obliged to sell her home at that time, because the inheritance was to be divided, she grew apprehensive, and thought that she would come to want, although, on quiet consideration, she saw that her fears were groundless. She complained of heat in her head and uneasiness at her heart, felt weak and excited, and was tired of life, especially in the morning. She says she could get no sleep at night, even with sleeping powders. Suddenly the thought came to her, 'What are you doing in the world now? Try to get out of it, so as to be at rest. It's no good any longer.' Then she hung herself up behind the house with her handkerchief, and became unconscious, but her son cut her down and brought her to the hospital. (Kraepelin, 1904, p. 6)

In the hospital she began to recover and was allowed to stay with her married daughter. Less than two weeks later her condition had deteriorated so much that she had to return to the hospital, where her recovery was slow and she suffered many setbacks.

From observing cases like this, Kraepelin arrived in the fifth edition of his *Psychiatrie* (1904) at a definition of involutional melancholia.

Melancholia, as we have described it here, sets in principally, or perhaps exclusively, at the beginning of old age in men, and in women from the period of the menopause onwards ... About a third of the patients make a complete recovery. In severe and protracted cases, emotional dulness may remain, with faint traces of the apprehensive tendency. Judgement and memory may also undergo considerable deterioration. The course of the disease is always tedious, and usually continues, with many fluctuations, for from one to two years, or even longer, according to the severity of the case. (Kraepelin, 1904)

The heat in the head might have been the vasomotor disturbance of menopause, which the widow misinterpreted because she did not know that it was a common and unpleasant but meaningless symptom; likewise the 'uneasiness at her heart' might have been palpitations, unnerving at first, but equally insignificant. The poor woman was truly unlucky to lose her husband and her home during the immediate post-menopause; twenty-four years of marriage and four children are not the best preparation for living on one's own. Running one's own home is not the best preparation for living in someone else's either. Struggling to make the new adjustment, to come to terms with a set of circumstances over which she had absolutely no control, the widow broke down. If she really decided to die, those who observed her decided that her decision cannot have been rational. If she was threatening suicide as a form of protest, she was behaving hardly less irrationally. She was sick. Unable to treat her situation, the medical establishment had to treat her. The treatment itself could be expected to produce derangement.

The treatment of the malady cannot, as a rule, be carried out, except in an asylum, as thoughts of suicide are almost always present. Patients who show such tendencies require the closest watching day and night. They are kept in bed and given plenty of food, though this is often very difficult, on account of their resistance. Care is taken to regulate their digestion, and, as far as possible, to secure them sufficient sleep by means of baths and medicines. Paraldehyde is generally to be recommended, or, under some circumstances, alcohol, or occasional doses of trional. Opium is employed to

combat the apprehension, in gradually increasing doses, which
are then by degrees reduced … Visits from near relations have a
bad effect up to the very end of the illness … (Kraepelin, 1904,
pp. 9–10)

… when presumably the patient decides that enough is enough, and
resumes control of her own life. Kraepelin found in her case evidence for
the existence of a specific climacteric syndrome, but by any common-
sense assessment the widow was undergoing a series of catastrophic
shocks when she was least able to bear them. An uncomfortable
menopause complicated by mourning, not in itself a rare phenomenon,
together with protest, placed her in a madhouse and in the psychiatry
textbooks for the next fifty years.

Popular awareness of menopause as 'the dangerous age', already
high at the end of the nineteenth century, was itself a cause of anxiety.
Women themselves feared the coming alteration because of the
prevailing general impression that they would be transformed into
something monstrous, a bristling half-man, beset by lecherous urges
and bitter malevolence. Not only did middle-aged women fear that
they might be doomed to 'climacteric insanity', they also had to
deal with other people's prejudices based on assumptions about their
menstrual status. Whether they were actually undergoing the change
or not, they were treated as if they were. We are not surprised to find
in such cases that women become extremely frustrated and irritable as
a consequence. If any protest on the part of a middle-aged woman is to
be regarded as the widow's was, as evidence of a pathological condition
within her, middle-aged women are under more pressure than ever to
suffer and be silent. The only strategies available to them are either to
deny menopause to the only persons who will credit its denial, namely
themselves, or to develop symptoms that positively demand intervention
and treatment. The treatment was likely to be drastic, for not only did
the women unconsciously pressure doctors for destructive procedures
by conspicuously failing to respond to conservative treatment, the
doctors were only too willing to give it to them. Bleeding, cupping,
purging, and provoking issues in menopausal women are all ritualistic
mutilations that persisted despite the vociferations of a few professional
men and rather more women, who could see that there was no rational
therapeutic basis for any of them.

In 1798, in the midst of the furore about the introduction of 'man-midwives', S. H. Jackson, a distinguished London physician, took it upon himself to address female patients directly in his book *Cautions to Women*. Unusually he included remarks on the correct understanding of menopause:

> On the principle menstruation commenced, so it ceases … With
> these important changes, the constitution may sympathise, and be
> discomposed, if improperly treated; but by the laws of nature, the
> general health, both before and after these local alterations may be
> better than when under the influence of menstruation … (pp. 20–21)

In 1833 the American William Potts Dewees dismissed the notion that 'women at this time of life were all in danger' as a 'vulgar error' (p. 148). He argued, moreover, that if 45-year-old women are to be made to believe that their future is 'so replete … with horrors to come … we may very justly suspect apprehension to be the cause of some of the distressing symptoms which sometimes accompany this interesting process of the human uterus …' (p.145)

After a lifetime of delivering babies and treating their mothers, Marie-Anne Victoire Gillain Boivin declared in *Traité de Maladies de l'Utérus et des Annexes*, published in England in 1834 as *A Practical Treatise of Diseases of the Uterus*, that 'derangements of the catamenia, whether as causes or effects, very frequently occur in the early period of life, and it does not appear that the time of their cessation abounds in diseases' (p. 13). The English translator adds a note: 'M. Benoiston of Chateauneuf has proved by numerous extracts from burial registers, that mortality is not more considerable, from the fortieth to the fiftieth year, in women than in men.'

After many years dealing with the truly frightful sufferings of women in childbed, Mme Boivin was unlikely to treat as serious any disorder that did not result in increased morbidity or mortality. Though other practitioners seeking a lucrative practice among older women might write feelingly of the danger of severe mental derangement and permanent invalidism, Mme Boivin dismisses the entire climacteric experience in a few terse words:

> Sometimes irregularities occur, indicating approaching cessation.
> The catamenia may be, for once, insufficient in quantity and

fail shortly after; then at some indefinable period a copious and continuous flow may ensue: these evacuations may sometimes occur twice in a month, then several months will pass without any appearance. The persons who have been subjected to these irregularities for three or four years, have grown thin and been alarmed, but have afterwards perfectly recovered their health. (p. 14)

Samuel Ashwell, writing a *Practical Treatise on the Diseases Peculiar to Women* ten years later, includes a whole chapter on 'the Disorders attendant on the Decline of Menstruation'. He begins coolly enough:

It has become too general an opinion that the decline of this function must be attended by illness; but this is surely an error; for there are healthy women who pass over this time without any inconvenience and many whose indisposition is both transient and slight. (p. 196)

He acknowledges that women have their own ideas about the climacteric, but in his version they themselves are responsible for the spread of apprehension about it:

Females themselves anticipate this period as extremely eventful, denominating it 'the critical or dodging time', 'the turn of life' etc. ... There are women who have never been vigorous and well during the middle period of their lives and some who have suffered from protracted illness or chronic uterine maladies who after this time acquire what they term 'a settling of the constitution' and good health. (pp. 196–8)

Though Ashwell's common sense persisted in some quarters, a different view was being disseminated and, for no obvious reason, becoming an unquestionable certainty. In 1851 an anonymous author contributed an essay on 'Woman in her psychological relations' to the *Journal of Psychological Medicine and Mental Pathology*, in which the sinister changes attendant on the cessation of ovarian function were described:

With the shrinking of the ovaria ... there is a corresponding change in the outer form ... The form becomes angular, the body lean, the skin wrinkled. The hair changes in colour and loses its luxuriancy; the skin is less transparent and soft, and the chin and upper lip become downy … With this change in the person there is an analogous change in the mind, temper and feelings. The woman approximates in fact to a man, or in one word she is a virago … This unwomanly condition doubtless renders her repulsive to man, while her envious, overbearing temper, renders her offensive to her own sex. (p. 35)

One would imagine to read this nonsense that the author had never met a jolly, fat old woman. By 1874 John Milner Fothergill could insist, in *The Maintenance of Health*, that 'the records of the Divorce Court, the annals of asylums, the dates on the tombstones in the churchyard, all tell us of the severe strain put upon the system of the woman during the change of life' (p. 112), when in fact none of them do. Perhaps this irrational certainty derived from France, where in 1848 a story called '*La crise*' by Octave Feuillet was published in the *Revue des Deux Mondes*, and so captured the public imagination that it was immediately adapted for the stage and eventually played at the Comédie Française. The wife of a magistrate, from being utterly sweet and biddable, is suddenly transformed into a harridan who speaks 'a language full of sharp, bitter words, harsh and peevish maxims'. As the possibility that this behaviour might signal a justifiable revolt against the dictatorship of the family was quite unthinkable, the play concludes that the problem is simply her '*âge critique*' (Cooper, W., pp. 69–70).

Some commentators have seen in the heightened French awareness of the menopause evidence of a greater interest in scientific matters. The same interest, presumably, encouraged Georges Apostoli in 1856 to begin wiring up a selection of rods and knives to a battery, running an electric current through them and inserting them into the uterus, the cervix having first been dilated by uterine sounds 'to the diameter of a No. 10 bougie', and another electrode being placed on the abdomen (Allbutt, p. 316). The negative pole was used to disintegrate tissue, the positive where an astringent or condensing action was wanted. There was no lack of eager customers:

Everyone who has had an experience of any extent in the treatment of pelvic diseases by electricity must have noticed how often the

patient expresses herself as greatly benefited by the treatment long
before any definite change can be detected in the local condition.
(Allbutt, p. 317)

In 1896, when this was written, electrogynaecology was all the rage
and had generated a large body of research, principally relating to the
ways and means of setting up the equipment. Higher and higher charges
were being used; fibroid tumours were being pierced and electrocuted,
pelvic tissue was being burnt; patients were dying of shock, infection
and the untreated original condition. Meanwhile in more than fifty
years no direct beneficial effect of electricity on uterine tissue had ever
been demonstrated. There was no option but to abandon the method.
By 1920 it was no more than a bad memory.

In 1858 John Charles Bucknill and Daniel H. Tuke published the
first textbook of psychiatry, *A Manual of Psychological Medicine*, which
remained the authority for twenty years. They took the trouble to
investigate what Fothergill had merely assumed, and found that Dr
Webster's review of 1,720 cases admitted to Bethlem Hospital indicated
that change of life was the least common physical cause of insanity
in women. Far more important were childbirth and alcohol abuse
(p. 260). Bucknill and Tuke described a case of 'Suicidal Melancholia,
changing to Mania', 'Supposed cause of insanity the climacteric
period'.

A gentlewoman aged fifty. Has been a most active, intelligent
woman, exemplary in all the social relations, and ruling a large
family with much judgment and force of character … Insane three
months. Mental State: Much distressed, full of gloomy forebodings,
distressed about pecuniary matters, wondering how things are
to be paid for, thinks all her family are ruined, &c.; hears noises
which sometimes she wonders at and cannot understand; at others,
she recognizes them for the voices of her children, and then holds
conversations with them; has great weariness of life; begs to be
hung or otherwise destroyed, and makes constant efforts to commit
self-destruction; watches every opportunity to secrete articles to
tie round her neck, and grasps her throat with her hands until she
becomes black in the face: when baffled in this thrusts articles down
her throat … (p. 514)

The woman was admitted to hospital, where her head was shaved and anointed with a cooling lotion. All her symptoms became more acute when her bowels had not been opened, so opened they were, with calomel (mercury chloride) and jalap, Seidlitz powders and castor oil in pill form. Two or three times a week six leeches were applied to her temples. Every other night she was given a warm bath, and every night she was given morphia. After six months of such torture the poor woman was desperate to be allowed to go home; her only too understandable agitation was construed as mania. The violent purges having ceased to work they dosed her with tartrate of antimony, which caused explosive vomiting. She improved in the eleventh month but in the twelfth she began to misbehave again. Her behaviour seems more like protest than insanity but she was dosed with calomel just the same. By force of regular dosing with violent purges her bowels would not function without daily doses of castor oil. Nevertheless, eighteen months after she was admitted to the asylum, she was pronounced recovered and allowed to go home. So much calomel and tartrate of antimony must have caused lasting organ damage but history does not relate how long she survived thereafter. Though neither Bucknill nor Tuke believed the diagnosis of climacteric melancholia, the certainty of the mass of practitioners that such a thing existed was not shaken.

Bucknill and Tuke were comparatively merciful; they did not allow the mechanical restraint of patients no matter how violent, still less the beatings and cold-water duckings that were still practised in some institutions. Nor did they allow themselves to fantasise about the kind of woman who was most likely to encounter difficulties during the climacteric. Their work was the beginning of rational care for the mentally disturbed; it is the more to be regretted that their scepticism about the influence of the uterus on the brain was not more widely shared. Women obligingly produced symptoms of derangement which corresponded to their attendants' expectations, somatising their psychic distress in ways that are nowadays never seen. By the turn of the century gynaecologists were loudly insisting on a close relationship between the uterus and the brain, which they demonstrated by pointing to women whose insanity had been cured by correcting 'retroversions' and prolapses, and by oophorectomy and hysterectomy. Lunatic asylums began to appoint gynaecologists to carry out spaying and hysterectomy as an integral part of treatment for mental illness, long before such operations were safe.

In an introduction written for the first French edition of *The Dangerous Age* by Karin Michaëlis which was included in the English translation of 1912, Marcel Prévost claims that 'in all the countries of Central Europe the most widely read novel of the present moment is *The Dangerous Age*. Edition succeeds edition, and the fortunes of the book have been increased by the quarrels it has provoked' (p. 8).

Prévost considered that the novel owed much to 'medical science' and saw it as an important contribution to fashionable sexual psychopathology, yet when we put pressure on it what emerges is not a description of climacteric syndrome, and may even be a denial of its existence. The heroine, Elsie Lindtner, is forty-two when she leaves her husband, whom she married for his money, to live in a virginal house where her bedroom has a glass roof through which she can see the stars. She has a young maid whose emotional life is equally stunted by women's inability to follow the dictates of their own idealism and their enforced capitulation to male demand. The heroine's friends, though of differing ages and temperaments, are in difficulties too. One suicides; another runs away with a younger man. The heroine invites the only man she has ever loved to visit her, imagining that at last they will be lovers. He comes, but she is turning grey and has got too heavy for her favourite white dress. She sees at once that he no longer loves her and decides to go back to her husband, only to find that he is engaged to marry a nineteen-year-old. She and her maid decide to take a trip around the world.

From the outset Michaëlis's heroine and her friends are aware of the belief that women pass through a 'dangerous age'. Agatha Ussing, who eventually commits suicide, has bought the whole idea, including the notion of psychopathy consequent upon cessation of ovarian function, when she says, 'If men suspected what took place in a woman's inner life after forty, they would avoid us like the plague or knock us on the head like mad dogs ... The worst of it is I know my "madness" will only be temporary. It is a malady incident to my age ...' (p. 58). (Curiously, in December 2016, 59-year-old comedian Dawn French described her one-woman show as occupying the interval between 'menopause madness' and dementia.)

Another of Elsie's friends makes a suggestion with which I have a good deal of sympathy:

> Somebody should found a vast and cheerful sisterhood for women
> between forty and fifty; a kind of refuge for the victims of the
> years of transition … Since all are suffering from the same trouble,
> they might help each other to make life, not only endurable, but
> harmonious. We are all more or less mad then, although we struggle
> to make others think us sane. (p. 90)

Some such idea inspired many housing projects for single women in America and Europe; most of them have since been abandoned. After eighteen years of struggle, in November 2016 the Older Women's Co-housing group opened its first co-housing project of twenty-five mews houses and apartments arranged around a communal garden, in High Barnet, on a site once occupied by a convent. Their mission statement goes like this:

> We are a community in which members' skills and talents are
> valued, shared and developed. Our members have to be capable
> of independent living and both enjoy privacy and the company
> of like-minded women. We welcome women of any culture or
> background who are prepared to commit to the group's values and
> to be active participants in our life together.
>   Our values are: acceptance and respect for diversity; care and
> support for each other; providing a balance between privacy and
> community; countering ageist stereotypes; co-operating and sharing
> responsibility; maintaining a structure without hierarchy; caring for
> the environment; being part of the wider community.

Good luck with that, say I.

Though her friends might be so certain of the source of their distress, the heroine of Michaëlis's novel feels obliged to ask 'a woman's specialist': ' "When is the 'dangerous age'?" He looked seriously at me and answered: "Really there are no absolute rules as to age. I have had cases at forty; again I have known of them at sixty." ' (p. 122)

The key in all cases seems to be misbehaviour involving the rejection of a woman's lot. We might as well consider Nora's walk-out in *A Doll's*

House as a manifestation of the dangerous age. Michaëlis's heroine seized the opportunity to widen the application of the term:

> Thereupon we began to discuss the thousands of women who are saved by medical science to linger on and lead a wretched semi-existence. Those women who suffer for years physically and are oppressed by a melancholy for which there seems no special cause. At last they consult a doctor; enter a nursing home and undergo some severe operation. (pp. 122–3)

It might seem that Karin Michaëlis shares the general conviction that the vicissitudes of the uterus render women's lives a misery to themselves and others, but there is an undercurrent of scepticism that shows in this extract. Women were indeed having their bodies cut about in an effort to cure vague malaises of all kinds, and the procedures were apparently producing the right result, but Michaëlis leaves open the possibility that surgical sterilisations are simply destructive. It seems very unlikely a priori that natural menopause produced the same derangements that were treated in younger women by inducing artificial menopause.

One school of thought held that women became amoral at menopause, because their sexuality was liberated from its reproductive function and became like a man's. Michaëlis rejects the common notion of the virilisation of older women for an opposite notion of her own: 'Hitherto nobody has ever proclaimed this great truth; that as they grow older – when the summer comes and the days lengthen – women become more and more women. Their feminality goes on ripening in the depths of winter'. (p. 91)

In fact Michaëlis's heroine has broken out of a cool and passionless marriage, not because of rejection of her sexuality but because of a realisation of the injustice that she and women like her must be doing themselves, only to discover that, as far as her male contemporaries are concerned, it is too late. Michaëlis dramatises her heroine's helplessness by having her educated by a rich old man who is rearing her to be his wife, only to be rejected by him when she fails to hide her disgust when he becomes ardent, then having her fall in love with a penniless artist whom she rejects for the solid loyal husband without whom she cannot survive. Her divorce sets her free. We may be permitted to hope that in her trip around the world she finds sexual and emotional fulfilment – not too tall an order for a well-preserved, well-to-do Danish woman of forty-five or so.

There were many attempts to debunk the notion of the dangerous age. In 1923, Laetitia Fairfield, first-ever female Chief Medical Officer for London, examined the data collected in a survey of the health of elementary schoolteachers in England, nearly three-quarters of whom were women. Her conclusions were published in the *Lancet* for 3 July 1923. At that stage menopause phobia had reached such levels that, in her words, one 'famous institution' had adopted a practice 'of getting rid of its women employees at forty-five years'. Fairfield protested against the injustice of such a system and the disincentive that it provided for the professional women of the future. She pointed out that ascribing a cluster of ills to menopause could obscure genuine pathology that needed treatment, and that the fear of menopause itself could cause illness. She found that women in the climacteric age group had less absenteeism than women in other groups, probably because most of their absenteeism in other age groups, which was conspicuously higher than men's, had been caused not by their own illnesses but by their children's, and that women's illnesses connected with menopause caused less absenteeism than any other factor. She thought it worth pointing out that she had found 'not a single case of insanity' through such a cause. Hers is the voice of common sense:

> No woman can be expected to like such a concrete reminder that
> middle age is upon her, and those of unstable and imperfectly
> adjusted temperaments will inevitably find adaptation to this
> new phase of life a difficult matter. Of the 'geyser-like eruption'
> of the emotions which is said to precede the physical signs I have
> been unable to discover any traces. As far as my observation goes,
> the neuroses due to emotional repression seem to be much more
> common in the middle thirties than in the forties.

Even other contributors to the *Lancet* did not take her point. H. Crichton Miller, writing on 23 February 1924 on 'The Physical Basis of Emotional Disorder', assumes that belief in menopause phobia is completely justified. He begins with an unfunny witticism.

> The menopause presents problems in every department of
> medicine, with the possible exception of orthopaedics. The

menopause has necessarily the most profound significance from an emotional point of view for the women whose maternal aspirations are unsatisfied ... we must not ignore the endocrine side, for the withdrawal of ovarian hormone has a repercussion on both thyroid and adrenals ... A temporary vagotonia ensures which, if it replaces a previous sympathicotonia, determines grave physiological changes. To ascribe the neuroses of menopause to psychic conflict is to express a partial truth ...

A sympathicotonia is the word health professionals use for the state of the autonomic nervous system when its equilibrium leans towards the sympathetic. If the balance shifts towards the parasympathetic the results may include low blood pressure, low heart rate, constriction of the pupils, often cold hands and feet, cold sweats, severe fatigue, and fainting fits.

Crichton Miller's exaggerated vision of menopausal derangement suggests that he had a remedy to promote. He had been treating thyroid deficiency with thyroid extract with great success for years, and in the current state of befuddlement about the endocrinology of menopause thyroid extracts are being touted again. His followers claimed success in treating all kinds of endocrine derangements with various animal substances, most of them completely inert. A huge business sprang up; every meat-packing company formed a medical division where the ductless glands of slaughtered animals were processed to provide the life-giving extracts. Professor F. S. Langmead, lecturing to students at St Mary's Hospital Medical School in 1922, pointed out to them that the extracts of ductless glands could not possibly be exerting any biochemical action to bring about the effects attributed to them, lamenting the 'pall of reckless assumptions and commercial enterprise in which endocrine therapeutics is now befogged' (the *Lancet*, 14 October 1922, p. 820), but the traffic in expressed ovarian juices kept on expanding.

The ovarian extracts given to women may have done no good, except as placebos, but at least they did no harm. The same cannot be said of the treatments offered for the heavy bleeding of the pre-menopause, which were often more dangerous than the bleeding itself. All kinds of symptoms, including giddiness, palpitations, delusions, nervousness, and general debility, were attributed by the learned gentlemen to anaemia resulting from such bleeding. The women themselves were

prostrated as much by terror as by lack of red corpuscles, until some
were apparently in actual danger of death, though no death from such
a cause was ever verified. The doctors, unable to replace the blood or
rapidly to correct the anaemia by any other method, resorted to all kinds
of techniques to stop the bleeding. The classic technique was curettage,
which stops bleeding caused by retained placental matter or overgrowth
of endometrium. Much of the uterine bleeding they saw was caused by
fibroids; one solution was to stop the bleeding by removing the bleeding
organ, by surgical hysterectomy. Many surgeons preferred this method,
which is still popular and used on the same slight justification. Others,
who noticed that fibroids shrink naturally at menopause, were in favour
of castration. Though surgical oophorectomy was practised for other
ills such as nymphomania or *furor uterinus* (which if it existed at all was
probably a manifestation of thyroid storm), it was not the method of
choice for bleeding in the peri-menopause.

In 1905 German radiographer Ludwig Halberstädter discovered that
bombarding with X-rays caused atrophy in the ovaries of rabbits. Within
months doctors began to use massive doses of X-rays to kill the ovaries
and induce menopause. There was little agreement about the amount
or the method, for the mechanism was little understood. The treatment
was lengthy and expensive and could be carried out only in a specially
equipped hospital. Other doctors favoured castration by the insertion
of radium rods into the vagina; this had the disadvantage of causing
local burns, and involving other organs, but the method was portable
and easier to administer than X-rays. Deaths from ulceration of the
bowel and intestinal burns certainly ensued. Though the response of
patients seems to have been highly idiosyncratic, gynaecologists began
to entertain the idea of irradiating the wombs of quite young women
in order to control heavy bleeding and bring about a normal discharge.
We can only wonder now at the flimsy rationale behind such drastic use
of novel and mysterious techniques. How much carnage resulted, we
shall probably never know. Many of the women who died had not the
faintest idea what had brought about their untimely demise.

To complain to a doctor is to demand treatment; to get treatment, of
any kind, sometimes persuades the suffering woman that her condition
is improving. The more ceremonious, dramatic and expensive a
treatment, the greater the placebo effect. Besides, climacteric distress is
of short duration; a treatment that takes six months or so may simply

coincide with the end of the business, especially as most women have waited for months or even years before asking for help. In the case of the unfortunate widow who was treated by Kraepelin for attempting suicide during the climacteric, the treatment for her melancholia may well have protracted her suffering. If it worked at all, it may have worked as aversion therapy. The contrast with her life in the madhouse may have been strikingly to the advantage of her previous life, which must have seemed utterly bearable by contrast. Women who attempt suicide are clearly experiencing life as unbearable, but we cannot decide therefore that it is the climacteric that makes life seem unbearable. Such distress is always 'multi-factorial'; to emphasise the element of stress due to menopause is to throw the woman back upon her own resources, which are plainly exhausted. Women can bear the unbearable just so long. Women who leave their husbands and/or children during that period do so not because they are finding the climacteric unbearable, but because they are finding their husbands and/or children unbearable. The woman who lashes out at menopause has found the breach in her self-discipline through which she may be able to escape to liberty. Many of the treatments she will be offered are simply ways of walling up her escape hatch and condemning her to quiescence.

There is of course an element of stress in menopause. Ageing is not easy for anyone, but it is easier for some than for others. For some women, some say one in three, others one in four, it is very much more difficult than for others. Studies of menopausal females in general, as distinct from women attending clinics, tell us variously that 95 per cent of menopausal women admit to feeling irritable (Neugarten and Kraines, 1965) or only 35 per cent (Jaszman et al., 1969) and only 21 per cent to feeling tired (B. Thompson et al., 1973) or as many as 93 per cent (Sharma and Saxena, 1981); either 78 per cent of all menopausal women experience depression (Neugarten and Kraines, 1965) or only 21 per cent (Thompson et al., 1973); insomnia affects either 67 per cent (Sharma and Saxena, 1981) or 27 per cent (Thompson et al., 1973). If the figures of the principal studies of the occurrence of symptoms in the general population are averaged out, we arrive at something like the percentages collected by Jaszman (1969), who concluded that women who are approaching menopause are likely to exhibit fatigue, irritability and depression, and those coming away from it, insomnia and mental imbalance. The first group of symptoms is taken to be the result of oestrogen deficiency; the second the consequence of ageing. On 6 December 2015 the *Mail on Sunday* announced that 'a quarter of women will experience menopausal symptoms that adversely affect their personal and working lives'. The prompt for the piece by staff reporter Nick Craven was a statement by Britain's 'health tsar' that 'women going through the menopause should be given time off work to deal with their symptoms and be provided with cooler workplaces'. The 'health tsar' was actually 66-year-old Professor Dame Sally Davies, the government's chief medical officer and first woman to hold the post. Apparently she stated that 'an estimated ten per cent of women had taken days off work because of the menopause'; who did the estimating was not revealed. Professor Dame Sally also apparently described the menopause as 'the last workplace taboo'.

The symptoms reported by women attending menopause clinics are often divided into three categories: somatic, psychosomatic and psychological. The first group comprises symptoms that are considered purely physical: hot flushes, cold sweats, weight gain, flooding, rheumatic pains, aches in the back of the neck and skull, cold hands and feet, numbness or tingling in extremities or crawling skin, breast pains, backache, swollen ankles, bloatedness, and bowel disorders. The psychosomatic symptoms include fatigue, headache, palpitations, dizzy spells and blind spots before the eyes. The distinction between physical and psychosomatic appears synthetic to say the least; deciding a priori that a headache is a psychosomatic symptom seems a suspect diagnostic procedure at best. If fluid retention is present, headache is to be expected as a purely physiologic response to the engorgement of the brain. As researchers have failed to relate hot flushes to oestrogen deficiency, or indeed a deficiency of anything, there seems to be no reason for deciding that it is a purely somatic symptom. Any woman could tell researchers that a hot flush is more likely to occur after frustration or embarrassment than when she is tranquilly proceeding with a task that presents no particular problems. Women often resent hot flushes that are otherwise bearable because they think that other people can observe them.

The psychological symptoms would be better described as behavioural symptoms: irritability, nervousness, feeling blue or depressed, forgetfulness, excitability, insomnia, inability to concentrate, tearfulness, feelings of suffocation, concern about health, panic attacks, 'mental imbalance', fear of nervous breakdown or insanity have all been reported by women complaining of climacteric distress. Some of these are clearly responses to existing physical symptoms; a woman who feels exhausted will not be able to cope with vasomotor disturbance, and will be kept awake by it at night and so becomes more exhausted, and expresses her exhaustion in whatever way is natural to her, by becoming weepy or irritable or infuriated. Older women react differently to climacteric distress than younger women, well women than sick women, happy women than sad women.

At all points along the climacteric continuum the health practitioner is invited to make judgments. She or he is drawn to decide whether the patient is a good coper, whether she is stable, whether she relates well to others, with only the foggiest notion, if any, of what she might have to cope with, what shocks may have rocked her stability, who the others might be to whom she is relating well or ill. Insomnia is always regarded as a symptom of psychological disorder, when there are clear changes to be observed in sleep patterns as a result of ageing. A symptom is more likely to be psychological if it is typical of the woman's response to other stresses not themselves connected with menopause, in which case it is properly not menopausal at all. If all clinicians were to take the attitude of Bodnar and Catterill that 'the emotional changes (during the climacteric) are of multi-factorial etiology, and the climacteric may only accentuate a pre-existing psychic insufficiency,' women would be ill-advised to ask them to help in handling the menopause. The concept of 'psychic insufficiency' is not only unscientific, but intensely moralistic, but many of the Masters in Menopause hold it, or something like it. Even the late Professor Christian Lauritzen could permit himself to observe in 1973 that 'the climacteric uncloaks many of the neurotic and psychogenic symptoms that women have managed to suppress until then'.

Lauritzen might as well argue that menopause corrodes the superego and reveals what has been hiding behind character armour for fifty years. Such attitudes lead directly to the implication, an implication that women all too readily pick up, that if you have a bad menopause it must be your own fault (see chapter 6). Women who sail through, on the other hand, can feel superior to women who don't, thus increasing the pressure upon distressed women to conceal or disguise their suffering. One of the psychogenic factors operating is anophobia (irrational fear of old women) on the part of the clinician, which has more to do with his relations with his mother and wife than with the demeanour of his patient.

Studies of the female population that attempt to establish the frequency of symptom development during menopause are few and mostly unsatisfactory. The first was conducted by the Council of the Medical Women's Confederation in 1933; 1,000 women whose ages ranged from twenty-nine to ninety-one, many of them institutionalised, were asked if menopause had incapacitated them. The study, as reported in the *Lancet*, concluded that 'in view of the general impression acquired from the literature on the subject it was somewhat surprising that approximately 900 of 1,000 unselected women stated that they had carried out their routine tasks without a single interruption due to menopausal symptoms' (the *Lancet*, 1933, 1, 106).

It would be thirty years before another attempt was made to study the occurrence of menopausal symptoms in the middle-aged female population; the number of symptoms that featured in these investigations varied from forty to eight (Greene, 1984, p. 43). Sometimes the point was to find which symptoms were properly menopausal, in which case sometimes younger women were included in the sample, and whether they could be distinguished from general symptoms of ageing, in which case sometimes men were included in the sample. Given the size of the 'constellation of symptoms' reported at menopause, it is not surprising that researchers have never been able to find sharp peaks in the prevalence of any of them 'at menopause'. No woman could have survived having all the symptoms, nor could she expect to endure them throughout the climacterium. Some of the studies seemed to show that certain symptoms were more likely to show up before menstruation actually ceased and others afterwards. The way that the women questioned interpreted menopause itself clearly has a bearing upon their reporting of the symptoms. If you think, as Mrs Thatcher's biographers did, that menopause is the kind of event that can be over in a month, you may well associate menopausal problems with some unconnected factor and you will be a good deal readier to decide that your efficiency remained totally unaffected. On the other hand, if menopause is presented as the cause of all the ills that afflict middle-aged females, unconnected symptoms may be interpreted as manifestations of menopause.

Agreement on the symptomatology of menopause is far from universal. Very few studies, for example, mention menopausal acne, yet some women who have never ever had any kind of skin eruption get a crop of pimples during the climacterium. Dutch researchers include carpal tunnel syndrome among the symptoms caused by autogenic dysregulation; if I had known that in 1992, when I had surgery on both hands for progressive loss of sensation as well as pins and needles and painful numbness, I would have taken oestrogen before undergoing surgery which resulted in an infection and permanent weakness in one hand. The symptoms were serious, the muscles in one hand were already wasting, and I might have had to have the surgery in any case. And I might not.

The characteristic symptom of menopause is 'vasomotor instability'; this is understood to be a direct result of the cessation of ovarian function, but no one can yet be sure what the connection is. As Barbara Evans wrote in *Life Change* (1988):

> Of all the troubles that women experience at the time of the
> menopause they complain most bitterly and most frequently about
> the hot flush. Flushing occurs when the nervous mechanism which
> controls the blood vessels is impaired and, in medical terminology,
> 'vasomotor instability' results. (p. 15)

This sounds like an explanation, until we begin to examine its terms. What sort of thing is a 'nervous mechanism'? What does 'control the blood vessels' and why should menopause impair it? Can it be mended?

At last it seems that we are on track for an answer to these questions. As some had long suspected, the received account of hormonal activity in the human female as exemplified in the above extract was way too simple; there were powerful agents operating in a complex synergy which had yet to be identified. Anatomists had known for some time that in the centre of the lower region of the part of the brain called the hypothalamus there was a site particularly rich in a variety of neurons, to which was given the name 'infundibular nucleus'. In animals – and a great deal of our new understanding of the complex activities of these neurons is derived from animal studies – it is called the arcuate nucleus. Some of the neurons are involved in the secretion of prolactin in lactating females, some stimulate or inhibit the activity of gonadotropin-releasing hormone. Some synthesise kisspeptin, a peptide that is a major regulator of the secretion of luteinising hormone-releasing hormone.

A brain hormone called neurokinin B has been found to be involved in the secretion of gonadotropin, in the timing of puberty and in pregnancy. It was also found to be one of the contributing factors in pre-eclampsia during pregnancy, and for more than a decade it was this aspect of its activity that drew most of the research attention. The ways in which neurokinin interacts with the other tachykinin peptides are complex; we now know that in post-menopausal women there is an increased expression of tachykinin neurons in the infundibular nucleus. In 2015 a cohort of endocrinologists at Imperial College London carried out a pilot study to see whether infusion of neurokinin B during the follicular phase of the menstrual cycle could induce flushing symptoms in healthy women, and found that it could and did. The release of neurokinin B is triggered by, among other things, a fall in the supply of oestrogen. Eureka! We are on the way to understanding the biochemistry of the hot flush; finding a medication that will help control it without too many undesirable side-effects may take some time but, at last, the race is on.

For the time being however women will have to make do with the little help that is currently available. Surveys of menopausal women in the general population to see how many of them suffer from symptoms give varying results. Hot flushes, for example, are experienced by anything from 61 per cent to 75 per cent of all women at menopause. This would be depressing information if it were not for the fact that the seriousness of vasomotor symptoms is very variable. Some women feel a sensation as if they had been sprayed with hot oil, which quickly passes and can easily be ignored. Others find that as the sensation of heat fades they are seized by shivering and cold sweats; still others suffer palpitations, panic attacks, or feel their skin crawling. At night the same dysfunction can cause disturbance of sleep and night sweats so copious that the sufferer must change her nightclothes and her bedding. Some women find that a hot flush can be expected after dealing with a crisis or making a concerted physical effort; others find the recurrence of flushing completely unpredictable. Some women will have only a few hot flushes during the climacteric; others will have them several times a day for years on end. A quarter of all the women who experience flushes will experience them for more than five years. 'Hot flush' is the name given to the phenomenon in British English; in America the usual term is 'hot flash', which gives a better idea of its suddenness.

Next in order of inevitability are the problems related to the atrophy of the tissues of the vagina and urethra. These literally do dry up when ovarian function ceases.

> In atrophic vaginitis … the vagina loses its texture, becomes smoother and thinner and its cells suffer from loss of a carbohydrate substance called glycogen. This, in turn, leads to a reduction of the protective secretion of acid, so predisposing the thinned vaginal lining to infection … Pruritus, or itching of skin around the vaginal opening, can also be troublesome, even maddening. In addition, as the vagina becomes less well lubricated, more sore, and less distensible, sexual intercourse becomes increasingly difficult and is often painful … (Evans, 1988, p. 16)

Since 2014 the preferred name for atrophic vaginitis is genitourinary syndrome of menopause (GSM); 45 to 63 per cent of post-menopausal women are thought to suffer from it and it gets worse with age. Glycogen is produced by the vaginal epithelium; what is referred to in the quote as the secretion of lactic acid is actually the making of lactic acid by bacilli that feed on the dead glycogen cells. These are called Döderlein's bacilli because they were first identified by German gynaecologist Albert Döderlein in 1892. Unlike other inconveniences of menopause GSM does not go away but is likely to get worse with ageing and even to appear for the first time long after the peri-menopause. All kinds of topical preparations are available, both hormonal and other, but as health practitioners seldom prompt a discussion of GSM and as women are actively discouraged from introducing unrelated matters in the usual rushed consultations which are all they can expect these days, a painful and disabling condition that can be successfully treated remains 'under-diagnosed and under-treated' (Palma et al.).

Evans also noted in 1988 that 'the urethra is subject to the same atrophic change as the vagina, and this may affect the sensitive base of the bladder …' What is true of GSM is also true of what is too often called 'sensitive bladder', which too is likely to remain untreated until the sufferer finds herself in aged care, by which time it may be too late. Meanwhile fortunes are made marketing incontinence pants, usually, given a target audience of sedentary older women, on TV and well before the watershed. There is no public service ad that urges women to ask their doctor about 'overactive' or 'sensitive' bladder.

As far as the individual woman is concerned, the symptoms of ageing don't need to be separated out from the symptoms of menopause, for she experiences them together. They're not simply concurrent, however; they interact. Typically, women carry out their busy lives without too much reflection about the rate at which they might be ageing. The first hot flush can come as a thunderclap. One of the commoner reactions to menopause is resentment that it has come so soon, when in fact it has come in its due season. This kind of expression of resentment needs to be decoded into a protest against the swiftness of the passing of our own youth, and the childhood of our children. The woman who feels regret to the point of bitterness is not necessarily exhibiting a pathological symptom of deep maladjustment. Most of us are carrying loads of stress too heavy to be borne without hurting; we may have struggled, through the years when our children were growing up, to provide all the things that we were given to understand were necessary, only to find that they are grown and gone without our having had the joy of them. Consumer society exists to diddle people; many a woman at menopause comes to realise that she has been gypped. There may be a period of turmoil as she comes to terms with this; there should be a period of turmoil, for coming to terms with disappointment is not easy. Women, left to their own devices, will handle it as they handle all the other upheavals that make up women's lives, if they have room to manoeuvre.

Younger women have been shown to have more negative attitudes to menopause than older ones (Eisner and Kelly, 1980; Dege and Gretzinger, 1982); women who regard themselves as menopausal are less negative. The finding shows women coping; it probably also shows that as menopause fades into the general spectrum of ageing, ageing is perceived and experienced as more difficult. The higher a woman's educational level, the more positive the attitude to menopause:

> Family members of women of lower educational status had many more negative attitudes and beliefs about the menopause, thought there was much less communication about these within the family and tended to be less supportive. These families also saw the events occurring around the woman at that time of life as involving mainly

loss, and discontinuity, resulting in emotional instability ... The authors regard these negative attitudes as primarily determined by social class, being based on a subcultural stereotype of the role and status of the postreproductive woman. They also add that 'those who had the most life stress and the least control over it were those who had the most negative attitudes to menopause'. (Greene, pp. 140–1)

So much for the common prejudice that labouring women do not carry on about the menopause as much as pampered middle-class ones. It seems obvious that if your life is hard, menopause will make it harder.

Lev Tolstoy married in 1862; he was thirty-four, his wife eighteen. He was mostly uninterested in her and in her children, of whom he gave her thirteen. Though he preached chastity, he used his wife whenever he needed to, despite his own feelings of repugnance, and afterwards pushed her away. In 1895, when she was fifty-one, she wrote in her diary:

> ... his biographies will tell of how he helped the labourers to carry buckets of water, but no one will ever know that he never gave his wife a rest and never – in all these thirty-two years – gave his child a drink of water or spent five minutes by his bedside to give me a chance to rest a little, to sleep, or go out for a walk, or even just recover from all my labours. (p. 126)

In 1897 she moved out of their bedroom but Tolstoy continued to have intercourse with her whenever he wanted, using her as coldly as a rapist. In the last year of his life he did not even want her for sex. By this time Countess Tolstoy was virtually demented; she was diagnosed as 'paranoiac and hysterical, with a predominance of the first'.

The woman who relates primarily to her husband, whose husband relates with her primarily through sex without tenderness, is psychologically battered; though her husband may never have struck her she has terrible internal bruising. Her ego is already so undermined that cessation of ovarian function removes the last shred of self-esteem that she has. If her husband makes clear that though he uses her for sex her old body (in Sofia Andreyevna's case bearing the marks of thirteen pregnancies) is unattractive, her insecurity will reach the critical stage at which Countess Tolstoy, aged forty-six, wrote desperately in her diary that she feared her husband would cast her out altogether. Countess Tolstoy was married to a great artist, a hero. The demands of his ego, and his guilt about his own sexuality, would have crushed the life out of a stronger woman than Sofia Andreyevna, even if she had not had to make fair copies of all his work, run his estate, his business affairs and his household, bring up his children and educate them herself, and submit to his compulsive sexuality, while he paraded himself before the world as a celibate. The verdict of history is that she was a bad wife.

Many women feel during the climacteric that they are changing personality; these changes occur so spectacularly that it is almost as if one person, the person you know, is being stuffed inside a new one. The most unnerving, even terrifying, change is a sudden horrible propensity to blind rage. The smallest frustration can reduce a woman struggling with the climacteric to gasping fury, so that before she knows what she is saying, she has said the unforgivable. She finds herself calling down horrible vengeance and uttering mad threats, which seem to be throttled out of her, as if she was being squeezed in a giant hand. Sometimes the outburst is accompanied by a feeling of physical anxiety, amounting to pain, or a feeling of unbearable pressure in the head, or behind the eyes. This is the reality behind what doctors refer to rather prissily as 'irritability'. Such an access of choking rage is usually followed by exhaustion, helpless guilt and a futile wishing that whatever it was had not happened, that the victim had not been abused or slapped, that the recalcitrant object had not been thrown or smashed, that the cat had not been kicked or the dishwasher knob torn off.

Very little organised observation of these mood swings has ever been attempted. Until women keep diaries of the climacteric, and chart their own course, we will not be able to form any idea of what causes them. They seem on the face of it to be connected with vasomotor disturbances, for hot flushes very often coincide with stress, and stress is often associated with other people. Consciously trying to keep calm simply adds to the stress. Sometimes the hot flush and the ungovernable feelings come after a prolonged effort, as if some internal monitor had suddenly turned itself off.

There may be another more sinister explanation of personality change at menopause. People in the developed world are exposed to relatively high levels of lead pollution; it had been thought that most of the lead that finds its way into our bodies was safely locked in the bony matrix and could not escape into the bloodstream. In May 1989, researchers at the University Hospital at Lund, in Sweden, found that accelerated bone loss at menopause causes release of lead stored in the long bones into the bloodstream. At menopause childless women, who have not disposed of accumulated lead, are more likely than others to exhibit significantly elevated levels of lead in their blood, up to 20 per cent higher than the pre-menopausal level. Research with rats at the University of Rochester has shown that the lead thus released from the long bones accumulates in soft tissues. The brain is one such tissue. Surges of lead into the biochemistry of the brain during the climacteric will cause brain toxicity, affecting intellectual function, memory, and mood control.

The best hope for preventing lead mobilisation was thought to have been offered by hormone replacement therapy; however with the negative results from the Women's Health Initiative, it was found that prevention of osteoporosis was not sufficient to neutralise the other negative effects of HRT. A 2003 study of 'Bone density-related Predictors of Blood Lead Level among Peri- and Post-menopausal women' in the US described added lead in the bloodstream as linked 'to a number of adverse health outcomes in adults, including increased blood pressure, reduced kidney function, decrements in neurocognitive function, and increased risks of atherosclerosis and cardiovascular disease mortality' (Nash et al., 2004). Just how real these risks are is impossible to quantify without huge cohort studies involving sophisticated and expensive techniques.

Despite the huge body of research into the frequency and the nature of symptoms at menopause, the sum of our ignorance still far outweighs our knowledge. We suspect that the climacteric syndrome is culturally determined, that its severity is mediated by other factors, pathological, environmental, socioeconomic and psychological. One thing, however, seems certain: the generations of women who imagined that the solution to the complex of problems they had to surmount during the climacteric could be supplied by the medical establishment have turned out to be the unluckiest of all.

5

All Your Own Fault

Oppressed women have got rather used to doctors, the only individuals most of them can turn to in time of need, becoming rather testy when faced with problems for which they can find no solution. Many women have given up complaining because of the prevailing response which implies that really they should just get on with it and stop feeling sorry for themselves. In 1983 Mary Anderson, MB, ChB, CBE, FRCOG, set forth 'the plain facts of the menopause' in a 'straight-forward and commonsense way' in a little book called simply *Menopause*. We can guess at just how sorely such a book was needed when Anderson tells us that she 'used to advise anxious women who might seek a consultation solely for the purpose of knowing "what to expect at the menopause" not even to learn to spell the word' (p. 36).

Such blithe condescension is shocking now and was probably hardly less shocking in 1983. Something like it can still be sensed in writing addressed to menopausal women. In a bad-tempered article on the flight from HRT, published in 2006 in a collection of essays on menopause, American gynaecologist Neil C. Boland delivered himself of this ill-written sneer:

> Chances are excellent that on any given day your doctor has already
> seen several patients that day that have stopped their hormonal
> therapy (HT) on their own. A lot of them are absolutely miserable,
> and felt much, much better taking their medication. They report
> they stopped because of 'the cancer scare' or they 'have heard horror

stories' or their cousin's dog groomer 'got breast cancer from that stuff'.

Dr Boland, self-described 'trusted expert in hormonal management', 'as well as a book author', deals in BioTe estrogen and testosterone pellets which, he claims, 'are exactly customised to you'. What cannot be found out from a visit to the website of the 'Treasure Coast Institute for Bio-identical hormone therapy' is just how much the whole work-up costs.

Anderson's confident assertion that two out of three women feel nothing of 'any importance to them' during and after the cessation of their periods strikes with a definite chill. Women are only too accustomed to not feeling very well, and are more likely to seek remedies for their children's ailments than their own, which have little 'importance to them'. The idea that most women over-report their symptoms is nothing but a medical prejudice founded on lack of interest in women's actual health status. Menstruation and contraception both affect the quality of women's lives; to many women menopause is just part of a continuum of not-quite-wellness that they accept. Anderson believed that it was 'the well-balanced, educated, contented woman who finds her family, sexual and professional life fulfilling' who was most likely to experience no symptoms of menopause whatsoever, which would seem to imply that the woman who has a bad time does so because she is a failure (p. 58).

Anderson's book is now out of print and she has been gathered to her eternal reward but a later generation can be just as pitiless. A woman called Doreen Morton was not afraid to append her name to this offering to an online menopause chatroom: 'Instead of expecting to feel like this after 50 get a life, exercise and think positive. I am way past 50 and am size 8, gym 4 times a week and never had a hot flush in my life'. Apparently Ms Morton has a life that allows her to visit a gym four times a week, that is, a life that affords her time and money. Some of us might think that this is more likely to be a matter of luck than good management. She has not been spared hot flushes because of anything she herself has done.

Thinking positive doesn't always make it so. Thinking positive, we are told, includes thinking 'of the number of highly successful, gorgeous women now in their 50's and beyond. The list includes Kim Basinger, Oprah, Vera Wang, Diane Sawyer, Patti Labelle, Goldie Hawn, Suzanne

Somers ... There's a reason they're saying that 50 is the new 30.' Fifty is not the new thirty; any woman who thinks it is is deluded. The women listed here are not simply fifty or over; they are all rich and famous, with an army of beauticians readying them for every public appearance. Even so the examples are not as reassuring as their publicists might wish. At sixty-two Kim Basinger is described by bloggers as 'a sex symbol who got old'; 'she can't exactly play oversexed/sex symbol type of roles anymore ... without it being looked at as creepy and/or unintentionally farcical.' There is little to be envied, you would think, in getting to play the older woman who introduced Christian Gray to a feeble amateur version of S&M in *Fifty Shades of Darker*. Patti LaBelle is nowadays selling her Sweet Potato Pie via Walmart and, at seventy-one, 'dating' her 41-year-old drummer.

Samuel Ashwell was probably not the first medic to decide that women who suffered at menopause had only themselves to blame. He was aware that there were women who noticed nothing amiss at menopause, and went on: 'That this does not more constantly happen, arises from the fact, that nature and health are often sacrificed to fashion and luxury ... habits unwisely begun, and still more unwisely continued' (p. 196). In other words, it's the suffering women's own fault.

A hundred years later, though the case had never been proved, the same point was still being made. In 1958 Norton issued a fourth impression of *Emotional Problems of Living: Avoiding the Neurotic Pattern* by two eminent psychiatrists, O. Spurgeon English, MD, Professor and Chairman of the Department of Psychiatry at Temple University School of Medicine, and Gerald H. J. Pearson, MD, Dean of the Philadelphia Association for Psychoanalysis. These eminent gentlemen believed that women who feel 'irritable, depressed, remorseful and pessimistic when the menopause appears' must have 'lived unwisely between the ages of twelve and forty-two'.

> Such a woman tends to be sensitive and to live a rather isolated
> social existence. She has not been warm and gregarious, rather one
> of those women who proudly declare they never visit around much
> but stay at home and mind their own business. In other words, she
> has made a virtue of the fact that she was afraid to associate with
> people or that she did not like people sufficiently to be friendly.
> Usually she has been strict and pedantic in training her children,

often excessively religious, meticulous about cleanliness, many times the excellent housekeeper in whose home no one can be comfortable. She has been sexually frigid, ungenerous and prone to be critical. Such women take little from and give little to the world, so that by the time menopause is reached they not only have no more activity of the sexual glands, but they likewise have become emotionally and spiritually impoverished. (pp. 431–2)

In short, women who suffer at menopause are bad people. In undue fairness, it must be pointed out that this is a picture of the typical sufferer from 'severe menopause neurosis or psychosis', whereupon it must also be pointed out that no such syndrome as 'severe menopause neurosis or psychosis' has been shown to exist. Clinical depression is no more common at menopause than in any other epoch of the female human's life, and the clinical depression observed at menopause has no features to distinguish it from any other depression. These men, who should have been helping the women who trusted them, abandoned their scientific method in order to vilify a kind of woman they didn't like. They note with satisfaction the high placebo response to the kinds of hormone replacement available in the fifties and go on:

In a problem of the menopausal syndrome the personality factor that has produced this menopausal symptom should be treated and the doctor should not depend upon ductless glandular preparations too much … Women who are not enjoying bringing up their children, who are working too hard and taking life in deadly seriousness, should have it pointed out to them that if they continue this course they are almost certain to be tired, disillusioned people at fifty. (pp. 433–4)

There is no group of women that has not been identified as courting disaster at menopause. Women who have not exercised their reproductive function in due time have been identified as a specially vulnerable group by some, while others have been equally convinced that women who were excessively attached to their mothering role tend to suffer more. Margaret Christie Brown, Consultant Psychotherapist at Queen Charlotte's and Chelsea Hospital, thought difficulties with menopause were to be expected 'where overvaluing, undervaluing or imposing of other attributes on the function of reproduction has occurred' (Campbell, 1976, p. 113). Brown's description of the woman least likely to suffer at menopause is disturbing to say the least.

> Surveys have shown that the group of women least likely to have menopausal symptoms are single women who have not suffered from dysmenorrhea. The reasons for this must be multi-factorial but one important factor is that these women have come to terms gradually over a number of years with non-fulfilment of a female role. It may have been a deliberate way to avoid the vulnerability of being female or it may have been by force of circumstances, in either case she is likely to have faced many of these issues many times and learned to tolerate them over a number of years. So that rather like living with a seriously ill member of the family, the mourning is done while the patient is alive and often death is welcomed as relief. (p. 114)

In *The Sexual Responsibility of Women* (1957) Maxine Davis MD chose to single out 'busy mothers or energetic careerists who are unwilling or unprepared to acknowledge the termination of the reproductive phase of their lives and the inception of a new era' as those most likely to be 'thrown into considerable turmoil by this event'.

Psychiatrists have no option but to blame people for their own suffering; admitting that unhappiness might be justified would undermine the entire rationale of medicating the mind. There can be no suggestion that feeling tired and disillusioned at fifty might be the appropriate response and that convincing yourself that you are happy and fulfilled might be self-deluding. 'Bringing up' children is not necessarily enjoyable; our children are not necessarily nice people and if they are it is not something we can congratulate ourselves upon. In any event, by the time we are fifty our children are likely to be relatively difficult of access.

Anderson's crisp statement implies that if you have managed your life correctly, that is to say you have a husband and children who all love you, and you have always enjoyed and are still enjoying sex with your husband, and have a fulfilling job as well, you are more likely, most likely, perhaps even certain, to whisk through menopause with your usual efficiency. (Anderson's faith is the more touching because, as

an unmarried professional, she herself had none of these advantages.)
Mrs Thatcher, according to her goofiest hagiographers, dispatched the
climacteric in a single month, namely February 1972, when she was
only forty-seven. The implication of Anderson's no-nonsense approach
is that if you can't do the same, then you're likely to be a moaning
Minnie. If you haven't managed to get a husband, let alone keep him
by your side until you are fifty, if you haven't borne any children or have
been unable to get the ones you have brought up to treat you decently,
if you didn't manage to get a decent education let alone a decent job,
then you'll probably make a hash of the menopause as well. The games
mistress reappeared when she talked of treatments for the misery of the
climacteric:

> Regrettably it is true to say that in all age groups throughout the
> Western world there is excessive drug use, leading to actual abuse
> of these drugs. They have become a household by-word – a music-
> hall (or TV) joke. Who is to blame? The drug firms certainly, the
> doctor certainly – but patients themselves must take a large share
> of responsibility. How often do patients go to the doctor's surgery
> specifically to seek a tablet to calm them down or to buck them
> up, because they are either anxious or 'stressed' or 'depressed' and
> feeling low? Modern life itself must take the main responsibility
> for all this with its stresses, anxieties and pressures. But do we not
> create the life we lead, are we not largely responsible for many of the
> situations in which we find ourselves and should not we be more
> able to find resources within ourselves to cope rather better without
> necessarily having recourse to drugs? (p. 71)

Though Anderson could vaguely see that modern life is not
particularly liveable, she still put the words 'stressed' and 'depressed' in
inverted commas; 'feeling anxious' is a pretty grudging way of describing
an anxiety state. The key to Anderson's attitude is in the question 'Do
we not create the life we lead?' Anderson would not accept my answer,
'Probably not, and certainly not if we are women.' From the time
women first come to consciousness their lives are strenuously moulded
by others; this conditioning has been so often described at length that
there is little point in reiterating it here but, as the point is so central, a
synopsis may be in order.

From the first weeks of life, when mothers feed boys who vociferate but soothe girls, feed boys more often and longer and praise girls for behaviour that they discourage in boys, and when the behaviour of fathers may range from total invisibility and distance to sexual abuse, women learn that their fate is not in their own hands. The pattern of responding rather than initiating is early set. If it is not, the chances of a female's life career following Anderson's ideal are slimmer rather than better. When sexual activity is initiated it is likely to be on the boys' rather than the girls' terms. Women do not understand the systems of self-promotion employed by men; they are not taught the ways in which from their boyhood men establish groups and contacts that will serve them in their professional careers. If women keep up in the professional race, it costs them a great deal more in terms of application and concentration, and yields them a great deal less in terms of human contact. Their male peers, on the other hand, will generally prefer women who do not compete with them.

Nearly a third of western European women will never marry; the higher a woman's educational qualifications and the better her job, the more likely she is not to marry. Unmarried men cluster at the bottom of the social scale; unmarried women at the top. Married men are the least likely to seek treatment for psychological disturbance; next come single women, next married women. The last, most vulnerable population, selected out of the marriage market, are the single males. Any discussion of menopausal women that assumes that all are or should be married and have had children is based upon a mythical paradigm. Of the women aged fifty or over in Great Britain, nearly half a million will be divorced and never remarried, while more than 3 million will be widows, and three-quarters of a million or more will never have been married; in all, nearly half the total number of British women are single. The largest group of households in Britain are the households with a single occupant. Incidence of divorce increases exponentially, while failure to marry is more and more often refusal to marry, not because the woman is immature or suffers from any other psychological blight, but because the institution of marriage is not designed for women's better health or optimal functioning. More divorces are initiated by wives than by husbands. There are rational grounds for eschewing or ending marriage; the women who choose to do so are taking control of their lives. Survival as a single woman is not easy, but the struggle is one's own struggle. Single women may be less likely to form symptoms that demand treatment simply because they have assumed responsibility for themselves. Even so, menopause doctors see as one of their chief functions the curing of ailing marriages. Despite all the evidence to show that celibates are no madder and often a good deal healthier than the rest of the population, health professionals and their ilk persist in the irrational belief that regular psychosexual release is essential for the proper functioning of all individuals.

The most obvious area in which a woman cannot be said to 'make her own life' is in marriage. Though she may choose her husband, she cannot make him choose her. She cannot control the pace at which intimacy progresses; though women nowadays initiate contacts more readily, they are as powerless as ever in pursuing them. Though a young woman may not shrink from telephoning a man she is interested in, there is little she can do if he doesn't return the call, or doesn't return it for a week. She can telephone again and complain, and in my experience usually does, but the result is worse than if she had let the matter drop. Eligible men live in a sellers' market, and they know how to exploit the fact. Ineligible men are just that.

Supposing a woman gets the husband of her choice rather than the man who chose her (and the man she gets is the man she thinks he is, though love be blind), she has no way of ensuring that he remains the man of her choice. Though she might conceive her babies at the right time and take all precautions to see they come out right, she will have very little to do with their socialisation and their enculturation, which has been taken over by an inadequate education system. She knows that she is more vulnerable to her children than they are to her. Chances are that, whether she wants to or not, she will have to work to service the family debt. The work she does outside her home is most likely to be poorly paid drudgery; inside the home, of course, drudgery is unpaid. Men nowadays are supposed to share housework; the extent to which they actually do so can be guessed from the activities of advertisers, who never, ever, show a man cleaning the lavatory.

What has been set up in the adult female is a pattern of response. She responds to the needs of her man, her children, her employer, her customers. The happier she feels in responding, the more successful she is likely to be in her roles as lover, wife, mother, secretary, waitress, saleswoman. What happens during the climacteric is that the people she has served all her life stop making demands on her. She becomes a moon without an earth. What she wants is to be wanted, and nobody wants her.

Unless of course she has the perfect husband, the perfect children and the perfect career. The woman who does have all those really cannot congratulate herself on her own good management; the woman who has none of them must not blame herself for what is after all a matter of luck. Luck is another name for privilege. Health, intelligence, beauty, educational and career opportunity are all positively correlated with affluence and social class.

Curiously, Anderson gave space in her 112-page book to a phenomenon that does not exist, namely, the male menopause. This happens to 'the male in his middle years', between the ages of forty-five and fifty-five when he is in the 'most active phase of his career', when, because of anxieties about ageing and what have you, he may suffer from impotence. Anderson did not enter into the vexed question of how many women have suffered from impotence all their lives or how much their failure to reach orgasm has had to do with the inconsiderateness of their partners. In the mythology of sexual monogamy in the leafy suburbs women reach orgasm with their husbands twice a week until something goes wrong in the middle years. 'What happens then very much depends on the personality of the man, his social and his economic status' (p. 100). (What has happened ever since a girl was married has depended very much upon the man's social and economic status.) 'He may react in a variety of ways' (p. 100). (Nothing new here either. The man has always had the choice of a variety of ways of reacting and his wife has had very little opportunity to influence his choice.)

> He may try to ignore what has happened and throw himself into his work even more. His partner who herself may be undergoing climacteric changes resulting in loss of sexual interest may be quite relieved, and so a state of relative contentment develops but without the fulfilment of sexual enjoyment. Occasional attempts at intercourse may cause vaginal pain to the woman … Then again his partner may become frustrated and angry and this can only result in greater reduction of his sexual drive and performance. If the man's personality is such that he is unable to work through this time of crisis he may become depressed and develop true psychiatric

symptoms – anxiety and what is called reactive depression. He may
sleep badly, he may begin to drink too much, he may gamble …
Extra-marital affairs are commonest at this age … (p. 100)

And on the other hand he may have done some or all of those
things all his life. Gamblers and alcoholics and philanderers usually
have an excuse for their social vice. Anderson did not devalue male
symptoms by putting them in inverted commas as she did with those
of the menopausal female; male misbehaviour itself is here elevated
to the status of a symptom. How different is this deference to the
contempt shown by Anderson for female people who feel 'stressed' or
'depressed'! Women too may drink during their midlife crisis, and for
them the health consequences of even a small and irregular intake of
alcohol can be catastrophic. Anderson did not think the problem of
female alcoholism or the ill-health resulting from it worth addressing.
The solution to male gambling, infidelity and even alcohol abuse,
as intrinsic a part as it is of male bonding, lies in the model wife's
behaviour.

With greater understanding of herself and her bodily changes at this
age, with adequate treatment of symptoms if they arise, it behoves
her to remember her partner also. To remain attractive, caring,
interested and interesting must be half the battle surely. (p. 101)

'*Only half*!' the exhausted woman cries.
The very notion of *remaining attractive* is replete with the
contradictions that break women's hearts. A woman cannot make
herself attractive; she can only be *found* attractive. She can only remain
attractive if someone remains attracted to her. Do what she will she
cannot influence that outcome. Her desperate attempts to do the
impossible, to guide the whim of another, are the basis of a billion-
dollar beauty industry. All their lives women have never felt attractive
enough. They have struggled through their thirties and forties to remain
attractively slim, firm-bodied, glossy-haired and bright-eyed. Now in
the fifties 'remaining attractive' becomes more than a full-time job.
Would Anderson recommend facelifts, mammoplasty, buttock-lifting,
aerobic dancing – what? Did Anderson not know what succulent young
bodies are available for the jaded executive's pleasure? Is a middle-aged

woman supposed to have the buttocks of a twenty-year-old? Such buttocks are displayed on advertising hoardings all over town. The man who is still making love to the wife of his youth may be thinking of other breasts than hers. Such imagery is available at every turn. The middle-aged woman who tries to compete with her husband's fantasy sex partners hasn't a hope.

The question whether there is such a thing as a 'male menopause' is now answered by the NHS website. 'The "male menopause" (sometimes called the "andropause") is an unhelpful term sometimes used in the media …' to describe 'depression, loss of sex drive, erectile dysfunction and other physical and emotional symptoms' in men in their late forties and early fifties.

> This label is misleading because it suggests the symptoms are the
> result of a sudden drop in testosterone in middle age, similar to
> what occurs in the female menopause. This isn't true. Although
> testosterone levels fall as men age, the decline is steady – less than
> 2 % a year from around the age of 30–40 – and this is unlikely to
> cause any problems in itself.

The NHS is evidently convinced that the female menopause results in oestrogen deficiency and that the notion of the male menopause is predicated on an imagined parallel, which is then denied. Elsewhere on the internet may be seen discussions of testosterone deficiency that are equally convinced that male problems in midlife are indeed caused by low testosterone. The NHS by contrast includes 'work or relationship issues, divorce, money problems or worrying about ageing parents', all of which would be affecting a man's female partner at least as much as it was affecting him.

The middle-aged woman whose husband has lost interest ought certainly to take care to look good, but not primarily to revive his flagging libido. A man who is depressed and frightened by the signs of his own advancing age may be panicked by the thought that he is 'matched with an ageing wife'. The behaviour of the young women around him convinces him that he is younger than his wife in mind and body. His wife can exercise till she has a heart attack, can spend all day being depilated, massaged, oiled, scented, coiffed and painted, until she beggars herself. Remain attractive indeed. Women might well ask,

'When in this life will I be allowed to let myself go?' Is one never to be set free from the white-slavery of attraction duty?

Having erected the cliff of remaining attractive and commanded her readers to scale it, Anderson remarked discouragingly: 'There is no evidence whatsoever that declining sexual pleasure is inevitable after the menopause' (p. 101). Something that is not 'inevitable' can still be probable, even overwhelmingly probable. Yet, though Anderson did not deny that lots, perhaps most, perhaps nearly all women, will suffer declining sexual interest after menopause, she nowhere suggests that they can be let off their conjugal duty. They have still got to appear 'interesting and interested'. Though never married herself, she had nothing to say whatever about women who have never had a proper partner, and now are less likely than ever to find one. She had no pity for the women who do not have desirable 'partners', or 'partners' of any kind, who might find pretty disheartening the news that they may be tormented by unfulfilled sexual desire all the way to the grave.

Though Anderson did fleetingly consider the possibility that by some mismanagement or another, a husband might just conceivably be dead or married to someone else, it never occurred to her that a husband might be unattractive. Or even that he might be maladroit as a lover, or coarse, or brutal, or demand peculiar rituals to keep his flagging interest up. The idea that a woman of spirit might reject the kind of sex her husband is offering never crossed Anderson's mind. Many a man who was attractive and amusing at twenty is a pompous old bore at fifty. Many men married to 'interesting and interested' wives are too dull to be interested in them or by them. Many a fascinating woman is stunned into silence by an overbearing husband who has never really listened to anything she has said. In Anderson's world no husband ever says, 'Shut up, dear.' Doubtless Anderson would argue in defence of her myth of the thirty-year-old monogamous marriage that a repulsive husband is his wife's fault, which is merely the corollary of her view that people with penises can do no wrong, whatever it is they choose to do. Yet Anderson would be astonished to find her writings compared to the Hindu scripture that enjoins women to accept everything a husband does and forgive it.

A more sophisticated version of the argument that seeks to blame the middle-aged woman for her own menopausal distress is offered by J. G. Greene, in *The Social and Psychological Origins of the Climacteric*

Syndrome (1984). After reviewing the evidence for a specific 'climacteric syndrome' and finding that the only symptoms that can be specifically connected with the cessation of ovulation are hot flushes and dry vagina, Greene is obliged to define a vulnerable group whose 'physical, psychological and social distress' will become apparent during this 'critical transitional phase of their lives'.

> Many of the characteristics and functions adversely affected during the climacteric are also at the same time declining with age, or may represent the accentuation of an existing problem or the recurrence of an earlier one ... the climacteric does not seem to act as a primary vulnerability factor per se, but tends to accentuate an already existing problem, accelerate the effects of ageing, or cause previous problems to recur. Nor, given the modest magnitude of the increase in, for example, non-specific, in contrast to the large increase in vasomotor symptoms, can these effects act equally on all women to the same extent. This raises the question of whether we can identify those women, or those groups of women, who, during the climacteric, are more vulnerable than others. The answer to this question seems to be a very definite 'yes'. (p. 211)

The accentuation of existing problems, acceleration of problems to come and recurrence of old problems at the same time as one is struggling with hot flushes, night sweats, painful intercourse, etc. may not constitute a climacteric syndrome to Greene's satisfaction, but they would loom large in the life of any woman, whether or not she is heroically trying to deny the existence of problems, whether or not she has any faith in the powers of doctors to solve the problems she has.

> ... when more personal and individual circumstances were examined, it was found that it was women with pre-existing problems or long standing difficulties, such as marital dissatisfaction, problems in early development, financial and economic difficulties, who reacted most adversely during the climacteric. (pp. 211–12)

This view might be called the 'last straw' view of the climacteric, in which the few symptoms actually caused by the cessation of ovarian function trigger off a string of others that aren't. Insistence on separate enumeration of symptoms under three categories, labelled somatic (bodily), psychosomatic (bodily-cum-mental) and psychological, distorts a basic reality, namely, that they are all connected. Fatigue, caused by sleeplessness caused by vasomotor instability, will cause many of the other symptoms in its turn, and carrying out hard physical labour in uncomfortable circumstances will make the fatigue much worse. Headache (labelled psychosomatic) and tearfulness (psychological) might well result. Greene's approach is analytic; he must separate out the elements and try to standardise them.

Greene does not quite reverse Anderson's argument that women who are 'well-balanced, educated, contented' are also likely to suffer less at menopause to read that women who have not been at the mercy of an unequal education system, unfair conditions in employment, the whims of men and the demands of their children, will suffer much less at menopause. Though he is more merciful than she, his analysis too is necessarily patient-oriented, so that rather than discussing the limited control women have over their lives, he tends to rate them as if they were solo performers. The idea that right attitudes will lead to the right menopause is the inescapable corollary of this kind of concentration on the patient as the treatable entity and the source of all her woes. Women who have 'adverse reactions' to marriage, for example, measured on a 'marital adaptability' score, can be expected to have 'adverse reactions' to menopause as well. They are 'adverse reactors' and hence problematic by nature. Likewise women who identify 'too closely' with their bodily and reproductive functions or are 'too dependent' on their mothering role are seen as asking for trouble at menopause.

Even Pauline Bart, writing in a feminist collection entitled *Women in Sexist Society* (1971), blames the middle-aged woman for her own depression:

> Women who have overprotective or overinvolved relationships
> with their children are more likely to suffer depression in their
> postparental period ... Housewives have a greater rate of depression
> than working women ... Middle-class housewives have a higher
> rate of depression than working-class housewives ... The patterns
> of black female role behaviour rarely result in depression in middle
> age. Often the 'grannie' or 'auntie' lives with the family and cares

for the children while the children's mother works; thus the older woman suffers no maternal role loss. Second, since black women traditionally work, they are less likely to develop the extreme identification, the vicarious living through their children that is characteristic of Jewish mothers. (pp. 109–12)

This could all have been put quite differently, so that it did not appear that depressed women had got it wrong, had over-invested in their children and therefore suffered inevitable rejection. The black woman who continues to fulfil a female role is not better at dealing with her empty nest, because her nest is not empty. Her children are probably still living with her, not because of tradition so much as poverty. Black women do not do the work they do because of tradition, but because of necessity. For the black matriarch, keeping all her children and grandchildren at school or in work and out of trouble is the most demanding kind of work. The fifty-year-old black woman is anything but unwanted; the fifty-year-old middle-class housewife-and-mother fiddling about in her empty house has no way of ignoring the fact that she is unwanted. These contrasting situations cannot be described in terms of choices, mistaken or otherwise.

All the arguments that attribute depression at menopause to failures and excesses in the individual woman's life career are essentially circular. This kind of argument says, for example, that a woman who becomes obsessed at menopause by an abortion she once had is not disturbed by menopause but by the abortion; therefore the abortion is responsible for her menopausal difficulties. These pseudo-arguments should be tossed out. Difficult menopause is not a punishment that a woman brings upon herself. It is a time of stock-taking, though, and some grieving that was not done at the appropriate time, usually because of the demands of others and the refusal of others to take the situation sufficiently seriously, might have to be done during the climacteric.

It is of no help to the menopausal woman to hear that her depression is the inevitable result of mistaken strategies and decisions taken long before. It must compound a woman's grief to hear that she has mismanaged her life for the last fifty years. It is not astonishing that a feminist commentator could permit herself such hostility towards her own mother; expression of such hostility is one of the ways women can begin to refashion their own images and roles. What is sinister is that a fundamentally irrational position here masquerades as argument and analysis. Women have not yet grasped the extent to which male authority rejects their protests and trivialises their real complaints; there is little hope that they will when feminist theorists use the same tactics.

If a woman's life does not live up to Anderson's British model or Greene's Scandinavian model, it seems only proper that she should be angry about it. Fortunately for society, if unfortunately for them, women's anger usually expresses itself in self-punishment. Obligingly, women internalise resentment which then takes the form of guilt. One of the most interesting results of any test made of the effects of replacement oestrogens on personality, most of which were inconclusive, was the conclusion reached by Schiff, Regenstein, Tulchinsky and Ryan in 1979.

> Schiff et al. included in their assessment three personality scales, the
> Clyde Mood Adjective Checklist, the Gottschalk-Gleser test and the
> Minnesota Multiphasic Personality Inventory. These tests assess in
> all some 26 attributes of personality but in only two of these were
> any changes observed. Following oestrogen women became less
> outwardly aggressive but more inwardly hostile. How this is to be
> interpreted the authors do not say. (Greene, 1984, p. 35)

Such an observation opens the intriguing possibility that women's submissiveness is mediated by oestrogen; deferring to the dominant male is clearly a necessary part of reproductive function. Hens hunker down before the rooster. Receptive she-cats present the nape of the neck to ingratiate themselves with the tom, but unreceptive she-cats turn and fight with as much ferocity as males. It is interesting to consider the famed 'mental tonic' effect of HRT as inducing a 'contented cow syndrome'. The possibility, ever so faintly adumbrated here, that menopause puts women back in touch with their anger after thirty-five years of censorship by oestrogen is delightful to contemplate. Interestingly, though replacement oestrogen facilitates sexual intercourse, it does not restore lost libido, which demands testosterone; in this at least oestrogen is clearly the biddability hormone.

Louann Brizendine graduated in neurobiology from Berkeley, studied medicine at Yale and psychiatry at Harvard. Thus forearmed, she entered the fray with a controversial book called *The Female Brain*

(2010). A contributor to theperimenopause blog quotes Brizendine as saying 'that during perimenopause there is a hormonal shift which occurs that actually "rewires a woman's brain" (my words) in such a way that she becomes less nurturing, less motherly, less willing to put herself second to the needs of others and much more apt to decide that she's had enough of many things that heretofore, she may have happily accepted with no fuss whatsoever.' This might be thought to obliterate the notion that women are responsible for their own difficulties with menopause, but the response of most feminists was angrily to reject the determinism of Brizendine's approach and to accuse her of the heresy of essentialism. Brizendine starts with the body chemicals and ends up with attitude; the feedback mechanism works both ways. If oestrogen suppressed rebellion, lack of it could free it, but not of course if we replace the oestrogen. Brizendine has since modified her position, which is no more outré than the mindset of those women who explain their mood swings as 'hormonal'.

It would be foolish to expect the male medical establishment, even when represented by those few female members who care to be associated with menopause, to encourage women to act out their anger or hostility or resentment in middle age. In this best of all possible worlds such feelings are never appropriate. We are only dimly coming to a recognition that the antisocial behaviour of demented old women might be an expression of justifiable rage too long stifled and unheard. When we find a frantic old lady in the nursing home cursing foully and soiling herself we are witnessing the end result of long corrosion of the personality. We should not be surprised to find that the most eldritch old hag was once the most self-effacing soul, nor should we assume that her present state has no connection with her earlier condition.

Some of our negative feelings about menopause are definitely the result of our intolerance for the expression of female anger. As little girls and adolescents we feared the anger of our mothers. We sensed that there was a debt of hostility in consequence of all that motherly self-sacrifice and self-effacement but; though we pretend that saying we had not required either self-sacrifice or self-effacement will stand in lieu of recompense, we know better. We are not really surprised when menopausal women spit out bitter home truths to their children, but we pretend that it is the hormonal imbalance that is speaking, turning anger into illness so that we can evade implication in it. Robert

A. Wilson embarked on a lifetime career of oestrogen prescription because of happenings that predestined his career, principal among them the decline of his 'gentle, almost angelic mother':

> At the time I could not understand it. What was a boy in his
> teens to make of a phrase like 'change of life' – especially if it
> were spoken in that tone of voice that in those days was used to
> mention any number of things then considered unmentionable.
> How could anything connected with my mother be spoken of in
> that tone of voice? Yet something terrible was obviously happening.
> I was appalled at the transformation of the vital, wonderful
> woman who had been the dynamic focal point of our family into
> a pain-wracked, petulant invalid. I could feel the deep wounds
> her senseless rages inflicted on my father, myself and the younger
> children. It was this frightful experience that later directed my
> interest as a physician to the problem of the menopause. (Wilson,
> R. A., p. 165)

Poor Mrs Wilson. If she was as ill as she seems to have been, it must have been particularly dementing to be denied treatment because everyone had a diagnosis – 'change of life'. Her eldest child was in his teens; how old could she have been? If she suffered from rheumatoid arthritis or early-onset Alzheimer's and was being tormented with nonsense about climacteric symptoms her rages would have been anything but senseless. Robert A. Wilson based a whole career on amateur diagnoses overheard in his youth. His mental anguish at his mother's rejection of him was exacerbated by another trauma, the sight of a woman's bloated body being torn open by a grappling hook as it was fished from a reservoir near his childhood home. Her suicide too was caused by (whisper, whisper) 'change of life'. Robert became a crusader. In fact he suffered from an acute form of anophobia (fear of old women).

> Anyone who has ever been employed in a business directed by a
> menopausal woman executive is familiar with another variant of
> this [menopausal negativity] syndrome. The work week becomes a
> futile, inefficient round of violent ups and downs, adult tantrums
> and pointless chicanery. The woman in a position of authority has a

ready-made means of side-stepping the passive kind of menopausal
negativism. She is presented with an irresistible and unlimited
opportunity to take out her frustrations on her poor employees.
(p. 85)

The middle-aged female manager, dealing with a workforce who
ignore everything she says because they have decided that she is
menopausal, is quite likely to have to think of a number of strategies to
get their attention. Criticisms of Margaret Thatcher's way of running
her cabinet reflected this mechanism, and doubtless she capitulated to it.
Anophobia is an accretive phenomenon; it causes the kind of treatment
of middle-aged women that they react to in a way that seems to justify
it. A good deal of the anxiety of the middle-aged woman is caused
by her awareness that she is turning into some kind of a harridan, a
scold, a jade, a drab, a fishwife, a beldame, but if you can't get attention
any other way, what are you to do? There is no way out after all; the
vituperative woman, the viper, the virago will be told that she has only
herself to blame for the negativity that surrounds her. Nagging is painful
utterance that the more it is repeated, the more resolutely it is ignored.

Railing has a positive value. Railing in literature, called variously
satire tragic or comic, lampoon, burlesque, invective, has been highly
valued, first as entertainment and second as a corrective to abuses,
yet though we have female poets we do not have female satiric poets.
Though there are hundreds of literary attacks on women by men, there
are very few attacks on men by women, and the few we have are almost
all answers to unprovoked attacks by men. It is almost as if women's
rage is, like women's sexuality, too vast and bottomless to be allowed
any expression. Despite the best efforts of feminists to awaken women's
anger and to turn their hostility outward so that it becomes a force for
social change rather than the procreator of symptoms, we have failed.
With one or two magnificent exceptions, no race of hilarious harridans
has appeared upon the earth.

The medicalisation of menopause is the last phase in the process
of turning all the elements of female personality that do not relate to
the adult male into pathology. Virginity is pathology; lack of interest
in heterosexual intercourse on demand is pathology; 'excessive'
involvement in mothering is pathology; middle-aged truculence and
recalcitrance are the most pathological of all. Now we have pills for all of

them and women are obediently taking them. Doctors cannot change social, cultural, economic or political conditions; they can only try to tailor the patient to fit better into her circumstances. We cannot blame the patient if she asks for help. We cannot blame doctors if they give the only help they can. We cannot blame the woman if she experiences the alteration in her responses as an improvement in her health, and chooses to ignore the underlying problems which she cannot solve.

If you are drifting around an empty house that no one wants to spend time in, the children being about their own mysterious affairs and your husband staying late at the office most days, you are oppressed. If you are stagnating in a dead-end job on a miserable rate of pay watching younger people rise past you through the promotion scale, you are oppressed. If you are a widow or a divorced woman struggling to adjust to a new life on your own in one of our unsafe and brutalised cities you are oppressed. If people take no pains to conceal their lack of interest in you, if people refuse to take you seriously because they have decided that you are menopausal, you are oppressed. If you believe that this state of affairs has been brought about by your inadequacy, and you have to add guilt to your emotional burden, you are not only oppressed, you will feel depressed. You will see yourself as dull, dumpy and grey and not blame the people who do not conceal their lack of interest in you. You are not, after all, interested in yourself.

If you are dumpy and dull and grey, how did you get that way? You might look to your family and your employer and ask as the neglected wife asks in Shakespeare's *Comedy of Errors*,

Are my discourses dull? Barren my wit?
If voluble and sharp discourse be marred,
Unkindness blunts it more than marble hard …
What ruins are in me that can be found
By him not ruined? (II.i.90–2, 96–7)

The evidence seems to show that the more dissatisfied you are with your life the bumpier the ride through the climacteric is going to be, as if your life is trying to jump the tracks. The only people who offer help, the medicos, can offer treatments that will keep you on the rails. They might smooth out the bumps but you need to be sure that you want to go on in the same direction. If you don't, there is no reason to feel guilty. There is no reason to feel guilty if your life has fallen to pieces all around you, either. If until this point your life has not been under your control, as is all too probable, you can now take control. Indeed, you may have no other option. Feelings of vertigo and panic are to be expected, and not to be apologised for. The truth behind the research that failed to find a significant increase in stress at the climacteric is that, though the new life may be more strenuous, it will not be more difficult than the old. Anxiety about ageing and worry about health are concomitants of menopausal uproar; when it is over the prospect of illness and decrepitude recedes once more to a manageable distance. Negative feelings are not your fault either. None of it, neither the mood swings, nor the weight gain, nor the loss of interest in sex, nor the insomnia, should incur the added burden of guilt.

6

The Unavoidable Consequences

Ageing begins before we are born and continues throughout our lives; the only cure for it is death. It is not a uniform process, however. Human beings age jerkily; not only do we become aware of gradual changes only when forced to take stock of ourselves, the actual degenerative changes of ageing are accelerated by unusual stresses and strains. When someone says that an experience aged her ten years or took ten years off her life, she is giving an exaggerated account of objective truth. Though it is never true to say that a trauma turned someone's hair white overnight, it is true that the loss of hair pigmentation can be accelerated by privation, shock or grief. Impaired vision may become obvious only when for some reason we are too tired to make the extra effort to focus; then a first pair of reading glasses may do for ten or twenty years, or not.

There is little that an individual woman in the throes of the climacteric can find out about her likely future career. The study of ageing is itself young, and has come to very few conclusions, but they are important for the menopausal woman who feels that the bottom is falling out of her life. In 1986, Nathan W. Shock of the National Institute on Aging summarised the results of longitudinal studies of ageing, that is, studies that follow the progress of a group of individuals over time, rather than contrasting the performance of older with other younger people. His enquiries resulted in a number of conclusions among which the first was 'that relatively few individuals follow the pattern of age changes predicted from averages based on measurements made on different subjects'. Ageing is so highly individual that average curves give only a rough approximation of the pattern of ageing followed by individuals or, in Shock's words:

> There is little evidence for the existence of a single factor that regulates the rate of aging in different functions in a specific individual. Because of the large range in the performance of most physiological variables among subjects of the same chronological age, it appears that age alone is a poor predictor of performance ... (pp. 739–40)

It is only with the greatest difficulty therefore that doctors can separate the symptoms of the menopause from the symptoms of ageing. This they need to do in order not to be accused of quackery, for the accusation that they offer hormone replacement therapy as the elixir of eternal youth is easily made. In an early Dutch study led by Dr L. Jaszman (1969), it was noticed that some symptoms that made their first appearance in the peri-menopause, including palpitations, joint pains and sleeplessness, persisted more than five years after the last menstrual period. These were taken to be associated not with the cessation of ovarian function but with ageing, and these are the symptoms unlikely to respond to attempts to correct oestrogen deficiency. The same conclusion was reached by Professor Carl Wood of Monash University (1979) in a study of Melbourne women: complaints of sleeplessness, joint pains, numbness, palpitations, dizziness and weakness were commoner in older menopausal women (Evans, p. 51).

When Dr Sergey Dzugan MD PhD, who heads up a US-based website called menopausewoman, undertakes to answer the question 'Why does Elle Macpherson (age 50) look more like 30 and Helen Mirren (70) look like she is 50?', he replies, 'Environment plays a big role, what you eat, diet and exercise. But, the problem is, we can stand on our head, drink carrot juice and do a lot of exercise and use any kind of diet. But unfortunately, until you restore hormones you will get decline. Hormones play a crucial role in keeping your metabolism in good shape. As soon as you lose balance between building hormones and destructive hormones you will start to have problems.' To find out what he means by 'hormones' it is necessary to buy his book *The Menopause Cure: Hormonal Health*.

The changes associated with ageing have been summarised as a continuous decrease at the rate of a per cent or so a year of basal metabolism, vital capacity, maximal breathing capacity, glomerular filtration rate, standard cell water and nerve conduction velocity. These are biologically more precise ways of saying what ordinary people mean when they say that when people age they slow down and dry up. The rate of decrease is affected by genetic and environmental factors; some people will age twice as fast as the mean, others half as fast. The slowing down may manifest itself in a disintegration of bodily function as messages take longer to get around the system; clumsiness, even dizziness and loss of co-ordination result. Organs do not age at the same rate; the heart beats more than two and a half billion times in a life of seventy years; no other muscle in the body can remotely approach this kind of efficiency. Thigh muscles, by contrast, tend to give up well before the age of seventy.

In a study reported in the *Proceedings of the National Academy of Sciences* in 2016 by the David Geffen School of Medicine at UCLA, 3,100 women who had gone through menopause gave blood samples which were analysed to provide information about the biological age of their cells, which was determined by examining a biomarker known as DNA methylation. Steve Horvath, professor of human genetics and biostatistics at UCLA, who led the study, pointed out that the evidence showed that women who went through menopause earlier were biologically older than women who went through it at a later age. The evidence also seemed to show that women who accepted HRT were biologically younger than women who did not, but without a more systematic study of biological age before and after menopause, no more definite conclusions were possible. A related study carried out by the Semel Institute for Neuroscience and Human Behavior at the same university found that disruption of sleep patterns in post-menopausal women was also connected to biological ageing. Researcher Judith Carroll is quoted as saying 'Not getting restorative sleep may do more than just affect our functioning the next day; it might also influence the rate at which our biological clock ticks' (Levine et al.).

It little avails the menopausal woman to know that the atrophic thyroid gland of the mature individual hypertrophies and increases its secretory activity ... that the ground substance of connective tissue increases ... that the collagen content in muscle declines, particularly in the limbs, not so much in the abdomen ... that of the endocrine glands, the gonads change first, then the pituitary, then the thyroid, or that the adrenal glands take over part of the function of the gonads until they too fail in what has come to be called the 'adrenopause'. A benchmark study of 1937 by Henry S. Simms and Abraham Stolman at the Columbia University Medical School found that tissues of people over seventy contained 'more water, chloride, total base, sodium and calcium' and 'less potassium, magnesium, phosphorus, nitrogen and ash' than the tissues of younger people. Older people sweat less and do not produce the kind of sweat that smells sharp.

With ageing, cardiac output declines. Renal function declines 35 per cent between ages twenty and ninety but some studies show that in particular individuals it improves. The liver gets smaller; from 2.5 per cent of body weight at middle age, it declines to 1.6 per cent by the tenth decade and the blood flow to the liver also decreases (Geokas and Haverback, 1969). Therefore it takes longer for drugs, etc. to be excreted. In 1973 researchers reported that they had found a significant fall in rosette-forming T-cells in blood occurring between forty-six and sixty years of age. What this means is that the body's defence against disease, its ability to produce an antibody response, begins to weaken (Hausman and Weksler, 1986). This may in fact be an advantage; the inflammatory response seems to be less violent in older people. They make take longer to recover from infection, but the course of the disease, say a cold, may be less violent. If the declining immune response in older people were to be bolstered or 'rejuvenated' we would expect to see an increase in autoimmune disease and inflammatory conditions like rheumatism and arthritis.

Menopause is a big blip on the ageing curve; the cessation of ovarian function is itself caused by ageing and is a part of ageing. The separation of management of menopause from the management of ageing, therefore, doesn't make sense. What happens to fifty-year-old eyes, hair, skin, ankles, feet, waistlines is at least as important as what is going on in the genito-urinary tract. The woman who comes hard up at menopause against the fact of her advancing age should have some way of knowing which of her symptoms is an unavoidable concomitant of ageing and which signifies ill-health. She may also have to consider whether or not she is ageing too fast, and why that might be. If she is overweight, smokes, drinks, and takes little exercise, she is piling on the burdens that the ageing organism has to carry; you are only as young as your most fatigued component, be it heart, lungs, liver, brain, skin or skeleton.

Fifty years ago, very few people had ever heard of osteoporosis. It was then understood to be a rare disease, mostly affecting people in extreme old age, whose bones had become so porous that they collapsed, resulting in fractures, particularly those of the vertebrae, resulting in the curvature of the spine that was called 'dowager's hump'. In fact elderly men too can become so bent that they cannot raise their heads. Nowadays osteoporosis is assumed to be an almost inevitable concomitant of the untreated menopause; from being rare it has now become a looming epidemic. Bone loss is part of the ageing process, but whether it is caused by a deficiency of oestrogen is far from clear, and whether replacement oestrogens will prevent it is also unclear, yet many otherwise well women are using HRT to ward off a debilitating condition from which they are unlikely ever to suffer. There is no evidence that upping your calcium intake will help either; the problem is that bone resorption begins to outstrip the making of new bone. If you munch calcium tablets, chances are the extra calcium will end up where it is not wanted.

We think of our skeletons as the solid framework upon which our bodies are built, a set of struts and girders that will endure unless they are twisted by some sort of earthquake or battered by other objects as solid or solider. In fact the human skeleton is alive; it absorbs and it excretes; it heals when it is injured, absorbing damaged bone and regenerating healthy bone. The skeleton constitutes 10–15 per cent of total body weight; calcium not only forms the mineral content of bone but provides the conductivity in nerves, is involved in hormonal activity, inhibits and activates enzymes, plays a role in blood clotting and in immune function. Vitamin D, available only from oily fish, eggs and sunlight, controls the calcium–phosphorus balance. There is a marked decrease in calcium absorption in middle-aged women, which is aggravated by inadequate Vitamin D exposure, impairment of kidney function and – menopause.

Bone loss occurs in all vertebrates with age; indeed, changes in calcium behaviour may be the principal mechanism of ageing:

> It is a matter of everyday clinical experience that the avidity of various tissues for calcium increases with age. This tendency

manifests itself in the formation of gross calcification in the cardiovascular system, cartilaginous structures, tendons, periarticular tissues, and lens of the eye (cataracts) as well as the development of calcareous concretions in such areas as the pineal gland, prostate and urinary passages. In addition ... there occurs with age a gradual increase in the chemically detectable calcium content of various organs ... It is generally held that calcinosis is a secondary result of 'decreased tissue vitality' and presents a 'dystrophic' phenomenon; yet a review of the literature shows that several investigators have considered the possibility that an increase in tissue calcium concentration may be the cause of many of the changes characteristic of senility. (Selye et al., p. i)

The particular form of rat torture devised by Selye, Strebel and Mikulaj to test their hypothesis need not concern us here. It is now generally agreed that as we age calcium migrates from our bones where it is useful to other areas where it is not. Menopause is thought perhaps to accelerate bone resorption because the lack of oestrogen allows unopposed action of the parathyroid, the gland responsible for inhibiting growth, so that trabecular bone in particular is rapidly resorbed, leading to the characteristic fractures of the wrist and the head of the femur, and the crush fractures of the vertebrae that result in 'dowager's hump'. Bone loss is most rapid within the five to ten years following the last menstrual period. The present state of knowledge is insufficient to show whether administration of replacement oestrogens over this period is sufficient to prevent this kind of bone loss. In fact there are no oestrogen receptors in bone, and nobody knows why HRT should affect osteoporosis (Guinan et al., 1987).

And there are some who insist that it does not. New Zealand health researcher Gillian Sanson spent years examining the evidence that oestrogen deficiency causes low bone-mineral density which then contributes to the risk of fractures. The first surprise was that the machines used to measure bone density were not standardised; the next that a diagnosis of low bone-mineral density was a poor predictor of fractures; the next that osteoporosis, so far from being inevitable in post-menopause, was rare; and the last that HRT could not be shown to exert any protective action whatsoever. There is no distinct group of individuals who can be identified as likely sufferers from severe osteoporosis.

> Osteoporosis is not a single disease entity, but it is the end result
> of a number of processes which become more common with
> increasing age and lead to the diminution of the amount of bone in
> the skeleton. (Exton-Smith, p. 524)

Increasing porosity of bone will manifest itself sooner in people whose skeletons at maturity were at the lower end of the percentile of body weight, whose diet has been deficient in calcium, who have been sedentary or, worse, immobile, and who have been given prolonged treatment with corticosteroids. Increased protein and phosphorus intake (as for example in a diet rich in red meat) accelerates calcium excretion.

Even vigorous young men will lose bone mass if they are bedridden or if they are weightless in space. The skeleton needs not only to be stimulated by the action of the sinews in order to maintain a healthy balance of accretion and excretion, but also, it seems, to be in contact with the ground. It would be interesting to learn if middle-aged women who habitually sit on the ground rather than in chairs ever display the characteristic fracture of the head of the femur that costs health authorities so many millions each year. When the facts that such women do not eat red meat and do eat yoghurt and green vegetables and walk for tens of miles each day usually carrying loads on their heads are taken into account as well, we would be surprised to find dowagers' humps among them. A hundred million or so such women live in the Indian subcontinent; a 2005 study of low-income women in India produced plenty of evidence of low bone-mineral density as a consequence of their diet, but no evidence of proliferating fractures (Shatrugna et al.). Osteoporosis does have a genetic component, but it is also a disease of affluence.

> Lanyon 1980, 1982 in animal experiments has demonstrated
> a fundamental relationship between bone mass and load-bearing
> requirements. Bone mass can be increased by exposing bone to
> strain changes which are well within the limits of normal daily
> activity. It appears that the frequency with which the strain

is applied is a more important oestrogenic stimulus than the
magnitude of the peak strain. (Exton-Smith, p. 529)

The salvation of the skeleton then, is the same as the salvation of the rest
of us: work, good, hard work that tires us but does not over-extend or
exhaust us. All the other treatments to delay bone loss have long-term
consequences of one sort or another.

There is no escaping ageing, which can be observed all around us, in
every living thing and many inanimate things, cars, houses, furniture
and clothes, but nobody quite knows what it is or why it happens.
The second law of thermodynamics tells us that a self-perpetuating
mechanism is impossible, but biologists have so far been unable to
enunciate a similar law for their own discipline. Cells, it seems, can
go on living and reproducing indefinitely, if the medium is right.
Nobody dies of old age; without an illness to knock her off an old
woman will stick around indefinitely. So some biologists have come
to the conclusion that, though death is inevitable, ageing is always
pathological. Death is biologically useful; ageing is not. Most creatures
don't hang about as they become gradually more and more decrepit,
but conk out smartly once they have passed on their genes. The human
female is unique among living organisms on this earth because she can
live twice the time of her reproductive span and more (see above p. 62).
Many a butterfly might like to continue sipping nectar once her eggs
were laid but the choice is not hers. The human female, having served
the species, is the only one that can build a life of her own; it is too bitter
a biological irony to think that she may not have the heart to do it.

One reason she may not want to live out her allotted span is that
the extra life is blighted by the consequences of ageing, so that it is not
life but half-life or shelf-life. No one seems to know whether human
ageing (as distinct from death) is avoidable or not. The best discussion
of the mystery of ageing is still Alex Comfort's first and best-written
book, *The Biology of Senescence*. Some have thought that we are born
with a biological timeclock inside us that counts down a lifespan which
can only be 'artificially' interrupted or lengthened. Their notion is
strengthened by the observable hereditability of longevity and by the
fact that most species exhibit a uniform maximum lifespan. Though
creatures may die of myriad causes before they reach the end of their
biological lease, they cannot live beyond it.

Discussions of longevity are difficult to keep out of discussions of human ageing, but they blur it impossibly. The Cumaean Sibyl lived for ever, but she was so wasted that she spent all of her unnatural life longing for death. The person who inherits arthritis along with longevity is not likely to be overcome with gratitude. The woman trying to understand what ageing will inevitably involve will find that the people who should be telling her (who are mostly younger than she) will waste her time babbling on about centenarians in Georgia or Kashmir. What they cannot prepare her for is what will happen to her in the fifty years before she turns a hundred. Most studies of ageing are studies of the already aged. The woman who is anxious not to become a member of the nursing-home population can learn little from studies of such populations. One of the worst fears of menopause is that bouts of confusion and memory loss are the first signs of Alzheimer's or senile dementia. The questions we all ask when we see the trembling old lady being buttoned into her coat are 'How did she get like that? How do you know when you are getting like that?' And when younger people treat us with pitying condescension we wonder if we have not already got like that.

Those of us who believe that dying is a service we should eventually perform in the interests of the ecosphere and the other people who arrive on the planet every day may be equally sure that ageing benefits nobody. Decrepitude is a source of pain and frustration to the decrepit and a dreadful oppression for those who care for her, in every sense of the expression. A woman who desires to remain vigorous for as long as possible, and take her leave quickly when she is too tired to go on, will not find much in gerontology that will help her to devise a strategy. For one thing gerontology is the study of old men. Alex Comfort would like to have replaced the word with geratology, the study of old age, but this would be merely window-dressing. Until relatively recently, women were despaired of. The menopause put them beyond help. The real impetus for the attack on ageing came from the ageing male élite, who wanted to enjoy the fruits of a lifetime's accumulated power, namely the love and adulation of young women. The result in that case was Viagra.

In case this should be thought to be mere loony feminist nonsense, let me summarise as briefly as possible the history of loony virilist nonsense. In 1889, 72-year-old Professor Brown-Séquard of the

University of Paris announced to a learned gathering of his colleagues that he had just been enabled to have congress with young Madame Brown-Séquard because he had injected himself with animal testicular extract. Brown-Séquard was the first of the hundreds of youth doctors whom Patrick McGrady, in his book *The Youth Doctors*, dubbed the Erector Set, led by Eugen Steinach, Serge Voronoff, John Romulus Brinkley and Paul Nichans, who treated 'popes, millionaires and potentates' and very few women. After Nichans treated Pope Pius XII, his fresh cell injections, never systematically investigated, were imitated by other doctors.

Clayton Wheeler, who 'addressed himself, with flowers and hand-kissing to a predominantly female clientele' (p. 49), was an out-and-out fraud. The glandular extract suppositories he supplied were desiccated hamburger. Nichans's therapy was practised in London by Peter M. Stephan, who treated women not for loss of sexual function, but for worry 'about their breasts', in treating which Stephan claimed to have 'about fifty per cent success'. McGrady's report of the conversation with Stephan unintentionally reveals how gross their shared assumptions about women and ageing must have been: Stephan replies to the question 'Can you really make something out of a pancake?' thus:

'Let's be logical … absolutely logical about it … there are drooping breasts and there are drooping breasts, are there not? I mean, don't give me an impossible case. Let's have a sensible case. A woman of fifty. All right, so they're drooping a bit and she has to wear all kinds of supports. That you can help. If they're pancakes, as you call them … no.'
'Can you get a breast to upturn?'
'I've done it.' (pp. 127–8)

The female equivalent of restoring erection in the ageing penis is understood by both men to be restoring turgidity in the breast. Unfortunately the sum of the evidence seems to bear out the impression that what men wanted from the youth doctors was the energy of youth while women were content with the appearance of youth. If men wanted to enjoy, women sought to attract. The youth doctor who treated women was, until Robert A. Wilson began the touting of hormone replacement in 1966, typically a cosmetician.

By contrast the decline of male erectile potency with age was serious business. When a group of researchers at the Pfizer plant in Sandwich, Kent tried out a new drug called sildenafil on sufferers from angina and hypertension, they could not but notice that, while it had no observable effect on the target conditions, it produced what have been described as 'marked' erections. Further tests involving portions of penile tissue exposed to electric impulses showed that the administration of sildenafil caused the blood vessels to relax as they would in a normal erection, and so was born the fastest-selling pharmaceutical product in human history. The drug was patented in 1996, approved by the US Federal Drug Agency in 1998, and by 2008 worldwide sales had earned nearly two billion dollars.

For women the issue was still attractiveness rather than potency. Most women first detect, and often remain obsessed by, the evidence of ageing in their faces, that is, wrinkles. Extraordinarily enough, nobody knows what a wrinkle is. The anatomy of wrinkled skin is the same as that of unwrinkled skin. Wrinkles are not only or even principally evidence of ageing; they are also evidence of repeated exposure, especially to the sun, but also to wind and cold (Kligman et al.). More than is usually realised, premature wrinkling of the facial skin is brought on by the prolonged use of our favourite drugs, alcohol, caffeine and nicotine. An Australian woman who lives in the sun, and smokes and drinks, has a face ten years or more older than her body. Even in the faces of women living in seclusion and using no stimulants, age shows its hand eventually; the facial muscles slacken and the skin loosens as the collagen layer is depleted. Though the faces of fifty-year-old nuns are pale and smooth by comparison with our weather-beaten Australian forty-year-old's, they are not young. Dry skins wrinkle sooner than oily ones, blond skin before olive, olive before brown, brown before black. Nevertheless black women die before brown women who die before olive women who die before blond women, and not simply because of the differences in their socioeconomic circumstances.

The fifty-year-old woman's face tells us not only that she has lived fifty years but where and how she has lived it. It is not in itself unattractive or attractive, beauty being after all in the eye of the beholder, but the woman herself may feel that it gives too much away. Women who have worn make-up all their lives are masked women: what happens as the years pile on is that the wrinkles burst through the mask; too often they are lines of frowning, pouting or tightening the lips. The shining girl-face begins to look serious or anxious, or even threatening. We cannot be surprised that ageing women look perpetually sad or worried or cross, or that they will go to some lengths to smooth out a face that invites an instantaneous negative response. To gain a temporary facelift the poor use Preparation H, which shrinks haemorrhoids; the rich go for the real thing. The doctors who make a fortune out of trimming away 'the debris of years' use the same pitch as the oestrogen replacers: 'You should have come to me years ago. Now you can never leave me.' A face lifted once has to be lifted again, and still the neck and the hands and the rheumy old eyes will give it away.

This is not the place to discuss ways of smoothing ageing faces, whether by peeling off layers of skin or cutting out the sag. There are literally hundreds of such procedures, none of which fools anyone but the woman who pays for it. Cosmetic surgery has been found to be of benefit with women who have very low self-esteem, and has been used to advantage on prison inmates, who identified particular features as stigmata, and saw the changing of their faces as essential to the changing of themselves. The woman who does not wish to dump or deny a part of herself will not try to junk her used face. During the climacteric she will be painfully aware of the changes in her physical appearance, which may be exacerbated by her mental state, but she will come to like her new face at least as much as she liked the one that, though young and vivid, seemed to need so much make-up to look good. One of the changes a woman ought to make at the climacteric is to change her make-up or perhaps, life being so short, to eliminate it altogether. If one's face is becoming something to look out of, rather than to be looked at, it does not need to be painted.

Why should skin wrinkle? Why should age spots appear on the backs of hands? Why do necks wattle and the skin over the breastbone turn into red chicken skin? Why do toenails grow thick and woody? Why does hair go grey and thin and, worst of all, fall out? Why do some people have bushy white hair and others a few colourless wisps? Why do joints get knobby and feet misshapen and knees and elbows horny? Why do eyes grow dim? These superficial changes are not the ones that biologists concern themselves with; there is no learned paper on relative changes in toenail density over a period of fifty years. Because, as one gerontologist put it, 'no one dies of old skin', most gerontology books do not discuss what happens to the skin as it ages. The truth is that the skin, the largest and most complex organ of the body, does age steadily throughout life.

The changes are complex and not well understood; at menopause a woman's secretion of sebum declines sharply until it is only half as much as that of a man the same age. Her skin suddenly gets perceptibly drier and thinner, though there is no alteration in its complex structure. As the years pass there is a gradual muting of the histamine response, which may be a blessing, because there is usually a gradual increase in sensitisation as the incidences of exposure mount up. Older people show allergic responses to more substances, but the responses are milder. Sensitivity to pain also decreases and the inflammatory response to a potential irritant is slower, so older people show a different pattern of reaction to skin contact with detergents or cosmetics or medication. The symptoms are slower to appear but may cause more damage and be less easily reversible. There are changes in the distribution of subcutaneous fatty tissue and the underlying vascular structure which in turn cause changes in heat retention. These changes are all too gradual for the changer herself to notice them, but at menopause she may become aware of them as sudden reversals. Your menopause summer may be the summer when you realise that you no longer tan the way you used to and the beach is no longer the place for you.

One tried and tested way of slowing down ageing is 'caloric restriction', which has been shown to regulate ageing and increase the healthy lifespan in a range of living creatures from unicellular yeasts to worms, flies, rodents and primates. The original study dates back to 1935, when Mary Crowell and Clive McCay of Cornell University showed that reducing the food intake without causing malnutrition almost doubled the lifespan of rats. The treatment is drastic; food intake is reduced by 20 to 40 per cent, and it comes with some undesirable sequelae. Hundreds of studies have produced the same result; variation of protein intake both within and without the restriction of diet has produced conflicting results. Human beings are not rats, who have millions of years of experience of feast and famine behind them; nevertheless it makes sense that people who are not growing or reproducing need less food than people involved in either or both. A slower metabolic rate simply cannot process as much food as fast as a faster one. Both the storage of the surplus and the elimination of the waste products involve effort, using energy which the ageing woman may well want to free up for something else. There is also some evidence that changes in the gut alter digestive processes so that a good deal of the vitamin and protein content is merely excreted. All the evidence seems to indicate that the ageing woman should eat less and better. She should also increase the proportion of bulk and fibre in her diet.

Two-thirds of sufferers from IBS or irritable bowel syndrome are women and most of them first encountered the problem in the peri-menopause. One of the theories of ageing that held sway at the turn of the century explained ageing as caused by the deleterious action of an unbalanced microbial population in the gut, which could be counteracted by eating yoghurt. In 1907 Elie Metchnikov, deputy director of the Pasteur Institute, declared that the longevity of Bulgarian peasants was entirely down to their consumption of fermented milk products, and it was he who believed that eating such products would establish the beneficial bacteria in the gut. These days the menopausal woman is more likely to be told to use a prebiotic such as 'A. Vogel's Molkosan, an organic lacto-fermented whey drink' which will cost her £5.99 for 200 ml. Diluted yoghurt is rather cheaper. The ingredient list of 'Primadophilus optima' marketed by Nature's Way at £16 or so for thirty one-a-day capsules is given as follows: '*Lactobacillus plantarum*, *Lactobacillus casei*, *Bifidobacterium breve*, *Lactobacillus acidophilus*, *Lactobacillus rhamnosus*, *Lactobacillus paracasei*, *Bifidobacterium longum*, *Bifidobacterium bifidum*, *Streptococcus thermophilus*, *Bifidobacterium infantis*, *Lactobacillus bulgaricus*, *Lactobacillus salivarium*, *Lactobacillus helveticus*, plus milk, soya and short-chain fructoligosaccharides, Potato starch, Stabiliser: Microcrystalline cellulose, Sodium alginate, Stearic acid, Fractionated coconut oil (non-hydrogenated), Oleic acid, Bulking agent: Magnesium stearate, Capsule: Hydroxypropyl methylcellulose, Antioxidant: Ascorbic acid.' The first thing to notice about this list is that no quantities or proportions are given. However, the solution may not be to bombard the natural bowel flora with thirteen varieties of introduced lactobacilli.

A more productive line of thought holds that it is not proliferation of the natural microbial population in the gut that causes problems but its depletion, such as results from antibiotic use. Many apparently autoimmune conditions respond well to the reintroduction of gut microbes. Faecal transfer, now more likely to be called a host of other names meaning the same thing, is now being re-examined as a therapy for a specific group of diseases that includes besides inflammatory bowel diseases like IBS, Crohn's disease and ulcerative colitis, chronic constipation and diarrhoea, myalgic encephalopathy, chronic fatigue syndrome, trimethylaminuria and recurrent *Clostridium difficile* infection, and even neurological conditions like multiple sclerosis and Parkinsonism. Some therapists have found encouraging results in the treatment of autism. In the US the FDA only recognised human faeces as an experimental drug, including freeze-dried in capsule form, as recently as 2013, whereas the Centre for Digestive Diseases in Sydney has been treating patients effectively with faecal transplants since 1988.

Nobody knows why women should be so vulnerable to IBS. The idea that it was a consequence of lessened motility of the gut muscles was not borne out by studies which showed no correlation between bowel motility and acute episodes, and no corresponding improvement when bowel motility was improved. Other studies indicate that the bowel becomes oversensitive and goes into spasm, but don't show how or why. Others have looked at the role of neurotransmitters like gastrin and serotonin. Even more surprising, though oestrogen is thought to play a role, nobody has been able to work out what it might be. Chances are that other neurotransmitters are involved and that stress plays a part in triggering painful episodes, but we have still to track the feedback mechanism that drives the phenomenon. In the meantime, avoidance of caffeine, nicotine and alcohol, plus salutary amounts of bulk and fibre, and perhaps the occasional dose of fleaseed (*Psillium psillium*) will go some way toward alleviating the inconvenience and discomfort of IBS.

The meaning of studies that have shown that the depression of body temperature in laboratory animals leads to longer survival is not easy to assess. It seems that chilling, as it were, is associated with delaying tumour development and depressing immune responsiveness. If autoimmune responses are involved in the typical diseases of ageing such as arthritis, it makes sense to depress or retard them, but the drugs that depress human body temperature, which include chlorpromazine, reserpine, L-dopa and THC, have other effects more spectacular and less desirable than a mean statistical extension of hypothetical lifespan.

Work on the restriction of calorie intake continues. Though it can be seen to improve longevity in some species, the effect on humans and other primates has been impossible to quantify. A substance called resveratrol, a phytoalexin found naturally in some grapes and nuts, that appears to mimic the benefits of calorie restriction, has been being investigated for nearly fifty years, but so far no safe level of administration has been identified and, while it appeared to slow some of the processes of ageing in laboratory mice, it did not improve their longevity. In the mid-Noughties resveratrol was publicised as an antioxidant, an anti-cancer agent and a phyto-oestrogen. In 2010 because of concerns about safety GlaxoSmithKline suspended a small clinical trial of its own proprietary form of resveratrol, and terminated the study later that year. GSK invested $720 million in a company with the intention of developing a version of resveratrol but virtually abandoned the project when it became clear that much of the data was concocted, notably by Dipak K. Das at the University of Connecticut. A year later, one of only two major foundations funding longevity research stopped making new grants for work on resveratrol and the amplifying proteins it was supposed to activate. Resveratrol is available as a food supplement, with the usual caveats that its effectiveness is unproven and the quality controls inadequate.

Rapamycin, made by a type of soil bacterium, named for Easter Island or Rapanui, has extended the lifespans of yeast, flies and worms by about 25 per cent. Nowadays better known as sirolimus, it has been shown to improve the longevity of laboratory mice as well as suppressing their immune response, and work continues to find ways of enhancing the one function and controlling the other. At present marmoset monkeys are being tested, while 1,500 pet owners have funded a 'Dog Aging Project' at the University of Washington (Harmon).

Since the 1990s, the middle-aged woman is more likely to be considering the role of antioxidants in retarding the ageing process, but the evidence is far from conclusive. When food is transformed into energy, the process creates by-products called 'free radicals', that is, unstable molecules that steal electrons from other molecules, and so damage DNA and cell membranes. An overload of these is thought to be a contributing factor in the genesis of some diseases of the heart and liver, of cancers, and even Parkinson's Disease, Alzheimer's Disease and arthritis. Vitamins A, C and E are thought to act as antioxidants, as are selenium, zinc and copper, as well as an array of phytochemicals such as the lycopenes in tomatoes, lutein in spinach and corn, and the anthocyanins in cranberries. The result has been the promotion of all kinds of substances as superfoods, which preceded any scientific verification of their mode of action. Our bodies can produce their own antioxidants, and taking supplements could knock out the natural process. Antioxidants present in fresh foods have been shown to be more effective and less prone to malfunction than those taken in concentration. Moreover, free radicals have their own function within the body as part of the armamentarium of immune cells. Large-scale epidemiological trials have so far failed to show that antioxidant supplements retard ageing or delay dying, and in some cases they appear to produce the opposite effect. Investigation of the health benefits, if any, of intermittent fasting also continues.

Ageing involves gradual mutations in many patterns of behaviour. As menopause is a jolt in this otherwise reasonably continuous process, permanent alterations may be perceived as sudden and aberrant. One of the behaviours that alter with age is sleep. Middle-aged women are not capable of the dormouse sleep of younger creatures (Miles and Dement). A pattern of eight or more hours' sleep may be turning into a pattern of napping. If the menopausal woman insists upon following an inappropriate sleep pattern she may find herself lying wide awake in bed for many potentially useful hours. The adjustment will be made more difficult if she is trying to fit her sleep pattern to someone else's, lying open-eyed in the dark alongside a snoring partner, say, whose snores never used to disturb her before.

Sleep comes in two basic kinds, REM and Non REM (NREM). REM stands for rapid eye movement, which is not to be observed in the onset of sleep, when the brain goes through various stages of activity that show characteristic patterns on an encephalogram, followed by a mixed stage, a stage showing two patterns called the K complex and the sleep spindle, and a third stage called slow-wave or delta sleep. In REM sleep the encephalogram shows a pattern similar to that of the waking brain and the eyes move rapidly in synchrony, while the reflexes that functioned normally during NREM sleep seem to be suspended. Nobody knows what the function of REM sleep actually is, though it seems to be physiologically necessary and is the first to be built up after a period of sleep deprivation. After about eighty minutes of NREM sleep, ninety or a hundred minutes of REM sleep ensue and the two continue to alternate during the total sleep time.

Middle-aged females in REM sleep exhibit the highest arousal threshold, that is, are the most easily wakened and the most sensitive to traffic noise in sleep. In the sixth decade of life a high proportion of people, about a quarter, have no stage 4 sleep at all. It looks as if slow-wave sleep can be increased by physical exercise and by fasting (Parker et al., 1972; MacFadyen et al., 1973; Karacan et al., 1973). However, although we have all learned to sleep for a single extended period at night, the circadian rhythm of sleepiness is biphasic and it is quite normal to have a period of drowsiness in the afternoon.

Nobody knows what particular function slow-wave sleep might perform. More important is the absorption of oxygen during sleep; deprival of oxygen during sleep, either by frequent apnoea or holding of the breath, or obstructed airways, is associated with daytime sleepiness, morning headaches and personality changes. Lifelong snoring is related to heart disease and hypertension. One out of every two women in her sixties snores.

Nocturnal wakefulness is not necessarily a disadvantage. Though one might occasionally yearn for the long, deep sleep of yesteryear, there is a sort of aptness in the fact that the older members of the human group are on watch at night, when the young are sunk in slumber. The nocturnal sleeplessness of older primates has an obvious function in ensuring the survival of the group and has probably been selected for. The wee small hours belong to older women; this is the time when the leprechauns come and sweep the kitchen hearth and polish the pots – not the leprechauns at all, of course, but their old mistress come noiselessly to get her kitchen just as she likes it, without guilt-tripping the younger members of her household. The world over, older women are up betimes. What they say is that they don't need much sleep; what they don't say is that they cherish those hours in charge of a houseful of sleeping people and feel a pang of regret when the bathroom door begins to slam and people sticky with the heavier sleep of the young begin to stumble about the house, complaining about having to get up at all. If they do not notice that yesterday's wet shoes have been carefully dried and the creases got out of yesterday's crumpled overcoat, so much the better.

It should not be forgotten, however, that sleeplessness is a feature of depression, and the sleep pattern of the elderly resembles the sleep pattern of depressed people. It is possible that some of the psychiatric disorders associated with ageing are aggravated or even caused by sleep pathology. During the climacteric temporary disturbances merge with, mask, or even exacerbate the gradual long-term change, so that the circadian rhythm can be prematurely and excessively warped. The middle-aged woman should give some attention to techniques of relaxation, so that she doesn't continue to wake herself up by holding her breath or by repetitive involuntary movements. She may need quieter circumstances, away from traffic noise; she may need more or fresher air, as well as rest and exercise; she may need a colder bed or a colder room. She does not need a heavy evening meal with lots of alcohol, coffee, and her own or other people's cigarettes. If the climacteric were respectable, she could expect such consideration as a matter of course. It was to find fresh air, rest, exercise and an appropriate diet that for centuries ladies in their late forties made their way to Aix-les-Bains or Buxton, and it is still not a bad idea.

Everything that is born must die. Death is the only certain outcome of birth. The born may not grow up to maturity, may not produce children of their own, may not grow old, but sooner or later they must die. When most people witnessed death in the immediate family, nobody would have been shocked by these statements. In the late twentieth century, when death had been driven underground and out of sight, dying was the only human activity that was regarded as obscene. Whereas once the dying individual occupied centre stage, surrounded by the members of her household, and gave her last energies to making a good end, she was now prevented from dying until she could no longer influence the manner of her death. A minority was trying to revive the old *ars moriendi*, the art of dying, by forming groups to press the case for giving the terminally ill a choice, but most people were content to have death happen out of sight.

That situation is now changing more rapidly than anyone could have foreseen. Proponents of euthanasia rights, arguing for the alleviation of suffering, and the preservation of bodily integrity, self-determination and personal autonomy, appear to be winning the day. Euthanasia is now legal in the Netherlands, Canada, Colombia, Belgium and Luxembourg. Where once support for the right to die was limited to fringe groups, it can now be found across the political spectrum from left to right; when the issue is to be decided, politicians are likely to be allowed a conscience vote. As the debate has become mainstream more and more people are having to consider how they might wish to manage their deaths. The medical profession is trying, hopefully vainly, to hang on to its right to decide who should live and who should die, but the current of public feeling is running against them.

At menopause as never before a woman comes face to face with her own mortality. In May 2012, Tracey Emin, RA, was forty-eight. She explained to Mark Brown of the *Guardian*, 'I am going through the menopause and I have been for ages. It is a nightmare, an absolute nightmare. It's horrible ... People don't talk about it, but the menopause, for me, makes you feel slightly dead, so you have to start using the other things – using your mind more, read more, you have to be more enlightened, you have to take on new things, think of new ideas, discover new things, start looking at the stars, understand astronomy ... just wake yourself up, otherwise it's a gentle decline. For women, it is the beginning of dying. It is a sign. I've got to start using my brain more – I've got to be more ethereal and more enlightened.'

Dame Tracey's readiness to acknowledge the face of death in 2012 shocked the *Guardian* interviewer, but she was as sincere as only she can be, and her vision of her future deserves serious consideration. Nothing she can do will wake her ovaries up again. It is now too late; that story is over. And so Emin married herself to a rock in the garden of her house in Provence.

The grief of menopause affects every woman consciously or otherwise. The feeling that one's day has passed its noon and the shadows are lengthening, that summer is long gone and the days are growing ever shorter and bleaker, is a just one and should be respected. At the turning point the descent into night is felt as rapid; only when the stress of the climacteric is over can the ageing woman realise that autumn can be long, golden, milder than summer, and is the most productive season of the year. The elegiac strain never quite fades from the middle-aged woman's consciousness, but it gives poignancy to the now rather than the bitterness of regret that is felt by some so keenly at menopause. When the fifty-year-old woman says to herself, 'Now is the best time of all,' she means it all the more because she knows it is not forever.

Simone de Beauvoir was infuriated to see how time speeded up in her middle age so that, just when she wanted things to slow down and let her savour the moment, the years sped past her. Awareness of time as flying has some advantages; it precludes boredom, for one thing.

It matters little that younger people find older people boring or slow. Older people have a right to resist being rushed, to stand and stare at the fragile world that has become so unspeakably dear to them. For the lucky ones, who will not have to leave while they are still in love with life, there will come a later time when that passion too will fade, but while one is still possessed by that great tenderness, it must be yielded to.

Death is the inevitable outcome of life, but ageing is a privilege. Ageing and dying are different processes but not distinct; the overlap in ageing and dying as fields of research is one of the reasons we can't understand what ageing necessarily involves and what aspects are avoidable. Subjectively, we don't experience ourselves as old or young. We can only assess our own age relative to other people's and that only vaguely. You are only as old as you feel, people say, and allowing yourself to feel old is wrong. Phooey, say I for, though in myself I feel neither young nor old, I know that I am old. If you are older than most of the people on earth, it seems more than a little silly to persist in claiming to be young. The young know that we are not young. If they murmur in disagreement when we call ourselves old, it is because they feel that we are denigrating ourselves. They certainly do not think it is for us to decide that young is what we are. If our society was based on age sets that knitted us into our own generation we might have objective markers by which to place ourselves on some sort of seniority scale. Then we might actually know what it means to 'be our age'. As it is, most of us simply cannot judge how old we are. In some things we are positively juvenile and in others virtually senile. We feel younger than many younger people and older than some people our parents' age. Many of us feel that we don't belong in the company of our own generation and seek to move in a younger circle, imagining that it keeps us young; for others it is the company of the thoughtless, graceless, self-obsessed young that makes us feel old.

As the populations of the developed worlds grow older and older, as a result of falling birth rates and death rates, they seem obliged to pretend that they are younger and younger. Though there has never been hard evidence that anti-ageing preparations actually work, the demand is inexhaustible, while the prices continue to mount to such a level that we might be pardoned for thinking that the cost itself should be enough to drive a placebo effect. For example, a mere £797 will buy you 50 ml of La Prairie Cellular Cream Platinum Rare, described by Selfridges as 'an extraordinary, transformative experience. Cellular Cream Platinum Rare is the height of luxury. From the first touch, it's a total immersion. La Prairie went to the ends of the earth to uncover the most beneficial ingredients for this cream. Colloidal platinum helps recharge skin's balance, increasing its absorption of nourishing ingredients. Climate-activated hydration adjusts to changing humidity levels and skin's temperature, releasing moisture as needed by the skin. Applying the most advanced cellular science discoveries, this rejuvenating cream preserves skin texture and tone and restores a radiant glow. There is nothing else like it. The pinnacle of art, science and luxury'.

Colloidal platinum, I learn from another source, 'is documented as one of the major rejuvenater's [*sic*] of the life force, working deeply with the DNA of the cell to create an internal environment necessary for the body to help reverse degenerative conditions'. Apparently a Japanese researcher used 'platinum nano-particles of the size 2–3 nm to increase the lifespan of the roundworm'; what relevance this interesting fact might have to the warding off of the ageing of human beings was not explained.

No woman, no matter how full of years, is supposed to admit to 'being old' regardless of her chronological age. In truth one's chronological age is usually obvious. If a woman of fifty or over is particularly vigorous or attractive, others will say that she is 'marvellous for her age' rather than wonder what her age might be. Nobody who is asked the question 'How old do you think I am?' ever answers the question honestly. The question that is answered is 'How old do you think I think you think I am?'

Nobody wants to be old. Most people don't want to be dead either, but there comes a point when one has to accept one or the other. If we were more aware of death, we would possibly be less resentful of ageing. If we were more familiar with older people we might not be so unprepared for the inconveniences that accompany the winning of extra years of life on earth.

7

Medical Ignorance

Women are born with all the ova they will ever produce. Until the menarche they are dormant. The young woman grows tall and strong, learns both to work and to play, and wonders about the day when she shall start having 'the curse'. When she is approaching physical maturity, but need by no means have arrived at her full growth and strength, hair begins to appear in her armpits and on her pubis, her body shape and complexion change and, often slowly, painfully and messily, she begins to menstruate. The one change among the changes of puberty that is actually welcome to the young woman is the growth of breasts, and this too can be irregular, painful and delayed.

Many a young woman at menarche wonders how she will cope with the rest of her reproductive life, when the beginning of it is so smelly and uncomfortable. The cyclical changes in mood control, the swelling of hands and feet, backache, headaches and depression that many women experience as a regular part of their menstrual cycle, represent a real deterioration in the quality of a teenager's life. Even at this stage she is likely to be given the idea that it is she who is making heavy weather of a natural process and she should look to her attitudes and sort herself out so that she is glad and proud to bleed once a month. The palliatives for cyclical distress are all inadequate, despite the cases their pedlars make for them.

The fourteen-year-old struggling with hormonal chaos is hardly likely to be consoled by the fact that she has only thirty years or so to endure her menstrual cycle. A few women, those for whom contraception has been an ordeal or a failure, or whose reproductive system never seemed to function smoothly, may look forward to 'menopause', and some actively induce it by undergoing hysterectomy long before ovarian function is due to cease, but for most women menopause is a word of fear.

In order to understand what happens when the menstrual cycle begins to falter we need to understand how it works. At birth the ovaries of the human female contain immature follicles, called primordial follicles, each of which contains a similarly immature primary oocyte. At puberty, a number of primordial follicles 'wake up' and, under the influence of a combination of stimulatory and inhibitory hormones, begin to develop and become 'tertiary' or 'antral' or 'Graafian' follicles. Most of the original group of follicles will die before a minority of them enter the menstrual cycle, in which they compete with each other until only one is left, the 'late-tertiary' or 'pre-ovulatory' dominant follicle, which ruptures and discharges the now 'secondary' oocyte. Complicated as it might seem, this is a simplified version of the sequence of events; even so there are visible gaps in the narrative. Recruitment of follicles occurs every month and takes thirteen cycles to reach the point where the oocyte is discharged into one or other of the Fallopian tubes.

Not only is the cycle cyclical in the sense that it passes through a series of phases each leading one into another, what is happening is a cycle of stimulus, secretion, reaction and abreaction. Most explanations interrupt the process rather arbitrarily at the point where a part of the brain called the hypothalamus or 'under-bed' sends a biochemical prompt via a peptide called neurokinin, the importance of which is only now beginning to be understood, to the pituitary gland to release chemicals of its own manufacture. The substance carrying the chemical prompt is called by what it does rather than what it is, either 'follicle-stimulating hormone-releasing factor' (FSHRF) or 'luteinising hormone-releasing factor' (LHRF). Because nobody knows how the prompt for FSH might differ from the prompt for LH, some sources prefer to call it GnRH, gonadotrophin-releasing factor. (There is disagreement about how to spell this important word, whether with or without an 'h'.) This message sent to the pituitary releases follicle-stimulating hormone, FSH, or the other, the luteinising or 'yellow-body-making' hormone, LH.

As the follicles ripen they release oestrogen, the hormone that women need in order to feel good. The oestrogen in its turn sends the signal back to the brain that it is time to turn off the FSH. As oestrogen levels in the blood rise and rise, the pituitary is stimulated to release more LH, and this is the chemical signal that causes the follicle to burst and shed the ovum. The oestrogen also prompts the uterus to rebuild its lining. However, it is important to remember that ovarian activity is not the sole source of oestrogen in pre-menopausal women. In the words of the Grand Master in Menopause, Wulf Utian,

> A most important concept to understand is that the total sex-steroid hormone production in the pre-menopausal female is made up of two components. There is a relatively constant base level of oestrogen, principally oestrone produced by peripheral conversion (extraglandular formation) from androstenedione. On this is superimposed the second component, namely, a fluctuating secretion of oestradiol from the developing graafian follicles and the corpus luteum. There is also a constant production of androgens with a small proportion contributed by cyclic activity. (Utian, 1980, p. 30)

The broken follicle turns into a dot of yellow matter, called the corpus luteum, which in turn secretes progesterone, the gestation hormone. Progesterone also acts on the lining of the womb, which thickens, accumulates blood vessels and forms glands filled with secretion, to provide the correct cultural conditions for an implanted fertilised ovum, should one drop in. The combination of progesterone and oestrogen is also the chemical signal that tells the brain to throttle back on the production of both FSH and LH.

If no fertilisation occurs, the secretion of oestrogen and progesterone ceases, the womb lining is starved and begins to drop away, to be shed and flushed out with blood. In the absence of oestrogen and progesterone, the hypothalamus starts up again sending out neurotransmitters to turn on FSH and LH, and off we go again. What happens at menopause is that these interlocking processes begin to misfire and slow down. The process is not uniform; the old mechanism often runs on irregularly under its own momentum, so that the default system can't stay switched on long enough to take over. Though our understanding of the role of neurotransmitters is improving, we still don't know what is happening to the relationship between the hypothalamus, the pituitary and the ovary when menstrual patterns begin to be disrupted in the run-up to menopause. Signals appear to be firing out of sequence, but why is more than we can at present explain.

There have been few studies designed to assess the amounts of circulating gonadotrophins and oestrogens in the bloodstream of untreated pre-menopausal women; examination of urine produced conflicting data (e.g., Pincus et al., 1954; cf. Furuhjelm, 1966). The paucity of hard information and the recurrent disagreements about the significance of what data we have can be explained by difficulties inherent in the subject itself. Nowadays hormonal activity can be measured in various ways, by radioisotopic tracer studies, by taking blood from peripheral veins or from the gland itself, or by taking urine samples over twenty-four hours, by bioassay of tissue receptors, or by a combination of methods but, as the synthesis and secretion of hormones vary according to all kinds of stimuli and respond to all kinds of factors, the results of these measurements are difficult to quantify. When hormones are bound to their carriers they behave in a completely different way from the free hormone.

It is this combination of variables that means that there is no blood test that can establish whether or not a woman is 'menopausal'. Even if oestradiol and LH and FSH are all measured, the tests would have to take place on different days, and even then they would not indicate which hormones were available at any particular time, or why. Gonadotrophin levels vary greatly from day to day and even during a single day in the peri-menopause. Over-the-counter urine tests to measure FSH are both expensive and misleading. Saliva tests too are unreliable.

The various techniques of radioimmunoassay that have been developed by pharmaceutical multinationals exist to assess the efficiency of various delivery systems of replacement hormones, as a necessary element in drug-testing. There is simply no one to pay the enormous cost of long-term investigation of the hormonal status of a group of healthy middle-aged women. Justification for mass studies involving expensive and time-consuming techniques of sampling can hardly be found, for they cannot be shown to save lives or directly to influence the incidence of life-threatening disease. It was against this background that the Million Women Study was set up, with the unlooked-for result that too many women lost all faith in HRT.

The belief that it is oestrogen deficiency that causes climacteric distress has never been substantiated by empirical proof, despite the best efforts of an army of clinicians and biochemists supported by the vast resources of the pharmaceutical multinationals. The usual account makes it seem as if only ovulation and menstruation can keep women feeling well. This is not what the young woman herself perceived, when after fourteen years or so of feeling as well as well can be, menstruation suddenly made her feel sick. It is a poor lookout indeed if mid-cycle pain, pre- and post-menstrual tension, cramps, bloating, backache, headache, and all the palaver of the cycle are the purest well-being compared to the physical condition of the female after menopause. The obstacle to understanding here is the defect that disfigures all gynaecological investigation; we do not know enough about the well woman to understand what has gone wrong with the sick one. Gynaecologists are like motor mechanics who have never worked on a car that actually went.

In order to understand the role played by oestrogen in keeping women healthy, energetic and optimistic, we need to know a great deal more about the systems of secretion of oestrogen, and the variability in the levels of circulating oestrogen in women of all ages. If oestrogen secretion knocks out another hormone which makes little girls feel well, perhaps we ought to be investigating replacing the little-girl hormone rather than oestrogen in older women. If this is impossible or inappropriate, then perhaps we should be considering stimulating oestrogen production from androstenedione instead of simply 'replacing' natural oestrogens with synthetic steroids in women suffering menopausal distress or post-menopausal deficiency. Unfortunately we don't know enough about the whole woman, whose anatomy is generally studied as if it were simply a man's body with a reproductive system installed in it, to have any clear idea of how the endocrine balance of well women differs from that of ill women, or, indeed, what degree of variability there is in endocrine function in both well women and sick women.

One substance produced by the pituitary gland whose role is not understood is prolactin. In pregnant women it primes the body for lactation, rising to levels which may be ten or twenty times what they were before conception. What prolactin is doing in the non-pregnant female is not known. Some women will produce excess prolactin; because nobody knows why this might be, the condition is called idiopathic hyperprolactinaemia, which gets us precisely nowhere. This would be less concerning if it were not the case that as much as 20 per cent of the population is thought to suffer at some time from hyperprolactinaemia. We know that heightened levels of stress can produce raised prolactin levels; in other species prolactin plays a role in such demanding activities as migration and nest-building. Some infertility in older, high-achieving women is thought to be caused by elevated prolactin levels. We know that secretion of prolactin parallels secretion of oestrogen, is stepped up at puberty and declines at menopause; we now know that neurokinin is closely involved in prolactin secretion but not what that might mean. Administration of oestrogen seems to trigger increased secretion of prolactin, which may not prove ultimately to be a nett health benefit.

After menopause the ovary changes in structure; the cells that excrete oestrogens and progesterone are gradually lost, and the cells in between, the stromal cells, become more abundant and active. It is now known that steroidally active stromal cells will produce androgens and, in extreme cases, produce a condition called hyperthecosis, with visible virilisation and hirsutism. Most of the work being done on stromal cells and androgens relates to the genesis of prostate cancer. Little is known of the sequelae of stromal cell steroidogenesis in women. An important study by Procope in 1968 identified two distinct groups of post-menopausal women; in one group the ovaries were completely atrophic and their removal made no difference to the women's levels of circulating oestrogens and androgens; in the other the ovaries were not completely inert, but showed 'ovarian cortical stromal hyperplasia' and were producing sex steroids. No subsequent studies were able to develop the revolutionary notion that 'women are not all the same' or to relate the difference in the ovaries to an overall difference in health status. Some such difference between post-menopausal individuals has been observed and recorded but no systematic examination of the phenomenon has ever been undertaken.

The theca cell which is crucial to the maturation of follicles has been described as the forgotten cell. Researchers simply argue about the processes, rather in the way that medieval natural philosophers sought to prove or disprove the existence of other worlds by debate rather than developing a telescope. As researchers from the Pomeranian Medical University in Szczecin observed in 2008, 'In everyday practice gynecologists are asked by their patients about the role of ovaries after menopause. Whether it is an irrelevant hormonally inactive tissue that can be excised during an operation or something more affecting women's health. If post-menopausal ovary produces a significant amount of steroid hormones that can affect women's health. We find it difficult to answer these questions mostly due to the scarce literature concerning structure and function of the post-menopausal ovary' (Laszczynska et al., 2008).

There is no way then that we can duplicate the intricate patterns of secretion in the pre-menopausal female in the post-menopausal female. Giving oestradiol by mouth, or transdermally, will apparently get women to feel well, but we cannot claim to be replacing the missing hormone cocktail. We don't actually understand why menopausal women should feel better when given oestradiol, but we have begun to suspect that we are replacing oestradiol in quantities far greater than those produced by natural secretion. If we give oestrogens by mouth most of the active substance will be degraded and excreted; we do not know by what biological pathway the active agent when taken by mouth reaches the target organs. It is at least possible, if not likely, that treatment with replacement oestrogen to ablate the fluctuations in menopausal levels may effect the switchover to a new pattern of secretion relying upon the stromal cells and the adrenals. The battering of this delicate mechanism with large amounts of exogenous steroids could have the opposite effect, and thwart its establishment. If so, the long-term outcome of dosing women with steroids during the climacterium would be to compromise their health and accelerate their ageing. This possibility is never discussed. By contrast, any suggestion that men displaying signs of testosterone deficiency should be routinely dosed with 'replacement' testosterone used to be swiftly rejected on precisely those grounds.

It is misleading to talk of the reproductive years as if they consisted of four hundred and fifty or so uniform cycles. The Menstrual and Reproductive History Research Program of the University of Minnesota, which began observing and testing a cohort of women in 1934, showed that during the ten years following the first menstruation cycles were often variable, and the variability decreased with age. Over the next two decades a steady decrease in cycle length was observed; women of twenty-five tended to have a thirty-day cycle, women of thirty-five a twenty-eight-day cycle. During the years immediately preceding menopause, marked variability was noticed again (Treloar et al., 1967). This transitional phase varied greatly in length and showed both unusually short and unusually long cycles.

It took twelve years for some of the same researchers to set up a preliminary study to determine whether they could establish a pattern in the variations of menstrual cycle preceding menopause; the job was made harder because although women could correctly recall the year of their menopause, they could not recall the details of the menstrual uproar that preceded it. A hypothesis appeared that late menopause was associated with greater variability of cycle patterns and therefore, as late menopause was also associated with a greater risk of breast cancer, greater variability in cycle patterns was thought possibly to be the crucial factor (Wallace et al., 1978). What was found was that women 'with a later age at menopause had a transitional phase characterized by longer intermenstrual intervals and greater cycle variability. Women who ceased menstruating before they were forty-four had an average cycle length of fifty-seven days in the two years before the last period; women who did not cease menstruating till they were fifty-five or older had a mean cycle length of eighty days' (Bean et al., 1979). The standard deviations in these figures were all fairly high, from forty-six and a half to sixty-four.

By taking the basal body temperatures during these cycles it could be seen that it was the follicular phase, that is, the period after menstruation and before ovulation, when FSH is circulating at a high level, that was prolonged. By the same evidence, in women whose cycles had reached their shortest duration, just before the transitional phase had set in, it could be seen that it was the follicular phase that was more quickly completed. The luteal phase remained constant throughout the reproductive years. However, during both the first and the last years of menstruation, cycles with no temperature blip signalling ovulation could be observed. Women aged between forty and forty-five by gynaecological computation (when age at first menstruation had been standardised) exhibited 34 per cent of anovulatory cycles (Sherman et al., 1979).

Several studies revealed, in the early phase of the cycle, in women aged forty-six to fifty-six, levels of FSH up to 25 per cent higher than in women aged between forty and forty-five. It seemed as if, as the follicles were proving less and less sensitive to FSH, the hypothalamus was stepping up the instruction to the pituitary, which was flooding the system with FSH which eventually succeeded in stimulating a follicle to push the process on to the next stage, until after the last menstruation, when finally no follicle would respond. This by its nature was something that could not be known until it had happened. The process by which increased levels of FSH are secreted begins much earlier than anyone had suspected and is well established by the time a woman reaches her early forties; it is followed by an increase in secretion of LH in the late forties. All kinds of explanation for these changes in hormone profiles have been suggested. The favourite is that the woman suffers some depletion of her oestradiol secretion, but no such depletion has been demonstrated. The next possibility was that there might be in women something like the substance called 'inhibin' in males, a follicle-stimulating release-inhibiting substance or FRIS (Van Look et al., 1977; Chari et al., 1979), which was secreted in diminishing amounts as women grew older. Perhaps the unknown circulating body chemical acts directly on the follicle. Others wondered whether it might be age-related changes in the hypothalamus and/or pituitary that produced the changes in the pattern of secretion. All observers knew that the older a woman who entered an in vitro fertilisation programme, the more FSH would be needed to get her to produce enough eggs for fertilisation.

Why follicles should become less responsive is not known. The degree and causes of variation in menstrual pattern were summed up at the Eighth Biomedical Congress of the International Planned Parenthood Federation, held in London in 1978, by Harry M. Sherman and Robert B. Wallace of the University of Iowa College of Medicine and Alan E. Treloar of the University of North Carolina in this fashion:

> The irregular episodes of vaginal bleeding in perimenopausal
> women can be interpreted as the irregular maturation of residual
> ovarian follicles. The potential for hormone secretion by the
> remaining follicles was diminished and variable. Menses were
> sometimes preceded by maturation of a follicle with limited
> secretion of both oestradiol and progesterone, but vaginal bleeding
> also occurred after a rise and fall in oestradiol without measurable
> increases in progesterone, compatible with an anovulatory cycle.
> (Sherman et al., 1979, p. 26)

So as women approach menopause they may experience normal cycles, longer cycles, and episodes of anovulatory bleeding. Moreover, 'because episodes of abortive follicular maturation and vaginal bleeding are often widely spaced, perimenopausal women may be exposed to persistent oestrogen stimulation that may be related to the dysfunctional uterine bleeding common at this time' (p. 28). In other words, the derangements of menopause are as likely to be caused by too much oestrogen as by too little.

The topic of the conference was 'Fertility in Middle Age'; the concern was to determine what contraception was appropriate for women in the peri-menopause. In discussing this, the researchers revealed that they could not actually know when menopause had occurred, although they had no scruple in asking women themselves to name a day. Most of the studies of age at menopause rely upon the recollection of the women in their sample, and seem to encounter no vagueness in their answers. Dr Helen Ware of the Department of Demography at the Australian National University, in response to a statistical paper on 'Factors affecting the age at menopause' in a sample of Dutch women, exclaimed,

> I am amazed that there were not many who replied to Dr Van Keep's postal questionnaire that they either did not know the date of menopause, or were not sure. In our experience of face-to-face interviewing in Australia only 24% of women knew both the year and the month of menopause, and even after probing only 26% could estimate either the month or the year although the oldest women in the sample were only 59. (Parkes et al., p. 52)

It is likely that women who have no periods for six months or more are certain that they have passed menopause. If a bleed happens after this time, they have to revise this impression, but the position is still the same; the woman simply verifies her prior conclusion. Given the anatomical confusion and the genuine vagueness of the phenomenon, what the woman probably recalls is her recognition of her menopause and her acceptance of it. In the absence of any other definition, she has to define it herself. Dr Ware was told that Australian women were probably less aware of the menopause than Dutch women, a suggestion to which she made no reply. The Dutch women probably filled in their postal questionnaire with assistance from family members, who may have more cause to identify a day and an hour for menopause than the women themselves.

The family planners at the IPPF conference had no joy from any of the papers attempting to establish firm statistical parameters for menopause and to declare a *terminus ad quem* after which ovulation could never occur.

> The hormonal studies confirm that the potential for ovulation during the perimenopausal period, while much reduced, is present. To prevent conception contraceptive practices, if desired, should be maintained until the onset of permanent menopausal amenorrhea. No basis was known, other than clinical experience, for judging whether a given interval without menses was likely to represent permanent amenorrhea. (Sherman et al., p. 30)

All that the statisticians could calculate was a set of unsurprising probabilities: the older you are the more likely it is that after six months without a period you will not have another – 52 per cent if you were aged forty-five to forty-nine and 70 per cent if you were over fifty-three. Ten per cent of the women in this sample, more than a year after the last bleed, had had another bleed which was not associated with illness or with taking hormones of any kind (Sherman et al., p. 30). This was a surprise. The received medical wisdom is that 'post-menopausal bleeding (i.e. bleeding occurring a year or more after your periods have stopped) is never normal. Thorough investigation of this important symptom involves a D and C (dilettation and curettage, or womb scrape), and you should never be persuaded to agree to less than this'. This medical opinion comes from health writer Caroline Shreeve (p. 4), who is both a GP and an alternative practitioner of herbalism and hypnotherapy. Conventional gynaecologist Mary Anderson agreed that 'post-menopausal bleeding', that is, bleeding a year or more after the cessation of menstruation, 'must be investigated by a specialist', explaining that 'one of the commoner causes [of such bleeding] is an early cancer of the endometrium of the uterus and if it is found it can be treated very successfully' (p. 32).

'Commoner' does not mean 'common'. The incidence of endometrial cancer is about 24 per 100,000 according to the US National Cancer Institute. In the UK in 2014 there were 9,324 new cases; the highest incidence was recorded in women aged between seventy and seventy-four. The analysts of the data from the Menstrual and Reproductive History Research Program of the University of Minnesota told the IPPF conference in 1979 that they did not find a single case of the 'commoner cause' in their sample of post-menopausal bleeders, although it might be hoping too much to assume that they bothered to look. What they said was:

> Moreover, even after one year (360 days) of amenorrhea, over 10 per cent of subjects recorded an episode of vaginal bleeding, apparently not associated with significant illness or exogenous hormone consumption. (Sherman et al., p. 32)

The word 'apparently' could be taken to indicate that D and Cs were not routinely performed in these cases. The researchers decided therefore that they could not be certain that follicular activity had actually ceased, and menopause could not reliably be said to have occurred, and so they came to the rather dispiriting conclusion that it would be prudent 'to maintain contraception, if desired, for a minimum of twelve months of amenorrhea'.

The possibilities are therefore two: if you bleed more than a year after your last bleed, you may have gone through menopause a year ago, or, conversely, you may not. Either following Dr Shreeve's instructions would involve you in an unnecessary D and C or it wouldn't. Raewyn Mackenzie, whose little book based on the questions sent to her New Zealand radio programmes met with international success in the Eighties, assures her readers, 'Most doctors now advise women over 50 to continue with contraception for a year after their last period and women under 50 to use contraception for two years after their last period' (p. 46). Provided of course they know which period is their last.

The greatest irony is that if you are on a contraceptive pill and in the peri-menopause, you can go on having regular breakthrough bleeds long after you have ceased ovulating. Then nobody knows if or when you have passed the menopause. Mackenzie advises her readers: 'It is difficult to know when a woman on combined oral contraceptives has reached menopause, and this necessitates her using another method while waiting to see if she is still menstruating' (p. 48). This process could of course go on for ten years or more. Mackenzie had already recommended that menopausal women continue using whatever contraception they have always used, provided it 'has always been acceptable and problem-free'. I know of no one who has used only one kind of contraception in her life and no one who has found any kind of contraception both acceptable and problem-free. No woman over forty-five should be using oral contraceptives in any case, because of the elevated risk of stroke, thrombosis and heart attack. An IUD would seem to be a better option for a middle-aged woman, unless she is not in a stable relationship, in which case she should reconcile herself to the use of condoms, 'acceptable' or not.

Despite the contradictoriness of her own argument, Mackenzie's book includes a cartoon of a smiling woman throwing caps, pills, pessaries and condoms out of a window, to illustrate her contention that 'Being free of the worry of contraception and conception is one of the pluses of the menopause' (p. 51). Curiouser and curiouser, for she has just spent a whole chapter telling us how the menopausal woman should continue to use contraception.

Somehow these practical problems of menopause management cannot be seen to go away. At a workshop on oral contraception for women over thirty-five organised by the International Health Foundation in Lausanne in March 1988, R. K. E. Kirkman of the Manchester Family Planning Centre asked: 'What about the IUD in the pre-menopause? Should we leave it in place until one year after the menopause?' He was answered by J. R. Newton of the Obstetrics and Gynaecology Department of Birmingham Maternity Hospital:

> In my view there seems to be no reason for leaving an IUD in
> place beyond the age at which the failure rate of the IUD is greater
> than the risk of unprotected intercourse. I prefer to remove the
> IUD before it becomes embedded after the menopause and would
> certainly not let an IUD remain there longer than six months after
> the last menstruation.

Wulf Utian interpolated:

> The presence of an IUD at this age often complicates the
> interpretation of clinical signs and this may be reason to remove
> the IUD.

Dr Newton answered:

> I could not agree more. I do believe in the value of the IUD as a
> contraceptive method after the age of 35. But even though the users

may be enthusiastic to retain the IUD we should know when to remove the device.

How they might go about deciding which menstruation is the last, given the frequent return of bleeding after more than six months, the learned gentlemen do not say. How long it takes the device to become embedded they do not say either (*Maturitas*, Suppl. 1, p. 97). In case it should be thought that thinking on this point has become clearer since 1988, in 2016 NHS Education for Scotland could manage no better than this:

Evidence suggests that the presence of these [intrauterine] devices may be a hindrance to investigations if the patient presents later; for example some conditions such as postmenopausal bleeding, which may necessitate an endometrial biopsy or ultrasound, may be difficult to diagnose. It is therefore recommended that if the IUD is no longer needed for contraception, it should be removed. However, the Clinical Effectiveness Unit (CEU) could find no published literature that retention of an intrauterine device would be harmful. An IUD should be removed after the menopause, but if it cannot be removed easily in an outpatient setting then consideration should be given to the benefits of surgery versus retention of the IUD.

This unhelpful offering was prefixed by a confession that 'this question was answered over 2 years ago. The answer may not be up-to-date and may differ from current research and practice.' An American website (fhi360) was unashamed to report:

Common practice is to remove an IUD in menopausal women after one year without menses. In cases where an IUD is not removed after menopause, ill effects have not been reported. However, no studies have been conducted on this to date.

It is small consolation to a woman who is flooding one week, and sees no periods for six months, and then has what seems a normal period, and then again nothing or a flood, that the medical establishment is nearly as muddled as her system appears to be. To the one question to which she really desires an answer, 'When will it be over?' there are only other questions: 'When did it begin? Has it begun? How long can it last? How short could it be?' Generally speaking the climacteric, or the peri-menopause, is taken to be ten years, from age forty-five to age fifty-five. Hormonal uproar will begin some time after forty-five, but it will not necessarily end before fifty-five. All the more reason then to cease talking about 'the menopause' as if it were a single event, and to resume referring to the period of change as 'the climacteric'.

In 2016 we are not surprised to find that in conclusion to his paper on 'The Menopausal Transition' delivered at the 1978 IPPF conference, Barry M. Sherman had to admit that 'knowledge remains very incomplete', even though 'the importance of events that occur during the perimenopausal and early menopausal years cannot be overestimated. In addition to the immediate problems of contraception during the perimenopausal years, and treatment of menopausal symptoms, the age-related problems of osteoporosis, hypertension, atherosclerosis, and carcinoma of the breast and endometrium are intimately related to the changes in the hormonal environment consequent to menopause' (Sherman et al., p. 32).

Sherman was then bombarded with questions. A professor of endocrinology from Bombay wanted to know whether there was any correlation between oestradiol levels and menopausal symptoms. Sherman answered:

> There are not many studies on the correlation between hormone levels and symptoms. Our studies show that individual women may have high menopausal levels of gonadotrophins and irregular cycles preceding any symptoms by many months. During continuous blood sampling over 24-hr periods we detected no change between changes in oestrogens or gonadotrophins and the individual episodes of hot flushes. The mediation of these symptoms is unknown. (Parkes et al., 1979, p. 94)

Sherman could have cited Hunter et al., 1973; Stone et al., 1975; Aksel et al., 1976; Studd et al., 1977; Chakravarti et al., 1977; Dennerstein, 1987; and Hutton et al. 1978, all of which did test plasma levels of ovarian hormones and failed to find a correlation, but for some reason he prefers to give the impression that the matter has not been investigated. He should have cited the example of Mulley and Mitchell writing in the *Lancet* in 1976:

> ... no correlation has so far been established between hormonal changes and menopausal flushing ... we contend there is no

clear-cut relation between hot flushes and oestrogen deficiency.
(p. 1397)

Even Utian has had to register the complexity of the case:

The mechanism of flushing has not been elucidated. The long
popular theory that flushes are due to increased gonadotrophins
is no longer acceptable. Nor does flushing appear to be related
to particular concentrations of plasma oestrone, oestradiol, or
adrenostenedione levels. This does not exclude the likelihood of
a declining level of oestrogen being responsible for the flushing
response; that is a changing state, rather than an absolute state.
(Utian, 1980, p. 110)

(At this point, we must stifle a shout of 'Bravo!' for it seems as if Utian
is about to emerge from blind adherence to the deficiency theory;
however, this flash of insight does not prompt him to desist throughout
his 1980 monograph from referring to symptoms as caused by oestrogen
deficiency.) Utian continues:

Sturdee and co-workers [1978] have reported the onset of the
hot flush to be associated with a sudden and transient increase
in sympathetic drive. This finding has been disputed [Ginsburg
& Swinhoe, 1978]. Hutton et al. [1978] have suggested that
catecholoestrogens may be involved, but this too is unproven.
Flushing is associated with endogenous adrenergic discharge and
exogenous catecholamines [Metz et al., 1978]. Further research
along this line will hopefully solve this puzzle in the near future and
perhaps result in suitable alternatives to oestrogen for treatment.

The Indian professor asked again:

What about sexual responsiveness and its relation to oestradiol levels?

Again Sherman could only reply:

I do not know of any data about the relationship between the
hormone levels in individual women and their sexual activity.

The head of research at the National Institute of Demographic Studies in Paris asked how 'one can recognise a cycle in which there is fertilisation but no implantation and in which the blastocyst dies after a few days'. His question was prompted by the consideration that among the erratic cycles of the middle-aged sexually active woman would be some which looked as if they were anovulatory and were not. He may have been wondering about the causes of very sudden and heavy bleeding in the peri-menopause. Sherman could only reply:

I do not know of any method.

A woman teacher of physical anthropology from Montclair State College in New Jersey brought up a 1975 study that showed 'that postmenopausal women still have a few remaining primary and secondary follicles although they are not in good condition. Is there any information on how long a woman can maintain primary follicles?' Again Sherman replied:

The studies are few and I cannot say how long primary follicles can remain.

John Studd, who set up one of the first menopause clinics in England, tells us in *Management of the Menopause* (2003) that 'the ovary contains the maximum number of oocytes (egg-cells) during the fifth month of foetal life. Thereafter the numbers decline and only one million are present at birth and as few as twenty-five thousand remain at menopause ...' To most of us 25,000 egg cells would seem more than enough. These numbers are not such that they explain anything. We are left wondering why fertility begins to decline before birth, and what the excess oocytes are for and what is different about the ones that stay behind, and whether anything could be done to slow the ageing of the ovary by, for example, lengthening menstrual cycles. Studd did not indicate any distinction between primary and secondary follicles, so his statement cannot answer the anthropologist's question.

Sherman had then to contend with the Professor Emeritus of Population Studies at Harvard Medical School, who wanted to know if there was any way a doctor could determine whether or not a female patient was past the menopause.

It used to be thought that a few days' treatment with human menopausal gonadotrophin would indicate whether or not a woman was past the menopause, depending on whether or not such treatment induced a rise in the level of oestrogen.

Sherman could not justify this procedure.

I have not used such treatment. Some of these women already have high levels of endogenous gonadotrophin. They can be followed for many months and suddenly they will have an oestradiol surge followed by menses, but we do not understand why it happens at a particular time ...

The problem seemed to be the basic one, as phrased by the Professor Emeritus of Obstetrics and Gynaecology from the University of Aberdeen:

What normally selects the population of primordial follicles to be recruited is not known.

We are not surprised to find that forty years ago medical researchers did not know why the menopause happened or when it happened, let alone why it caused a variety of symptoms from trivial to unbearable, or whether it caused these symptoms in a few, some, many or most women, but we are surprised to find that this ignorance can hardly be said to have dissipated. As demographers the learned men and women gathered under the auspices of the Galton Foundation and the Ciba Foundation in 1979 had to determine how to devise family planning strategies for the middle-aged, so they were understandably anxious to arrive at a basis for a statistical model, but no parameters were forthcoming. It is still true to say that if the statistics work one way they cannot be made to work the other.

Business and professional women tend to have an earlier menopause, according to some rather old studies, but in those days working women tended to be single and married women not, so other researchers considered that 'a physiological amount of sexual intercourse' fended off menopause (Kisch, p. 599). Others thought that marriage selected women less likely to suffer early menopause or 'dry up' like old maids. A woman's age at the birth of her last child and the number of children she has are both associated with a later menopause; the use of oral contraceptives at any stage in the reproductive career delays menopause according to some studies and not according to others. Late onset of menses is associated with early cessation, but the data is not reliable. Smoking accelerates all the ageing processes including the ageing of ovarian follicles, and smokers tend to have an earlier menopause; obese women have a later menopause.

The middle-aged woman who opts for sterilisation as terminal contraception, because she has already achieved her completed family size, presumably carries out her own cost–benefit analysis and should be encouraged to do so. In the 1990s female sterilisation by tubal occlusion was the most popular form of family limitation, but by 2000 the rate in the developed world had decreased by almost a third and the incidence of vasectomy surpassed it. Even so, far too many women are being sterilised when their fertility is already decreasing, and far too many women will undergo hysterectomy after sterilisation, some within months of the operation. If we were to tot up the number of times a woman in the developed world, especially an American woman, undergoes some form of invasive pelvic surgery – caesarean, laparoscopy, laparotomy, curettage, abortion, tubal cautery, cutting or ligation, oophorectomy, salpingectomy, surgery of the cervix, amniocentesis, hysterectomy, hysterotomy – we would notice a regular pattern of abdomen piercing and cutting that should be listed among the techniques of psychotic self-mutilation, with the chilling distinction that these are forms of self-mutilation in which doctors have been only too happy to cooperate. A woman who for no good reason wishes to extirpate her uterus will be given every assistance. Female castration has always been a popular procedure, carried out in a multiplicity of ways, some of which were widely practised even when they carried with them a high risk of subsequent illness and death. When we have understood the psychopathology behind both the practitioner's enthusiasm for destroying the female organs of generation and the patient's conviction that they are what is making her sick, we shall have taken one step on the road to restoring the female eunuch to her full vigour and potential.

No human organ has been so often operated on as the uterus and yet doctors do not agree if and when to perform hysterectomy. 'When in doubt cut it out' appears to be the policy generally followed, but even then surgeons and gynaecologists cannot agree whether to leave the ovaries or take them out. The removers say that retained ovaries can turn cancerous, that retained ovaries hardly work or do not work at all, and hysterectomised women too often present for further pelvic surgery. The preservers maintain that patients feel better after the operation if they still have their ovaries, that they will not suffer hot flushes and other symptoms associated with menopause, such as osteoporosis, and that continued oestrogen secretion protects against coronary heart disease. The removers say that exogenous sex steroids offer better protection against these undesirable outcomes. The patients themselves often proselytise for the particular form of devastation that they have undergone, convinced that after it they feel better than ever they did before.

One in four women will develop uterine myomas or fibromas, 'fibroids' as they are popularly known. Nobody knows why they form or how to treat them. Enormous ones can be asymptomatic, tiny ones symptomatic. They, or something else, may cause heavy bleeding in peri-menopausal women, especially if we include women in their early forties under this definition. At menopause myomas usually subside; in some women they continue to give trouble. Nobody knows why they should. Nobody has any idea whether there might not be a systemic medication that would shrink fibromas. There is after all no need to look for one, because a hysterectomy will finish them once for all, and take with it any prospect of cancer of the cervix or endometrial carcinoma. The fact that hysterectomy is a major operation, with an inbuilt risk of fever, infection and other complications, is neither here nor there. Fibromas should not be a justification for destructive surgery, but they are a counter-indication for HRT. Fibromas are oestrogen-dependent, and post-menopausal hormone-replacement therapy could interfere with their involution, but most menopause manuals make no mention of them at all. Wendy Cooper's book-long advertisement for HRT, *No Change*, mentions no counter-indications for HRT, as if none of her readers was likely to have suffered from either endometriosis or fibromas. This kind of omission encourages the woman who has fibroids to think that she has something grave and rare and to accept major surgery for a minor problem.

It would be quite wrong to imply that there have been no concerted attempts to establish the epidemiology of menopausal distress. As long ago as 1934, under the leadership of Allan E. Treloar, the University of Minnesota set up the Menstrual and Reproductive History (MRH) Study; it ran for seventy-five years. Data collection ended in 2009.

Initially, 2,350 University of Minnesota women volunteered to participate in the study; a second group of 1,600 women was enrolled between 1961 and 1963, and in 1965 a panel of 1,000 native Alaskan women was invited to participate. Women in the study range from their teens to mid-nineties and represent fifty states and twenty-five foreign countries. After Treloar's retirement, the programme was acquired in 1984 by the University of Utah's College of Nursing under the direction of Dr Ann Voda and renamed the Tremin Trust Program. Upon Dr Voda's retirement, the programme moved to Pennsylvania State University under the direction of Dr Phyllis Kernoff Mansfield; access to the raw data is now limited to accredited Penn State PRI researchers. In 1986 a prospective cohort epidemiological study called the Iowa Women's Health Study enrolled 41,836 women aged between fifty-five and sixty-nine years. Iowa was chosen because the population was relatively stable and so lifetime histories could be taken without undue wastage; the study is still used by researchers, but its usefulness is a great deal less than had been hoped. What years of study have failed to elucidate about the menopause, a condition which every GP now considers her/himself qualified to treat, is really quite extraordinary.

We don't know what is happening.

We don't know why it happens.

We can't tell in a particular case if it's about to happen, happening, or over.

We don't know why some women form some symptoms, others different symptoms in different combinations, and some no symptoms at all.

We don't know which symptoms are related to menopause, and which to ageing, and which to neither.

We don't know what a hot flush is, beyond the fact that it is the one symptom that everyone associates with menopause.

We don't know why some women sweat profusely during flushing, some after flushing, some not at all, or why some have feelings of panic and others do not.

Nobody knows why some women suffer intense joint pain at menopause.

Nobody knows why women have disturbed sleeping patterns during the climacteric; sometimes these are described simply as a consequence of vasomotor disturbance, but there are many cases where women who are unable to sleep are not suffering from hot flushes or dripping with sweat. They are simply awake. This symptom is sometimes described as 'psychological'.

We don't know which menopausal symptoms are primarily physical, which psychosomatic and which psychological.

We have no idea which symptoms might indicate distortion of a natural function.

We don't know in what measure ageing complicates menopause or indeed if ageing complicates menopause. Some studies show that early menopause, including surgical or radiation menopause, is the hardest to deal with, others don't.

The practitioners who deny that there is too much that they don't know are the most dangerous. Taking responsibility for your own health is the first step towards 'coping with menopause'.

8

The Treatments – Allopathic

Historically, doctors asked to prescribe palliatives for climacteric distress have done their best. They have let blood, prescribed violent purgatives, sent women to spas and mountain resorts, and dosed them with bromide, mercury, sulphuric acid, belladonna and acetate of lead. Suspecting that the problems women encountered were directly caused by the cessation of ovarian function, they turned to glandular extracts, plant hormones, and bits and pieces of the reproductive equipment of other species – dried corpus luteum from pigs, grilled ovaries from cows and sheep – but nothing worked.

When natural oestrogens were first isolated in 1923, their potential usefulness in treating menopausal distress was recognised but no feasible mode of administration was established. Robert A. Wilson dosed his patients with a 'crude extract made from dried sheep's ovaries' but the allergic reactions outweighed any improvement. In the 1930s stilboestrol was prescribed for menopausal distress, but the side-effects, nausea, headaches and skin reactions, were worse than the condition. In the late 1930s German chemists managed to synthesise oestradiol benzoate, which was effective in cases of climacteric distress but had to be given by injection. It was not until the 1960s, after the contraceptive problem had been solved to the satisfaction of the birth controllers if not that of the users, that the steroid manufacturers turned their research departments on to the problems of the peri-menopause.

The popularisation of oestrogen replacement in the 1960s was so successful that between 1963 and 1973 sales of oestrogen preparations quadrupled; half the post-menopausal female population was using HRT or, as the Americans call it, ERT, 'estrogen replacement therapy'. Then came the bombshell: incidence of endometrial cancer was up 10 per cent. The increase in incidence was much less than the increase in use of the hormones, and endometrial cancer was still rare, but the news media made nothing of that. The actual presence of cancer was not always confirmed. What rose by 10 per cent in ten years was the number of diagnoses of endometrial cancer. Though between the two national surveys, the one in 1948–9 and the other in 1969–71, the incidence of endometrial cancer had doubled, the death rate had halved. Given the extraordinary alacrity with which American doctors used to perform hysterectomies, nobody can know what the 10 per cent rise in diagnoses of endometrial cancer in twenty years actually represents, especially when the widely varying dosage patterns followed during the early years of HRT are taken into account. All genital cancers have become more common over the last fifty years; the causes may well be found to lie in environmental changes and lifestyle choices as well as in the use of hormones. American doctors could not afford to examine the data and investigate the case further. Out of terror of malpractice litigation they became overnight as reluctant to prescribe HRT as before they had been enthusiastic.

To ask for more rational approaches to women's health is to cry for the moon. The proponents of HRT were trapped by the logical weaknesses in their own position. They had never proved that there was an oestrogen deficiency, nor had they explained the mechanism by which the therapy of choice effected its miracles. They had taken the improper course of defining a disease from the therapy, and though the hysteria about the rise in incidence of endometrial cancer was no more logical than the case for oestrogen replacement, the whole shaky edifice collapsed. Sales of oestrogen preparations in the United States halved; and over the next two years diagnoses of endometrial cancer fell by a quarter. QED. Oestrogen replacement was too dangerous to use. To the women who said that they didn't care about the risk of cancer, their doctors, well aware of the legal implications, said that they could not allow them to run it.

Enter the British. In 1976, Stuart Campbell, then Senior Lecturer at Queen Charlotte's Hospital in London, summarised the HRT experience:

The American experience has been none too reassuring and
an apparent alliance between feminist movements and certain
gynaecological interests has produced the 'feminine forever' cult
which implies that oestrogens should be prescribed from the cradle
to the grave. This specious therapeutic approach to therapy has
unfortunately not been accompanied by adequate epidemiological
and follow-up studies and now from the USA there is evidence of
a major reappraisal of hormone therapy due to the findings of two
poorly documented retrospective studies (*NEJM*, 1975) that there
may be an association between postmenopausal oestrogens and
endometrial cancer. This syndrome of therapeutic overkill followed
by overreaction can only be avoided by a deep understanding
of the psychological, hormonal and other pathophysiological
changes of the perimenopause … we are at the moment a long way
from this …

If Campbell had known more about feminists, he would have been
aware that feminist movements have from the outset been deeply
suspicious of steroids. In 1969 Barbara Seaman published *The Doctors'
Case against the Pill* and led the campaign to force the Nelson hearings
on the safety of the contraceptive pill to take evidence from women;
for the next nine years she studied the effects of exogenous steroid
use on women's health and then published *Women and the Crisis in
Sex Hormones*, a seminal text of the feminist health movement. The
National Women's Health Network lobbied successfully to force the
drug companies to include a list of all side-effects and contra-indications
in every package of steroids and replacement oestrogens that is sold.

The feminist position on oestrogen replacement is vigorously
summarised in an article of 1977 by Rosetta Reitz, 'What doctors won't
tell you about menopause':

They didn't tell me my estrogen supply continues even though
I'm not producing eggs. They imply it stops cold in order to
sell me their estrogen-replacement-therapy. But I'm not buying
that … I know if I don't put any foreign estrogen into my body,
my endocrine glands will regulate my hormonal activity and my
adrenals will step up their estrogen production. The doctors don't
know how this works or which unidentified glands also rally

into this activity, but they admit it is so when they speak among themselves. (Dreifus, pp. 209–10)

Campbell's extraordinary misunderstanding of the feminist position is less forgivable than his diplomatic vagueness about 'gynaecological interests'. The International Conference at which he was speaking in 1976 was sponsored by some of the most important marketers of steroids for the dosing of women, namely Ayerst Laboratories, manufacturers of Premarin, the US market leader, Schering Chemicals Ltd, Syntex Pharmaceuticals and Abbott Laboratories.

Campbell must have known that the 'forever feminine' cult was not the product of an unholy alliance between feminists and gynaecological interests but of Robert A. Wilson MD (FIS, FACS and FACOG), Consultant in Obstetrics and Gynaecology at three New York hospitals, Diplomate of both the American Board of Obstetrics and Gynaecology and the 'International College of Surgeons', fellow of four more learned societies, member of seven more, and President of the Wilson Research Foundation, New York and, it would appear, for many years recipient of funding from Big Pharma, notably Wyeth. Wilson administered oestrogen therapy over forty years to 5,000 patients before he began his public preaching in 1962. In 1963 he and his wife Thelma together worked on articles pleading for 'adequate estrogen from puberty to the grave', offering to 'eliminate the menopause'. By 1965, when he wrote the seminal text *Feminine Forever*, he had authored or co-authored thirteen publications on oestrogen therapy and accumulated the twenty-one titles listed on p. 177 of the English edition of 1966. *Feminine Forever* is intended to impress the common sense out of the laywoman. A ringing preface by another of the American Masters in Menopause, Robert B. Greenblatt, declared:

Woman will be emancipated only when the shackles of hormone deprivation are loosed. Then she will be capable of obtaining fulfilment without interrupting her quest for a continuum of physical and mental health. (Wilson, R. A. p. 15)

Whatever that may mean; most of us would be surprised to discover that we were involved in any such quest. Greenblatt's rhetoric seems to imply that sanity and well-being are for most women as far-off and mysterious as the Holy Grail.

THE TREATMENTS – ALLOPATHIC

While it is most gratifying to find that learned medical gentlemen have at last come round to the idea that women should have rights, it is rather less gratifying to discover that the Masters in Menopause see those rights as within their gift. In 1966 Wilson calculated that the recipients of oestrogen replacement therapy numbered 'between six and twelve thousand'. He is not troubled by his own vagueness in the matter, which seems to indicate some inadequacies in follow-up. Instead he tells us that we can recognise these women just by looking at them.

> The outward signs of this age-defying youthfulness are a straight-backed posture, supple breast contours, taut, smooth skin on face and neck, firm muscles, and that particular vigour and grace typical of a healthy female. At fifty such women still look attractive in tennis shorts or sleeveless dresses. (pp. 17–18)

What woman could ask for more? Wilson was certain that the menopause was 'a serious, painful, and often crippling disease' (p. 29). He had 'known cases where the resulting physical and mental anguish was so unbearable that the patient committed suicide' (p. 39).

> I have seen untreated women who had shrivelled into caricatures of their former selves. Some had lost as much as six inches in height due to pathological bone changes caused by lack of estrogen. Others suffered sweeping metabolic disturbances that literally put them in mortal danger.
> Though the physical symptoms can be truly dreadful, what impresses me most tragically is the destruction of personality. Some women, when they realize that they are no longer women, subside into a stupor of indifference. Even so, they are relatively lucky. The most heart-breaking cases, I feel, are those sensitive women who witness their own decline with agonizing self-awareness. (pp. 39–40)

We can only hope that Dr Wilson's utter faith that the dread disease menopause was the sole cause of every physical and mental symptom in the middle-aged women he saw did not involve him in too many misdiagnoses. In his enthusiasm to eliminate menopause Wilson was soon prescribing replacement sex steroids for women before menopausal symptoms made their appearance, in some cases long before. He invented for himself a stereotype of the 'estrogen-rich' woman who was a perfect companion for man, taut-breasted, sexually responsive, free of menstrual tension. Wilson saw as his enemies 'old wives' who whispered that his wonder-drug caused immorality and cancer; his first publications addressed themselves to the second of these irrational fears. The discovery of increased incidence of endometrial cancer in women on HRT brought the whole bonanza to a halt.

The British were already ahead of the game. In 1978 Stuart Campbell and Malcolm Whitehead published the results of their own study. Of 167 women attending their clinic at King's College Hospital in London they found that three already had endometrial cancer, and no fewer than eleven already exhibited the precancerous condition known as uterine hyperplasia, or overgrowth of the womb lining. When the latter eleven were given progesterone the womb lining returned to normal. Campbell and Whitehead then devised sequential dosing systems for forty-six patients, in which they were given oestrogen opposed by a progestogen in the second half of a monthly cycle; in other words they decided to imitate the secretory rhythm of menstruation and induce breakthrough bleeding. Out of the forty-six there was only one case of hyperplasia instead of the three to nine that would have been expected on an unopposed oestrogen regimen. This improvement was considered to justify the imposition of breakthrough bleeding and the other side-effects of progestogens on all forty-six (Whitehead, Campbell et al., 1978; Whitehead, McQueen et al., 1978; Campbell, McQueen et al., 1978).

In 1980 John Studd reported on a series of 745 patients at Dulwich Hospital and the Birmingham and Midlands Hospital for Women. Almost 10 per cent, seventy-two of the 745, at some time developed uterine hyperplasia. The condition comes in three kinds, cystic hyperplasia, adenomatous hyperplasia and atypical hyperplasia. The last is the most worrying, for about half the women who show this kind of overgrowth of the endometrium will develop uterine cancer. Only four of Studd's cases were of this kind; sixty were of the least worrying kind, cystic hyperplasia, and all of these cases returned to normal after taking progestogens; six of the eight women with adenomatous hyperplasia also returned to normal after taking progestogens, and even two with the atypical type. However, the treatments were not all the same; some of the women who had been given implants, and were more likely to develop uterine hyperplasia than the others, did not take the progestogens prescribed for seven days each month, and more than half of them developed hyperplasia, compared to 15 per cent of the others. When the progestogen regime was lengthened from seven days to ten days that percentage dropped to 3; when it was lengthened again to thirteen days it disappeared altogether (Studd et al., 1980, 1981).

This is the kind of evidence upon which the prescription of progestogens to oppose the action of oestrogens on the womb lining is based. It doesn't do to ask about the more than nine out of ten women in Studd's sample who didn't develop uterine hyperplasia when given unopposed oestrogens; everyone must take the progestogens because of the minority who will exhibit uterine hyperplasia if they don't. Evidently nobody knows how to identify the one out of ten. Nobody knows just how little progesterone you can get away with, whether you need to slough the womb lining every twenty-eight days, or every six months or once a year. This would not be a problem if taking progestogens was fun, but progestogens make many women feel sicker than ever menopause did. It is unlikely that a British woman will be allowed to make her own assessment of the cost–benefits of taking progestogens however, as British doctors will not sanction the use of oestrogen unopposed by progestogens, even though progestogens are thought to undo a good deal of the beneficial effect of oestrogen.

Progesterone is the hormone that acts upon the lining of the womb in the second half of the menstrual cycle, the secretory phase. It blocks the accumulation of oestrogen in the endometrium, and it promotes the formation of an enzyme that changes oestrogen so that it prevents the overstimulation of the endometrium that is thought to lead to an increase in endometrial cancer in women taking replacement oestrogens. It will be noted that uterine hyperplasia was initially dealt with by administration of progesterone to counteract the action of oestrogen on the womb lining. When it came to devising a dosage regimen 'progestogens', that is synthetic steroids resembling progesterone, were used instead. These are equally likely to be called 'progestagens' or 'progestin', all of which argues a lack of attention to detail at the very least. Progesterone itself is inactive if taken by mouth, because it is broken down by the digestive juices; for oral administration the synthetic progestogens norethisterone and norgestrel were developed. If oestrogens can make women feel good, progesterone can make them feel terrible. As Barbara Evans explained, 'it increases the use of energy by the body and affects the amount of salt which the kidneys excrete. It may make the skin greasy and may induce acne. It may also be responsible for breast-tenderness, depression, backache and abdominal cramps as well as "bloating"' (p. 45).

Oestrogen is thought to confer some protection against diseases of the heart and blood vessels; the likelihood is that progesterone and/or progestogens reverse this. A conference on 'Prevention and management of cardio-vascular disease in women' held in July 1987 found that while oestrogens exert a protective effect by increasing triglycerides, decreasing low-density lipids (the risk factors) and increasing high-density lipids, progestogens reverse the protective effect. The association of the contraceptive pill with an increase in the incidence of deep-vein thrombosis and pulmonary embolism is undeniable; it used to be thought that the oestrogens were the culprit, but it seems far more likely that the progestogens are the risk factor that makes a woman on the pill five times more likely to suffer from either than a woman who has never taken it. The Royal College of General Practitioners' Oral Contraceptive Study of 1977 found that the incidence of arterial disease in women who had used oral contraceptives was not related to the variations in the doses of oestrogen to which they had been exposed but to the amounts of progestogens in the pills they had taken. Women wanting to take responsibility for their own health ought to balance the increased risk of heart disease and deep-vein thrombosis against the increased risk of endometrial cancer in women taking unopposed oestrogens, but they will find the statistical evidence inscrutable.

The American experience contrasts sharply with the British experience; attitudes to cyclical progestogen vary from sceptical to downright suspicious, and unopposed oestrogen is much more readily considered as a viable option. The copious instructions to prescribers and patients included with every pack of Premarin by order of the US Food and Drug Administration in the 1990s noted tersely that 'although the evidence must be considered preliminary, one study suggests that cyclic administration may carry less risk than continuous administration … If concomitant progestin therapy is used, potential risks include adverse effects on carbohydrate and lipid metabolism …' John Studd, the very man who gave progestogens over thirteen days of the cycle to prevent uterine hyperplasia, is still saying in the foreword to the revised edition of Barbara Evans's book *Life Change*, published in 1988: 'We must also determine if there is a cancer risk and, if so, what balance of hormones must be used to avoid overstimulation of the lining of the womb.' While they are determining, many women are obliged to give up HRT because they cannot tolerate the progestogens that they may not need.

Who is likely to develop endometrial cancer from oestrogen replacement? No one. The chances of getting the disease at all are one in a thousand or less, so likely is not the right word. If you already have a tumour that produces oestrogen, in another site, for example the ovary, your chances of also having an endometrial cancer are as high as one or even two in five. Women who develop endometrial cancer are more likely than others to develop a breast tumour and also to suffer from high blood pressure. Women who have a late menopause and women who are obese run a higher risk of endometrial cancer than thin women who have a relatively early menopause, but women who have had children are less likely to have an endometrial cancer than women who have had none.

Though everyone is terrified by the least risk of cancer, and doctors devoutly believe that no risk of developing a potentially fatal condition should ever be run, no one seems unduly concerned about the much greater likelihood of post-menopausal women developing heart disease or circulatory disorders, which together cause four times as many deaths as all cancers of the womb, cervix and breast. In the statistical analysis the rise in the number of diagnoses of endometrial cancer was nowhere balanced against the decline in the number of deaths from heart attacks. A group of researchers from South California School of Medicine examined the case histories of all the women in a large retirement community who died of coronary artery disease and found that women who had been treated with oestrogen were less than half as likely to die of heart disease. Heart attacks in American women declined more than 30 per cent between 1976 and 1981 when oestrogen replacement became common practice.

Age-adjusted deaths from I[schaemic] H[eart] D[isease] in white females in the US are over four times the combined death rates of breast cancer and endometrial cancer. If the protective effect of oestrogen replacement therapy on the risk of fatal IHD is real, this benefit would far outweigh the carcinogenic effects of oestrogens. (Ross, R. K., et al., p. 2)

In an article in *Geriatrics* (May 1990), Lila E. Nachtigall, Professor of Obstetrics and Gynaecology of the New York University School of Medicine, and her daughter Dr Lisa B. Nachtigall review the evidence presented by Burch et al. (1974), Gordon et al. (1978), Hammond et al. (1979), Pettiti et al. (1979), Bush et al. (1983, 1987), Barrett-Connor et al. (1989) and Knopp (1988) and come to a conclusion which is heard more and more often, that protection against cardiovascular disease should be the prime reason for prescribing oestrogen replacement, with relief from vasomotor disturbance and mitigation of osteoporosis as mere fringe benefits. In the words of Cummings et al., 'even a small beneficial effect of estrogen therapy on the risk of coronary heart disease would far outweigh any increased risk of deaths from either endometrial cancer or breast cancer' (p. 2448).

Under the heading 'HRT may prevent heart disease' the British Menopause Society website includes the following, with a dateline of 4 May 2016:

> The role of HRT in the prevention of heart disease continues to cause confusion. While the recently published NICE guideline on diagnosis and management of the menopause stated that HRT does not increase the risk of heart disease when started in women aged under sixty, it did not recommend the use of HRT to prevent heart disease since the evidence was not conclusive enough.

The NHS guideline would have been less confusing if the BMS headline had not been so utterly misleading.

The supporters of HRT see distress at change of life as the result of a deficiency, as diabetes is a result of a deficiency in insulin. If, as Barbara Evans says, 'It is unwise to take oestrogen without clear evidence of deficiency, because the risks may not be justified', it must always be unwise to take oestrogen, for the evidence of deficiency is anything but clear. For the evidence to be clear, we would have to have found out something about the levels of oestrogen in women who are not finding the menopausal transition unmanageable. The studies described by Barry M. Sherman and his colleagues showed that 'the menopausal transition, by irregular menses, is not a time of marked oestrogen deficiency ...'

> ... very low oestradiol concentrations characteristic of menopausal women may not occur until six months or so after the onset of amenorrhea. Because episodes of abortive follicular maturation and vaginal bleeding are often widely-spaced, perimenopausal women may be exposed to persistent oestrogen stimulation in the absence of regular cyclic progesterone secretion, a situation that may be related to the dysfunctional uterine bleeding common during this time.

In other words, menopausal women may be suffering from too much oestrogen rather than too little. We are not surprised to find that the first question Sherman could not answer in discussion was:

> Is there any correlation between oestradiol levels and menopausal symptoms? Some of our patients with menopausal symptoms have quite adequate amounts of oestradiol and other oestrogens. (Parkes et al., p. 48)

Sherman was obliged to answer:

> There are not many systematic studies on the correlation between hormone levels and symptoms. Our studies show that individual women may have high menopausal levels of gonadotropins and irregular cycles preceding any symptoms by many months. During continuous blood sampling over 24-hr periods we detected no relationship between changes in oestrogens or gonadotropins and the individual episodes of hot flushes. The mediation of these symptoms is unknown.

So much for 'clear evidence of deficiency'. It seems at least as likely that climacteric distress is caused by too much oestrogen as by too little.

Though a good deal of work has been done since that of Sherman and his colleagues, the mechanism by which administration of oestrogen relieves climacteric distress is still unknown. Older women do not suffer from hot flushes and night sweats, because, it is assumed, their bodies have become used to functioning on the low level of oestrogen derived from the androstenedione secreted by the adrenals supplemented by a much smaller amount secreted by the ovaries, which together amount to no more than a fifth of the pre-menopausal level (Vermeulen, 1983). Women who accept HRT, on the other hand, may have more than five times the amount of oestrogen in the bloodstream that they had before menopause, so it is small wonder that when they come off it their symptoms can recur with a vengeance. What is puzzling is that this does not happen for all of them. If the climacteric syndrome is actually a deficiency disease it ought to last as long as the deficiency. The truth is that it is nothing of the kind.

By the 1990s the array of replacement steroids was impressive – and confusing. If you prefer to take medications by mouth, you had the choice of the oestrogen preparations Premarin, Harmogen, Progynova and the generic ethinyloestradiol. These are by no means all versions of the same thing. The oestrogen in Premarin is derived from the urine of pregnant mares. There are twenty-six ranches in remote areas of South Dakota and Canada where mares are impregnated and kept for the duration of their eleven-month pregnancies attached to rubber collection bags in stalls where they cannot turn around. They may be kept this way for as many as twelve pregnancies. There were three strengths, signified by three colours; the yellow pill is twice the dose of the maroon, and the purple is twice the yellow.

Harmogen, piperazine oestrol sulphate, was discontinued in the UK in 2010. Progynova is oestradiol valerate, suitable for short-term treatment; it is marketed in two strengths. The generic ethinyloestradiol is also sold in two strengths. The array of choice here was not offered to consumers, of course, but to their doctors. They would decide whether the patient should take the pills continuously, whether she should take them for three weeks and then rest, whether she should take them for three weeks and then take a progesterone preparation, to oppose the effect of the oestrogen on the lining of her womb, or whether she should take them for three weeks, take progestogens as well in the third week, and rest in the fourth week.

Eleven different kinds of progestogen preparations were available, using seven different hormones, all of which had different modes of operation and different side-effects. The permutations of oestrogen plus progesterone plus posology amount to hundreds of options, all slightly different. The chances of any doctor, even in a specialist menopause clinic, knowing his way round even half of them are nil. Progestins are sometimes prescribed for women who cannot tolerate oestrogens as a preventative of osteoporosis and hot flushes, although why they should be able to do this if the climacteric syndrome is caused by a deficiency in oestrogen is unclear. One of the most urgent requirements for successful HRT would seem to be the development of better progestogens, and better ways of administering them.

In Britain in the 1990s women had the choice of three kinds of sequential HRT packages: Cycloprogynova, which offers eleven tablets of oestradiol valerate (white) followed by ten tablets of the progestogen norgestrel (orange) followed by seven days of no tablets at all. This was recommended by the manufacturers for long-term use. Prempak-c, on the other hand, offered uninterrupted twenty-eight-day cycles of Premarin, supplemented over the last twelve days by additional tablets of norgestrel. Trisequens came in a circular calendar pack; the patient worked her way round it through twelve blue tablets containing oestradiol and oestrol, ten white tablets of oestradiol, oestrol and the progestogen norethisterone, and six red tablets that contain lower doses of the same. During the red phase the patient is supposed to see breakthrough bleeding.

The climacteric syndrome could also be treated by injections of depot testosterone. Schering withdrew their combined testosterone–oestradiol valerate preparation, Primodian Depot, from sale in the UK on grounds that have never been explained, but it is still available online. The combination was intended to avoid some of the undesirable effects of unopposed oestrogens, listed as haemorrhages, fibroids and breast problems, and androgens alone, namely virilisation. The side-effects listed by the manufacturers included increase in libido, feeling of fullness, nausea and vomiting, anorexia, dizziness, irritability, breast tension, gain or loss in weight, and allergic skin reactions and, in some susceptible female patients, deepening of the voice. The hormones were in esterised form, held in an oily solution; they dispersed over a period of weeks, when the injection was repeated.

Eventually implants that lasted six to nine months came to oust injections in popularity. These are pellets of oestradiol, or oestradiol and testosterone, or testosterone alone, inserted under the skin; for some reason this technique of administration works best in restoring lost libido. Certainly the administration of testosterone will bring about an instant increase in genital sensitivity, but the patient is very aware that this touchiness is unrelated to sexual response as she knows it. If a peri-menopausal woman is not part of a heterosexual couple, she will not be offered this treatment, for the diffuse genital tension she will feel can only lead into dangerous and compromising situations or humiliating bouts of masturbation. Lack of libido in a single woman is not a ground for treatment.

Women who have an implant are advised to take progestogens by mouth for ten to twelve days a calendar month, in order to induce a small bleed; indeed, they are not simply offered the progestogen but must promise to take it as a condition of getting the implant, which is known to exert a stronger effect upon the womb than oestrogens taken in other forms. We know from the behaviour of the women in Studd's programme at Dulwich that they found the effects of the progestogens disturbing and that they tended to stop taking them. Oestrogen absorbed from an implant does not affect blood lipids; progestogens absorbed by mouth do. Some of the symptoms that caused the women at Dulwich to stop taking the progestogens may have signalled quite serious side-effects of progestogens unopposed in the bloodstream. The evidence seems to show that women who have suffered from thromboses in pregnancy should certainly not be given oral progestogen to oppose non-oral oestrogen, and probably should not be given progestogens at all.

In some cases, menopausal symptoms like the itching and painful intercourse caused by the atrophy of the vagina are treated by the local application of hormone creams. Curiously, though these are the symptoms most obviously associated with oestrogen deficiency, they do not always respond to oestrogens taken by mouth, and sometimes the creams are prescribed in addition to oestrogens by mouth. The worry here is that oestrogens are readily and rapidly absorbed through the vaginal wall to act directly upon the uterus. (Some experimental programmes running at the moment are trying vaginal delivery for contraceptives, with good results.) Oestrogen vaginal creams and pessaries can cause uterine hyperplasia, therefore, and oral progestogens may be prescribed along with them. Other creams and gels have been devised for absorption through the skin, and are meant to be rubbed on the abdomen. One of the most curious aspects of HRT in England is that the method most used on the near continent was for many years to all intents and purposes unavailable. Oestrogel, manufactured in Belgium by Besins, is an oestradiol gel which is rubbed into the skin of the upper arms. The rationale behind transcutaneous methods of administration is to lower the dose of oestrogen and still achieve an adequate level of oestrogen in the bloodstream, bypassing the liver, where the effects of stored oestrogen are anything but good. They are so successful that the continued preference for oestrogen by mouth must be seen as irrational.

The fastest riser through the HRT popularity charts in the 1990s was the patchet, originally developed by Schenkel et al. in 1985. These are small round transparent purses containing tiny amounts of the oestradiol dissolved in ethanol; the patchet is simply stuck on to the belly or upper thigh and the gel is absorbed gradually through the permeable layer next to the skin. Patchets for delivery of HRT were developed by Ciba Geigy using Alza's transdermal delivery system. The Ciba Geigy regimen offers three strengths of oestradiol, calculated to deliver three dosages over four days, all very much less than would be conveyed in an oral oestrogen pill. Within a very few years Ciba Geigy had perfected a system of delivering a progestogen along with the oestradiol, so relieving the users of the necessity for a breakthrough bleed. Patchets are expensive and these days doctors are not anxious to include them in their prescription budget.

In 1988 a new synthetic steroid appeared on the market in the Netherlands; this was tibolone, marketed under the names Livial and Tibofem. It has oestrogenic, progestogenic and weak androgenic actions, is used mainly for endometriosis and is being investigated as a possible treatment for female sexual dysfunction. It appears to be of use in treating persisting symptoms in post-menopausal women, who will not need to take progestogens to prevent uterine hyperplasia if they are on tibolone. One study found that while tibolone appeared to slow down bone loss and prevent fractures, it was associated with an unacceptably high risk of stroke, and the study was called off. Tibolone is one steroid that is associated with improvements in mood and libido, however. It has not been licensed for use in the US.

So many studies claiming to have proved the protective action of HRT on practically every organ of the female body appeared year on year in the 1990s, it seemed there could be no justification for denying the treatment to any woman, or for ceasing the treatment once she was on it. However, other studies of the actual take-up of the therapy and its duration indicate that the rate of usage remained stubbornly low. Campaigners accused doctors of being unsympathetic, or conservative, or indifferent to the sufferings of older women. Pressure groups formed to raise the profile of HRT and the level of patient demand utilised the rhetoric of women's rights, claiming that all women have a right to HRT which antifeminist doctors were withholding. Certainly doctors' behaviour appeared neither consistent nor logical; most British doctors prescribed HRT only for the shortest time and for the severest symptoms, as if it were a kind of pain-killer-cum-tranquilliser. Some, mostly American, doctors prescribe HRT before menopause symptoms appear and try to keep the patients on it for the rest of their lives. The German Master in Menopause, Christian Lauritzen, believed that HRT must be continued for a long period:

> With regard to osteoporosis 10–15 years treatment seems
> necessary to prevent the disease for life. Lasting positive effects
> on cardiovascular diseases are noticed after five years medication.
> However substitution for life is seldom and most patients drop out
> for various reasons. (Lauritzen, 1990)

(Once again we encounter 'poor compliance', this time in 'most' patients.) In fact no preventive effect of HRT on the development of osteoporosis has actually been demonstrated, because the longitudinal cohort studies have simply not been done. Attempts to establish an epidemiology of low bone density were tried and abandoned; the likelihood of bone fractures in elderly women remains unknown. It is a hard sentence indeed to be obliged to take a daily medication for a disease that one may never suffer from.

Pauline Kaufert and Penny Gilbert pointed out that doctors in Manitoba, like doctors in Montreal in an earlier study by Margaret Lock, were found to follow 'a diverse collection of clinical models, some giving oestrogen to virtually all their patients, others being more selective in their prescribing habits. The one common factor was that each physician believed absolutely in the correctness of his own approach.' Such was the confusion and the level of unease that a large-scale attempt to assess the efficacy and usefulness of hormone replacement therapy was called for as a matter of urgency, if only because so many women were trying the therapy only to abandon it, despite widespread pressure to conform.

In a Danish study of ten years of HRT, a questionnaire was sent to all women born in 1936 living in four Copenhagen suburbs. Of a total of 597, 526 replied. Of these 37 per cent had had HRT at some time; 22 per cent were still using it. Of the 40 per cent of women who had deliberately interrupted the treatment, 28 per cent claimed they had got no relief of their symptoms while 44 per cent reported adverse reactions such as weight gain, nausea, irregular bleeding and engorged breasts, 7 per cent had become ill from unrelated causes and 12 per cent had negative attitudes; they either disliked the bleeding, or were afraid, or found the drug too expensive. The average duration of use by the ones who stayed until the end of their course was twenty-three months; two-thirds of the women used only one preparation, although one woman tried six (Koster). This pattern of use, with a high drop-out rate, and a short duration even among the people who claim to be benefited by the treatment, is fairly typical of the countries with the highest rate of take-up.

In 1991 the US National Institutes of Health embarked on the Women's Health Initiative, consisting of a set of clinical trials and an observational study involving 161,808 unhysterectomised post-menopausal women aged fifty to seventy-nine. With an age-span of such breadth, there was no way of separating sequelae of menopause from the processes of ageing. One group using Prempro, a combination of Premarin and a medroxyprogesterone acetate (Provera), was matched with a group on placebo. By 2000 it was clear that the Prempro users had more heart attacks, strokes, pulmonary embolism and deep-vein thrombosis than the control group. When it became as clear that incidence of breast cancer was 26 per cent higher in the Prempro group, the study had to be called off. In July 2002 a press conference was held to announce that the trial had been abandoned, and women warned against continuing use of combined HRT.

In 1996 Cancer Research UK, the NHS, the Medical Research Council and the Health and Safety Executive joined forces to run the 'Million Women Study' of the effect of HRT use on women's health, with a particular emphasis on the incidence of breast cancer. From 1996 to 2001 women attending breast cancer screening centres were invited to participate. Within a very short time it became apparent that HRT use was associated with a higher incidence of breast cancer. Users of combined oestrogen–progestogen formulae had twice the breast cancer risk of non-users. Rates of endometrial and ovarian cancer too were so much higher for HRT users that it was clear that the use of HRT as a first-line treatment for osteoporosis prevention could not be justified. The official conclusion is that 'because HRT use is linked to higher rates of breast and other cancers, and of stroke, it is now recommended that HRT should be generally used for a few years only to relieve menopausal symptoms such as hot flushes' with the proviso that 'the balance of risks and benefits of HRT still needs to be considered for each woman individually', which takes us all the way back to square one. The Million Women Study congratulates itself on saving lives, but the logic is questionable, to say the least:

> In terms of direct impact on women's health, use of HRT has fallen by about half over the past few years, both in the UK and across the world. It is very encouraging to see that fewer breast cancers are now developing in women in their 50s and 60s – the age group most likely to use HRT. While other factors have also to be considered, it is thought that the fall in numbers of breast cancer cases and the fall in use of HRT are linked, and that as a result of the changes in HRT prescribing, many thousands of breast cancers have been prevented.

Between 2001 and 2005 sales of HRT fell by half. Current guidelines now suggest that women who need HRT should try to use a low-dose oestrogen-only preparation for as short a time as possible. It should be remembered that transdermal application involves much lower doses than formulae taken by mouth, but for some reason even now this is seldom made clear to British acceptors of HRT.

Both the American and British cohort studies were meant to illuminate a confusing state of affairs. Both have been criticised for poor design and lack of stringency. Both suffer from the weakness of the categories that have had to be used, and from the oversimplification of their accounts of causation. Ten years after the shutting-down of the Women's Health Initiative, Wulf Utian, the original Master in Menopause, felt able to condemn it in the roundest terms:

The real story of the WHI may turn out to be incalculable damage wrought on younger peri- and early postmenopausal women who discontinued their therapy and who are now several years beyond menopause and off hormones. Not only have they suffered through menopause-related symptoms, but the very women who might have been protected from heart disease, the single biggest killer of women over 50, and osteoporosis, one of the most significant causes of long-term disability, are the ones potentially most damaged by the WHI.

What follows is speculative at best.

Women who discontinued postmenopausal hormone therapy (PHT) have significantly increased risk of hip fracture compared with women who continued taking hormone therapy (HT). Indeed, there are estimates that discontinuation of PHT may have resulted in over 43,000 bone fractures per year in the USA. The number of increased cardiovascular events in young women who discontinued ET may be even more staggering. Publications from the WHI clearly demonstrate no increase in cardiovascular risk in women aged 50–59, and indeed, for the first time ever, an intervention, namely estrogen, has been demonstrated to actually reduce calcified plaque burden in the coronary arteries of these women. Even statins have not been demonstrated to be this effective in women.

Now a new scientific study recently released online ahead of print reports that over a 10-year span, starting in 2002, a minimum of 18,601 and as many as 91,610 postmenopausal women died prematurely because of the avoidance of estrogen therapy.

The pendulum continues to swing back towards enlightened acceptance of HRT not only as useful in specific circumstances but as having the potential to prevent disease and prolong life. In the US, PBS hired 69-year-old Goldie Hawn (who is supposed to keep fit and looking good by using meditation) to narrate *Hot Flash Havoc*, a documentary meant to 'set the record straight' about HRT, which was released in the US in March 2016. The film 'makes the case that hormone therapies not only treat the symptoms of menopause, but prevent disease and have the potential for prolonging life'. PBS promoted the film online as the 'most provocative and revealing documentary ever made about menopause', which would not be saying much, and goes on:

> For the first time this documentary sets the record straight about the U.S. government sanctioned Women's Health Initiative (WHI) study released in 2002, which misrepresented that the hormonal replacement therapy being used by millions of women to treat the symptoms of menopause, could actually increase the risk of heart attacks and cancer.
>
> This misinformation caused confusion, hysteria, and fear among women as well as healthcare providers, endangering the health and well being of millions of women, many of whom flushed their hormones down the toilet.

The case appears overstated. The evidence of actual use of HRT does not show enthusiastic long-term use, but what its promoters complained of as 'poor compliance'. The case of Barbara Metcalfe is not particularly unusual: to deal with the devastating hot flushes that followed her surgically induced menopause, she took what the doctor ordered.

> I went down the conventional route, and, full of hope, began a course of HRT. Within days, my breasts felt painful and engorged. I became depressed and confused and – worse – the sweats and flushes didn't even abate. I gave it some time for the tablets to kick in – during which my already huge bosom went up a full cupsize – but I only became more bloated, itchy and frankly miserable. So, about six months later I came off it. I tried red clover and other natural remedies but quickly realised nothing was going to work. So I took nothing.

PBS remains unembarrassed by its unsupported belief that women succumbed to 'confusion, hysteria and fear' when the WHI programme was abandoned, and goes on to solicit donations, rather as the Amarant Trust did in the bad old days of optimistic oversell.

When you watch *Hot Flash Havoc*, executive produced by Heidi Houston and directed by Marc Bennett, you will have the opportunity to donate to PBS and receive a DVD of *Hot Flash Havoc*, plus a DVD series called *MENOPAUSE TALKS* (Think Ted Talks with menopause experts), a copy of *The Menopause Makeover*, AND *Change your Menopause* by Dr Wulf Utian.

Not everyone will be delighted to know that the Grand Master in Menopause is still in business at the old stand. According to one website reviewing the documentary, hotflashhavoc.com, the 'storyline' is as follows:

> When the U.S. government-sanctioned Women's Health Initiative Study was released in 2002, a nationwide panic resulted – causing women to flush their hormone medications down the toilet. As a direct result in the United States alone, tens of thousands of women have died from heart attacks. This is an insightful documentary that reveals fact vs. fiction surrounding menopause and the controversy around it through the world's leading experts. The medical information contained in this film could save your life ... or the life of someone that you love.

It was not the release of the study that caused the reaction, but the curtailment and abandonment of the study. The number of women who die of heart disease each year in the US is in the region of 290,000; to maintain that a mere 'tens of thousands' of these deaths might have been prevented by the use of hormone therapy is footling at best.

British TV doctor Miriam Stoppard is another who is firmly committed to the notion of menopause as signalling the onset of a deficiency disease, as befits someone who was once managing director of the pharmaceutical arm of Syntex, manufacturers of norethisterone, the first oral highly active progestogen.

Meanwhile women are still faced with the conundrum of how best to take care of themselves as they traverse the fifth climacteric. An apparently immovable fixture on which internet search engines home in at the first click is the great Oprah Winfrey, and in particular the Oprah TV show of 29 January 2009, which was devoted to HRT, in particular to so-called 'bioidentical hormones' for which Winfrey alleged almost magical effects. 'After one day on bioidentical estrogen, I felt the veil lift,' 55-year-old Winfrey, who claims never to have experienced a hot flash, told her audience of forty million or so. 'After three days, the sky was bluer, my brain was no longer fuzzy, my memory was sharper. I was literally singing and had a skip in my step.' 'Bioidentical' is a coinage adopted for the replacement hormones synthesised from yam and soy that had always been preferred in European practice to the conjugated equine steroids derived from the urine of pregnant mares that were and continue to be market leaders in the US. The FDA rejects the whole 'BHRT' category, but its statements appear to be based on a misconception, that 'bioidentical' products are typically 'compounded in pharmacies'.

'Unlike commercial drug manufacturers, pharmacies aren't required to report adverse events associated with compounded drugs,' says Steve Silverman, Assistant Director of the Office of Compliance in FDA's Center for Drug Evaluation and Research. 'Also, while some health risks associated with "BHRT" drugs may arise after a relatively short period of use, others may not occur for many years. One of the big problems is that we just don't know what risks are associated with these so-called "bio-identicals".' In fact bioidentical replacement hormones are simply those that are plant-derived, and they have been commercially available since before the appearance of equine hormones and subject to the same evaluation processes.

Sharing the stage with Winfrey in January 2009 was 62-year-old one-time TV actress, now author and health campaigner, Suzanne Somers. Every morning Somers rubs her upper arms with a bioidentical hormone preparation; for two weeks a month she adds progesterone cream, and once a day she injects estrogen directly into her vagina. In her books she claims that she starts each day by injecting herself with human growth hormone, vitamins B12 and B complex. She boasted on a radio show that she has sex with her husband twice a day. In 2001 she was diagnosed with stage 2 breast cancer, underwent lumpectomy and radiation therapy, and now says she would have treated her cancer differently. She does not consider the possibility that overdosing herself with steroids may have triggered the cancer.

In 2014 55-year-old writer Jeanette Winterson, who was struggling with sleep disruption, dry skin, hair loss and general malaise, was advised to seek assistance from Dr Marion Gluck, whom she describes in an article for the *Guardian* as 'a world pioneer in the prescription and preparation of bio-identical hormone therapy for women and men'. Gluck was trained as a GP in Germany, began her practice in Australia, has been using her own therapy for fifteen years and treats 13,000 patients a year. As we have seen, bioidentical hormones are available in standardised versions from Big Pharma, but Gluck prefers to have individually tailored versions compounded for her patients, describing other doctors as 'the robot arm of the drug companies'. After being prescribed a regime that contains much lower doses of hormone than would have been available in standardised doses, Winterson ends her article: 'I feel at home in my body again.'

What Winterson doesn't tell you is how much her treatment at Gluck's clinic in Wimpole Street actually cost her, though she acknowledges that it was expensive. Another practitioner offering the same services charges £590 for the initial consultation, in addition to the costs of the various tests and £45 a month for the treatment itself. There is considerable disagreement about the usefulness of blood tests and the possibility of arriving at 'a complete hormonal profile' as the Gluck clinic is said to do. Dr Nick Panay, consultant gynaecologist at Queen Charlotte's and the Chelsea Hospital, told the *Daily Mail* that Gluck's prescribing did not make sense. 'It is not possible to work out the level of hormones based on a blood test. First, because your levels fluctuate all the time and second, because you can't predict what a person needs from the test result.' Nevertheless GPs and gynaecologists do send menopausal patients for blood tests and do act upon the results.

British TV performer Denise Welch suffered from depression for many years. When she was approaching fifty the depressions became so acute that she feared for her life. She told the *Mirror* in 2011: 'I was about to go to America in the hope I might find someone there who could treat me because for years I had been pushed aside and told this wasn't hormonal and I was being ridiculous. But then I heard about a specialist called Professor John Studd so I went to see him. He quickly discovered I was almost completely deficient in oestrogen. When he prescribed it for me, alongside the low-dose anti-depressants I was taking, everything got better.'

John Studd, the British Master in Menopause, runs his clinic on the other side of Wimpole Street from Dr Gluck. Much as we might like to know how he discovered that Ms Welch was 'almost completely deficient in oestrogen', her account gives us no clue. Stung by the

American notion that bioidentical hormones are some sort of novelty, Studd describes on his clinic's website the approach he had been using for more than twenty years:

> It is important to realise that bioidentical hormones in the form of oestradiol, testosterone and progesterone have been used in Europe, particularly France for at least 20 years and I have used nothing else during this time.
>
> The best method of taking bioidentical hormones would in my view be Oestrogel 2–3 measures daily with the possible addition of transdermal testosterone gel and then Utrogestan 100 mgs daily for the first 7 days of each calendar month. This would bring about a regular scanty bleed on about the 10th day of each calendar month.

What he doesn't say is that, in applying oestrogel from the pump pack provided, the user can vary her dose. If her breasts become tender she can reduce it.

For some years now British women complaining of heavy irregular bleeding in the peri-menopause have been likely to be offered the Mirena coil, which was first used in Europe in 1991. This was originally designed to function as part of an intrauterine contraceptive system. It works by releasing levonorgestrel, a synthetic progestogen, to thin the lining of the uterus so that a fertilised ovum cannot implant, as well as thickening cervical mucus to slow down sperm. In some women, it inhibits ovulation altogether. In menopausal women the levonorgestrel is thought to control and eventually eliminate problem bleeding, but in fact nobody knows why or how the Mirena coil actually does this. Doctors are paid £70 for each coil they fit, and each coil costs the NHS £88; once in, the coil is meant to function for five years. For some women the progestogen will cause bleeding or spotting for six months or so, but this is thought to be manageable. Since 2000, when the Mirena coil was approved for use in the US, there have been more than 47,000 adverse incidents, of which about 21 per cent involve heavier bleeding. The manufacturer, Bayer Pharmaceuticals, has been accused of intentionally selling a dangerous product, deceptive advertising and concealing the risk of complications. There are 500 actions now pending. In the only cases I know of women of menopausal age being fitted with Mirena coils to end problem bleeding, the bleeding continued for more than six months and the coils were eventually removed.

Dosing suffering women with excess oestrogen may represent inadvertent homeopathic prescribing by committed allopaths. The principle of homeopathic prescribing is to supply more of the element that is causing the imbalance, so that the body stops secreting it and equilibrium can return when the added substance is gradually withdrawn. It could be that by dosing women with much more oestrogen than their bodies had produced, their endocrine systems are persuaded that there is no need to pump out oestrogen to fend off ovarian failure. What this means is that when the exogenous steroids are withdrawn, the endogenous hormone cannot kick in, and the patient suffers menopause with a vengeance.

What if those female bodies that fight menopause by flooding themselves with FSH and keeping up oestrogen secretion are robbing other vital functions in the process, so that the organism has to go short of endorphins and corticosteroids? Some such dysfunction would explain some of the strangest manifestations of menopause, for example, joint pains and crawling skin, and even the famous hot flushes. In that case the deficiency would be seen not in oestrogens but in other body chemicals. Nevertheless prescription of oestrogen would relieve them, if only temporarily, because it would take the pressure off the hypothalamus to produce more and more FSH and oestrogen, and let it revert to its usual patterns.

Until we know if women without symptoms have something that women with symptoms do not, we have no logical ground for describing menopausal distress as a deficiency disease. It would make more sense, in view of the fact that older women adjust to very much lower levels of oestrogen, to ask what the biochemical trigger is that facilitates the switchover, and try to prime that pump. As we are not within thousands of research hours of doing that, we prefer to treat the problem symptomatically. What we are really doing is denying the process that is trying to occur, and pushing the woman off the rung of the life ladder that she has arrived at, to a lower one, where she will wait indefinitely to complete the fifth climacter.

Heaven knows what the future holds for the woman seeking help in managing her menopause. One technique that has been seen by some as a way of postponing menopause is ovarian transplant, which was first used to restore the fertility of a patient post-cancer treatment in Belgium in 2004. In 2012 (5 July) *Marie Claire* published details of a conference where 'leading doctors' described how twenty-eight babies had been born to women who had ovarian tissue removed and later replaced or had been donated ovarian tissue by a twin. Some such procedure could enable women to avoid menopause altogether by having slices of living ovary removed, cryogenically stored and then surgically replaced when the plundered ovary began to fail. The need for some such procedure was emphasised by Sherman Silber, director of the Infertility Center of St Louis MO, who explained that 'a woman born today has a 50 per cent chance of living to 100 … they are going to be spending half their lives in post-menopause'. Tim Hillard, a gynaecologist and trustee of the British Menopause Society, entered a caveat: 'You would have to balance it very carefully, the higher risks of breast and womb cancer that go with having oestrogen circulating for longer against the increased risk of heart disease, osteoporosis and maybe dementia that go with the menopause,' adding that the technique could be used as an 'alternative to hormone replacement therapy'. Current estimates of the probable cost do not bear out this possibility.

In 2015 the journal *Human Reproduction* (Jensen et al.) reported on forty-one cases of Danish women who had ovarian tissue transplanted back into their bodies after treatment over as much as ten years for cancer. Six of the women underwent the procedure to avoid menopause; thirty-two were hoping to have a baby. Ten of them succeeded; altogether thirteen babies were born. It was not plain sailing for everyone; the ovarian tissue remained active for less than a year for four of the women, for more than ten years for two. Several women needed two or three transplants.

Rather less spectacular and a great deal cheaper is likely to be a new treatment for hot flushes. That such a thing is eagerly awaited might be concluded from a heartfelt lament by British commentator Vanessa Feltz (aged fifty-four) writing in the *Daily Express* (15 March 2016).

> I don't want to read stuff about a pill to stop menopausal hot
> flushes. I want a packet right now delivered into my outstretched
> palm. I don't want to read: 'If all goes well it could be in routine
> clinical practice within five years.'

Five years! That means five years of taking my cardigan on and off 36 times an hour – I know, my young male producer counted. It means five years of having to stand seminaked in the garden at three in the morning.

It means half a decade of veering from tropical heatwave to the ice age and plastering a grin on your boat race as if nothing has happened.

For heaven's sake don't dilly-dally. Have mercy on the menopausal damsels of the universe and shove this straight into the file marked 'EXPEDITE'.

Now that the role of neurokinins in triggering hot flashes has been understood, the chances of an effective treatment to be available soon are much better than had been hoped. In March 2016 endocrinologist Dr Julia Prague of Imperial College announced that her team was looking for thirty menopausal women to help them trial a new treatment for hot flushes in which the release of neurokinin could be counteracted by a neurokinin receptor antagonist called AZD4901, originally developed to treat schizophrenia. This had already proved of interest as a potential treatment for polycystic ovarian syndrome.

Just how far Dr Prague will get in pioneering a whole new armamentarium of drug treatments for some of the most challenging of the symptoms of the 'climacteric syndrome' will depend on whether she can find funding for the large-scale cohort studies that will eventually need to be carried out. If Big Pharma succeeds in rehabilitating HRT from the damage done by the WHI and the Million Woman Study, such funding will be slow in coming. Every day brings new evidence not simply that HRT works, but that only HRT works, but it is hardly more reliable than the distortions of the mass trials. In 2006 the US federal government funded a one-year, double-blind, randomised, controlled trial comparing the effects of three formulations of Black Cohosh with hormone therapy and placebo for relief of hot flashes and night sweats, which was reported in the popular press as follows:

… 351 women aged 45 to 55 were given a variety of botanicals or HRT, in a study called Herbal Alternatives for Menopause (HALT). One group received black cohosh (*Cimicifuga racemosa*); a second group received a multi-botanical consisting of black cohosh, alfalfa, boron, chaste tree, dong quai, false unicorn, licorice, oats, pomegranate and *Eleutherococcus senticosus* ['Siberian ginseng']; a third group received the multi-botanical plus dietary counseling to increase the consumption of soy-based foods; a fourth group received estrogen, with or without progestin (HRT). Finally, a fifth group received placebo. After one year, all groups except those on HRT had no fewer hot flashes or night sweats. Only HRT gave significant relief.

In fact, all groups experienced a fall in the number and frequency of symptoms, including those who were given nothing but the dummy pill. The conclusion was that most women would be feeling much better after a year in any case, even with no treatment at all (Newton et al.).

9

The Treatments – Traditional

When Philippa, fourteen-year-old daughter of William the Good, Count of Holland and Hainault, landed at Dover in 1327, on her way to meet her proxy husband, Edward III of England, she brought with her her mother's herbal. All women, even the grandest, were then expected to doctor their households. Most of them were illiterate and used recipes that they had seen their mothers use, varying them according to time and place. Philippa, far from her homeland and her mother, would have to rely on her beautifully lettered book, which included descriptions of the properties of herbs in Latin and in English, little diagrams of the affected parts, and drawings of English wild plants (British Library MS Add 29301).

Philippa bore her husband seven sons and five daughters, so we are not surprised to find her herbal to be full of medications 'for to bring out the secundyne' (afterbirth) and 'provoke menstrues', to 'deliver the dead child' and 'cleanse the mother' (i.e. the womb) as well as for the 'flux of the menstrue' and for 'women that have their terms too much or too often'. There are one or two that might be thought to relate to older women, the use of myrrh, for example, 'for to comfort the mother in a woman and waste the humours that are in her', or 'calametum' (a corruption of calamint) 'to draw the superfluity is in a woman', but her remedies are more likely to apply to infection in breeding women than to the discomforts of menopause.

Queen Philippa was unusual among self-medicating women in that she had a written text to go by which makes at least nominal use of a male authority, for it includes a version of 'Circa instans' by the

Salernitan physician Matthaeus Platearius. The secular scholars of the Italian school were not shy of prescribing for women's troubles; the monks who made copies and translations of their works for use in the infirmaries and dispensaries of their monasteries left out much that referred to women and their organs of generation, for reasons which are fairly obvious. The nuns who cared for women were poorer and less literate and made do without great parchment tomes. Once the eminent gentlemen, monkish or other, had established their authority, they had to defend it, not against women or practitioners but against their male rivals.

The early documentary history of medicine is largely a hierarchy of texts, with very little empiric evidence of how remedies worked in practice. Most of the people on earth at the same time as the most famous of the ancient practitioners were dosed for what ailed them, not by the likes of Hippocrates, Galen or Paracelsus, but by their mothers and their mothers' mothers, who did the best they could with what they had. The 'old women' set bones, washed wounds, let blood, delivered infants, drove out infestations, anointed buboes and chafed sore joints, with an array of embrocations, vulneraries, electuaries, tinctures, syrups and tisanes that altered from place to place, from climate to climate, from season to season. Despite the activities of male scholars, this vast body of knowledge was never systematised. The written herbals that survive represent only a minute fraction of medication as it was always and everywhere practised.

Sometimes the women cured; mostly they did not interfere with healing. Much of their activity soothed and comforted the patient rather than fighting the disorder. There was a marked element of psychoprophylaxis in the magical and semi-magical rituals that attended much of the dosing. What nostrums there are for menopausal distress are hidden in general prescriptions for sleeplessness, lethargy, melancholy or fits of the mother.

Few or none of the hundreds of specifics to bring on menstruation listed in all the ancient pharmacopoeiae should be understood as treatments intended to delay the cessation of the menses. The 'obstruction' or 'suppression' of the menses in younger women was regarded as a serious symptom, principally because menstruation was considered a necessary evacuation of superabounding blood together with evil humours; the treatments vary with the suspected cause and the somatic type of the individual. A few of the treatments for excessive blood loss could be profitably used by older women, but the metrorrhagia of the menopause, though inconvenient, can be easily observed to be a self-limiting phenomenon that did not threaten life. Haemorrhaging in younger women was all too often a cause of death; the high visibility in the old herbals of treatments to stay or allay women's courses principally relates to this greater need.

One of the ancient herbal treatments for treating the climacteric syndrome is 'Agnus Castus'. According to Dioscorides (I. 103) and Pliny (*Naturalis Historia*, XXIV, 59), Athenian women anxious to avoid lascivious dreams in the absence of their husbands put the leaves of Agnus Castus in their beds; for its known anaphrodisiac property it is also known as 'chaste tree'. Because monks ground it and sprinkled it on their food in an attempt to suppress sinful desire it was called 'monks' pepper'. The Cistercian monk Andrew Boorde, writing *The Breuiary of Helthe*, of which the first of many editions appeared in 1547, includes Agnus Castus in 'a receipte to kepe a man or a woman lowe of corage', that is, free of concupiscent desires: the whole recipe is worth citing, for it bears a family relationship to nostrums for climacteric syndrome:

> To keep one low, is the usage of eating or of drinking of vinegar or smelling to it, and so daily used, Rue and Camphor for this matter is good to smell to it. And Tutsane otherwise named Agnus castus and Singrene otherwise named Houseleek, and strong purgations, watch and study … (Boorde, Fol. xxxvii^v)

Tutsane was not Agnus Castus but a St John's Wort, namely *Hypericum androsaemum*; the confusion probably comes about because both plants were used in much the same way. (Secure botanical labelling does not begin before Linnaeus.) Both the St John's Wort and the Agnus Castus could be grown only where the winters were mild; in most of Britain both herbs would have been available only from an apothecary. We can be fairly sure that the houseleek mentioned by Boorde is a Sempervivum. As such it had the common name 'Sengreen', i.e. evergreen.

Taxonomic confusion continues into the twenty-first century. Dr Christiane Northrup and her American colleagues refer to Agnus Castus as 'Vitex', the current botanical name for 'Agnus Castus' or 'chasteberry' being *Vitex agnus-castus*, the name given it by Linnaeus in

208

Species plantarum in 1753 (p. 638). The genus Vitex of the Verbenaceae contains about 250 species, nevertheless American herbalists appear happy to refer to one species by the non-specific generic name. On numerous websites we read 'Vitex is a good choice when trying to boost progesterone levels' and that 'relief is often found using traditional women's herbs such as … vitex'. Jessica Godino of Red Moon Herbs tells us on her website that she uses 'Vitex as a supreme hormonal tonic for women. Both extensive clinical studies, as well as over two thousand years of use in folk medicine, have proven the effectiveness of this remedy.' Be that as it may, *Vitex agnus-castus* disappeared from the British pharmacopoeia at the beginning of the eighteenth century and did not return until the mid-twentieth.

Another common native herb that older women found useful was the Greater Periwinkle, *Vinca major*, which like Agnus Castus and Tutsane could be grown in sheltered cottage gardens; the extract of the flowering plant has been found to have a marked effect upon smooth muscle. As it also reduces blood pressure and dilates both coronary and peripheral blood vessels, it is useful for women in whom menopausal distress is complicated by hypertensiveness. The 1826 edition of Culpeper's *Herbal* says that 'the French use it to stay women's courses. It is a good female medicine, and may be used with advantage in hysteric and other fits.' Culpeper advises either an infusion of the green plant or the expressed juice of it, 'to the quantity of two ounces for a dose', which seems excessive.

Another of the few herbs named in connection with the menopause specifically is *Alchemilla mollis* or Lady's Mantle. Prolonged use of the dried leaves, taken as an infusion, relieves both metrorrhagia and menopausal distress. The little sister of *Alchemilla mollis*, *Alchemilla alpina*, is considered more effective but is correspondingly more difficult to come by. Culpeper suggests sitting in a warm bath in which Lady's Mantle leaves have been steeped to prevent miscarriage; the same uterosedative effect could be useful for menopausal symptoms. Unfortunately when Culpeper assures us that it is also useful for 'such women or maids as have over-great flagging breasts, causing them to grow less and hard, being both drank and outwardly applied', scepticism creeps in.

Perhaps the most important if least mentioned of the plants used in treating menopausal symptoms is Henbane, *Hyoscyamus niger*. This poisonous member of the Solanaceae has been used since antiquity as an ingredient in anaesthetics and in potions designed to produce hallucinations. As 'Herba Apollinaris', it was used by the priestesses of Apollo to inspire their oracles. John Gerard's *Herball* of 1597 states: 'The leaves, the seeds and the juice, when taken internally cause an unquiet sleep, like unto the sleep of drunkenness, which continueth long and is deadly to the patient. To wash the feet in a decoction of Henbane, as also the often smelling of the flowers, causeth sleep.' Older women have used Henbane as a medication since ancient times. It is known to be sedative, analgesic and anti-spasmodic; powerful alkaloids, hyoscyamine, atropine and hyoscine, all of which have useful therapeutic function, are to be found in the leaves. Gustav Schenk, who roasted the seeds and inhaled the vapour in the course of research for his *Book of Poisons* (1955), suffered a series of extraordinary hallucinations, which culminated in the distinct impression that he was soaring high above the ground.

Henbane has been used successfully in modern times to treat hysteria (Osol et al.). In Boorde's *Breuiary of Helthe* (1547), insomniacs are advised 'to make a dormitary of henbane, and lay it to the temples' (Pt. II, fol. xxiv). Like the herbs discussed above, Henbane is not truly native to Britain, but it can be found growing wild in areas where it is likely to have escaped from cottage gardens, often on chalk. In 1910 Dr Crippen used it to kill his first wife. In the 1930s a derivative of Henbane was used to cause labouring women to drift into 'twilight sleep'; at the same time it was used in asylums to control mania. The old wives who used Henbane have left no record of what they used it for; it is thought to have been an ingredient in witches' flying ointments, by those who believe that witches could fly; it may have been used to induce shamanistic ecstasy. All we can be sure of is that it was used.

Almost none of the medical texts refers directly to the psychological stresses of the climacteric. Though works on hysteria and melancholy abound, and each is a portmanteau term that describes a wide variety of conditions, none concerns itself specifically with the mental sufferings of the menopausal woman. The classical notion of hysteria derives from Hippocrates, who considered that the womb was no mere organ like other organs, but an imperious, mysterious, rebellious, in-dwelling creature that could torture the woman who did not satisfy its demands by rising upwards in her body and suffocating her (Jorden). The withering away of the womb represented, if anyone considered it at all, a liberation from its tyranny and its furious hunger, which forced women to risk their lives again and again in the lottery of pregnancy and childbirth. The view that the stresses of menopause represented the death-throes of the wild womb lingered on in some quarters until the mid-eighteenth century. We find French anatomist Moreau de la Sarthe, for example, in *L'Histoire naturelle de la Femme* (1803), arguing that if a woman survived to the climacteric, the womb rebelled against the forced relinquishment of its power over the organism. The menopausal uterus 'overthrows the whole system and brings about nervous afflictions and a profound alteration in the digestive functions' (p. 180). For adherents of this theory menopausal anxiety, sleeplessness, palpitations, and even hot flushes, which were observed in younger hysterics as well, were variants of hysteria, and to be treated in the same ways.

A systematic discussion of women's diseases in the vernacular medical texts is, alas, too much to hope for. Though accidents and plagues befalling men's organs of generation may be discussed at length, the 'privities' of women are considered improper subjects. Even in Queen Philippa's herbal the generic patient is referred to as 'a man'; the early printed texts follow the same convention. When a woman is writing, for example the 'woman-physician' Mary Trye in 1675, reluctance to discuss female ailments is, if anything, more marked. At the end of *Medicatrix, Or The Woman-Physician*, Mary, whose generic patient is also 'a man', after an advertisement for her own practice and the medications she had learned from her father, remarks of the 'Diseases attending Women', 'As Historical Fits, or Fits of the Mother, Green-Sickness, Wastings, barrenness, Obstruction, Fluxes of Several Kinds &c. The Diseases incident to this Sex are many, and not proper here largely to be discoursed on; therefore I purposely omit them ...' (Sig. K4ᵛ)

Similarly the theoreticians of melancholy saw little to distinguish menopausal depression from female melancholy in general. The classic theory of melancholy explained the condition as the result of a superfluity of one of the four humours that make up the human constitution, namely black bile. The word 'humour' began its career in English as meaning a bodily fluid, gradually took on the association with a state of mind, until the anatomical constituent of the idea eventually perished, leaving only the secondary meaning. Texts like

Robert Burton's *Anatomy of Melancholy* move freely back and forth along a psychosomatic continuum, so that biochemistry is seen as causing mental and spiritual distress, which in turn aggravates the biochemical imbalance. It would seem then that we might expect a better understanding of the complex nature of climacteric syndrome from the students of melancholy than from the medical theorists, if only they would concern themselves with older women; in fact they were only mildly interested in female melancholy of any kind.

A Treatise of Melancholie (1586) written by physician and clergyman Timothie Bright suggests a treatment for depression that is one of the few that could be taken to apply to older women:

> If this melancholy falleth unto maidens, women, and their ordinary course fail them, the veins of the hams or ankles are to be cut, and drinks of opening roots, fennel, parsley, Butchers' Broom, madder and such like, with germander, golds, Herb Grace, mugwort and nep are to be much used, with sittings and bathings in mallows, camomile and nep, pennyroyal, bay leaves, fetherfew ... decocted in water, wherein so much honey has been dissolved, as will give it a taste of sweetness. (p. 264)

Bright's ingredients are nearly all commonly available in the wild or in the cottage garden. Dried roots of Dandelion, Yellow Dock, Licorice, Angelica and Burdock were all used in laxative infusions. Fennel is *Foeniculum vulgare*, Parsley *Petroselinum crispum*, Butcher's Broom *Ruscus aculeatus*, Madder *Rubia tinctorum*. Germander is the name of any of the Teucrium genus, probably *T. scorodonia*; golds are Marigolds, *Calendula officinalis*; Herb Grace is Rue, *Ruta graveolens*; Mugwort is *Artemisia vulgaris*; Mallows are *Althea officinalis*, often called Marsh Mallow; Camomile is probably but not necessarily *Matricaria recutita*; Nep is *Nepeta cataria*; Pennyroyal is *Mentha pulegium*; Bay is *Laurus nobilis*, and 'fetherfew' is Feverfew, *Chrysanthemum parthenium*.

Though the opening medicines Bright names in the first part are not the ones usually recommended for older women, the baths he recommends, but for the inclusion of Pennyroyal, are sedative and anti-spasmodic. He adds, moreover, that the venesection should be performed at the new moon for the younger women but at the full 'for the elder sort'. Similar spasmolytics appear in the recipes for the soothing baths for melancholy that feature in several surviving receipt-books, such as the one kept by Mary Fairfax in 1632:

> Take mallows, pellitory of the wall, of each three handfuls, camomile flowers, melilot flowers, of each one handful; hollyhocks two handfuls, hyssop one great handful, fenugreek seed one ounce, and boil them in nine gallons of water, till they come to three, then put in a quart of new milk, and go into it blood warm or something warmer. (Fairfax family, p. 16)

A handful is a precise measurement: it is as many twelve-inch sprigs of the herb as may be held in the hand at once. One can hardly imagine an older woman going to all this trouble for herself; if a younger woman, a granddaughter perhaps, made up such a delicious bath for someone else, the evidence of tender care or 'cherishing', as it was known, must have constituted a large part of the effectiveness of the therapy. Pellitory of the Wall is *Parietaria officinalis*; Melilot is *Melilotus officinalis*; Hollyhocks are *Alcea rosea*; Hyssop *Hyssopus officinalis*. Fenugreek, *Trigonella foenum-graecum*, is not native to Britain and would have to have been bought from an apothecary, at considerable expense.

Though it might be fun, it is hardly realistic to try to reinvent the practices of the old herb women in our time. All botanicals behave differently in different circumstances, and exhibit different properties. Altitude, available moisture, sunlight or lack of it and soil type all affect the chemical composition of growing plants. To dry vegetable material in the sun is to destroy most of its most valuable constituents; to gather herbs by a roadside is to collect them with a full load of pollutants. There is more point in buying herbs fresh in a local market than dried and encapsulated in a shop, especially if you have consulted the sellers at the market as to how they use them. Herbs raised on a kitchen windowsill will be practically inert, and those grown in a greenhouse hardly better. Spot checks on commercially marketed herbs reveal them to be often out of date, and sometimes not at all what is claimed on the label. Most commercially available herbal preparations are inactive; the ones that are not can be downright dangerous. Camomile tea is drunk by many women in southern Europe as a specific for all kinds of female complaints; to swap the dust in the teabag for freshly gathered plant material is to run a significant risk of gripes and nausea, even supposing you chose the right plant. Vendors of teas called Camomile are very cagey about what they made it with. Camomile can be identified as any of several Matricaria species, or as an Anthemis, or as Chamomilla or as Chamaemelum or Scented Mayweed. It can be called German, Italian, Hungarian, English, Roman, Scotch, wild, genuine, garden, lawn, sweet, true or common Camomile.

Most women have no realistic option but to seek the aid of the medical establishment in dealing with difficulties encountered at the climacteric. A study of the treatments offered before the panacea of HRT became available provides little more, however, than food for thought. Though the name 'menopause' was not invented till Gardanne coined the term in 1821, the phenomena associated with the cessation of the menses were observed long before. At first the disturbances of the menopause were thought to result from the fact that menstruation no longer discharged excrementitious humours from the womb, and a good deal of the apprehension felt by women entering the climacteric was due to this notion. In *The Anatomy of Melancholy* (1628, 1632) Burton summarises the theory 'out of Hippocrates, Cleopatra, Moschion and those old *Gynaeciorum Scriptores*' in describing the melancholy of 'more ancient Maids, Widows and barren Women' whose

> … heart and brain [are] offended with those vitious vapours that come from menstruous blood … offended by that fuliginous exhalation of corrupt seed, troubling the brain, heart and mind; … the whole malady proceeds from that inflammation, putridity, black smoky vapours, &c and from thence comes care, sorrow & anxiety, obfuscation of spirits, agony, desperation & the like …, to Nuns and more ancient Maids … 'tis more familiar. (Burton, 1989, I, p. 414)

Burton accurately describes hot flushes and palpitations:

> The midriff and heart strings do burn and beat very fearfully, & when the vapour or fume is stirred, flyeth upward, the heart itself beats & is sore grieved and faints … they are dry, thirsty, suddenly hot, much troubled with wind, cannot sleep &c … so far gone

sometimes, so stupefied and distracted, they think themselves
bewitched. (I, p. 415)

An ancient, barren woman could hardly have put it better herself.
Though Burton was a bachelor and led 'a monastic life in a college', he
was quite convinced that the cause of these manifestations was 'enforced
temperance'. His observations bear out the impression that historically
the climacteric was associated with women who had not perished in the
lottery of childbirth, who were mostly virgins, widows and the sterile.
Burton, who would have been more familiar with labouring women who
were prevented from marrying by their servile status, had also noticed
that they did not manifest the same kind of distress: 'seldom shall you
see an hired servant, a poor handmaid, though ancient, that is hard kept
to her work, and bodily labour … troubled in this kind …' (I, p. 416)

Burton's ideas, which have as much to do with the history of pre-
menstrual syndrome as that of climacteric syndrome, are no more than
the sum of medical orthodoxy of his time. In 1683, in a letter written in
Latin to his colleague, William Cole, Thomas Sydenham, MD, declared
that menstrual blood was none other than the sustenance supplied for the
foetus in the womb, which had to be shed if impregnation did not ensue
in due season. In the letter, which was published in his *Opera Universa*
in 1685 and in a translation by John Pechey, a Licentiate of the College of
Physicians, in 1701, Sydenham had little to say about older women except
to offer a treatment for excessive blood loss during the climacteric:

But as to the Flux … [that] … comes most commonly a little before
the Time the Courses are about to leave them, *viz.* about the Age of
Forty-five if they flow early, but about Fifty if they come somewhat
later; from these as it is said, a little before they quite go away (like
a Candle burnt to the Socket which gives the greatest light, just as
it is about to go out) they flow impetuously, and subject the poor
Women almost continually to Hysterick Fits, by reason of the
quantity of Blood which is continually evacuated … (p. 337)

Sydenham began his therapy by letting blood:

Let eight Ounces of Blood taken from the Arm, the next Morning
give the common purging Potion, which must be repeated every

third day for twice and every Night at Bedtime through the
whole Course; let her take an Anodyne made with one Ounce of
Diacodium.

Sydenham does not give his reason for letting blood or for the
purging which was also universally prescribed for climacteric syndrome.
Both were intended to reduce the tendency to 'plethora', which is what
was thought to cause the symptoms in the first place. Plethora, as the
name implies, was 'a morbid condition generated by excess of blood';
some considered that the blood itself was of poor quality, being 'full
of excrementitious matter' by reason of defective excretion of wastes
whether by inadequate sweating, salivation, defecation, urination or
menstruation. Purging and bleeding were to be practised if plethora was
suspected, in order to avoid haemorrhage, and as a measure to reduce
the violence of what was considered to be not the menstrual discharge
of blood without fibrin, but a haemorrhagic flow of whole blood. The
hysterics Sydenham describes was probably a reaction of sheer terror,
for heavy bleeding in younger women was too often a precursor of
death. Diacodium, by the way, is syrup of poppies.

John Pechey had already, in 1698, published Sydenham's therapy
as his own in *A Plain and Short Treatise of an Apoplexy, Convulsions,
Colick, Twisting of the Guts, … and several other Violent and Dangerous
Diseases*: his intention in doing so as stated in the Preface was that 'This
little Book may be an assistant to Charitable ladies and Gentlewomen
in the Country … here they may find plain directions, and the most
celebrated medecines.' He spells out the recipe for the 'common purging
potion' which is identical with that to be found at the beginning of
another translation of Sydenham's prescriptions, published in 1694 as
The Compleat Method of Curing Almost All Diseases:

Take of Tamarinds, half an Ounce, of Senna two Drams, of
Rhubarb one Dram and a half; infuse them in a sufficient quantity
of Fountain-water, and in three ounces of the strained liquid,
dissolve of Manna and Syrup of Roses solution, each one ounce.
(p. 23)

By 1701 Pechey was advertising his own purging pills at the end of his
translation of Sydenham's *Opera Universa* for sale at the relatively high

price of one shilling and sixpence. His were the antecedents of a long line of 'female pills' for self-medication which continued to be sold at high prices until the middle of the nineteenth century (Brown, 1977).

Though Sydenham's anatomical understanding was empirical and scientific, his prescribing seems to have been affected by the Paracelsian doctrine of sympathies; the most effective aspect of the ball of medicinal nougat that he instructs the apothecaries to confect for middle-aged ladies suffering heavy and continuous blood loss is that it is the colour of blood.

> Take of Conserve of dried Roses two Ounces, of Troches of Lemnian Earth one Dram and a Half, of Pomegranate-peel and Red-coral prepar'd, each two Scruples, of Blood-stone, Dragon's-blood and Bole Armenick, each one Scruple; make an Electuary with a sufficient quantity of simple Syrup of Coral; let her take the quantity of a large Nutmeg in the Morning, and at five in the Afternoon … (p. 338)

Earth from the island of Lemnos was not only considered to be astringent but was quite evidently red; nothing has more red colour than pomegranate; coral has no medical property beyond the associations of its fresh redness and the fact that in water it is an animal but exposed to air becomes a stone; syrup of coral is probably a herbal preparation, perhaps of coralwort, *Dentaria bulbifera*, which was taken as a powder in wine to stay fluxes; bloodstone, Pliny's heliotrope, was a kind of jasper streaked with red that was thought to have the property of staunching blood; dragon's blood, which was the red resin of a Mediterranean species of palm, is to be found in Queen Philippa's herbal as 'Sanguis draconis for women that have their terms too much'; 'bole armenick' was a pale red earth from Armenia used internally against fluxes of all kinds. Interestingly, when the recipe for this electuary appears in later pharmacopoeiae derived from Sydenham's, it is not recommended specifically for the metrorrhagia of menopause. What is striking about this list of ingredients is not just their colour but also their cost; all would have been available only from apothecaries and at very high prices.

With her red electuary the patient was required to drink 'six Spoonfuls of the following Julep' made up of workaday local materials in use for hundreds of years.

Take of the Waters of Oak-buds and Plantain, each three Ounces,
of Cinnamon water bordeated and of Syrup of dried Roses, each
one Ounce, of Spirit of Vitriol a sufficient quantity to make it
pleasantly acid. (338)

The product of distilling the buds of the oak tree just before it comes
into leaf had long been used by herbalists to 'stop all manner of fluxes in
man or woman' and 'The juice of plantain clarified … stays all manner
of fluxes, even women's courses, when they flow too abundantly'
(Culpeper, 1826). Sydenham's syrup of roses, cinnamon water and
vitriol was intended merely to disguise his julep's humble origins.
Time, effort and money were not to be spared in treating the sick lady
whose still-room must have been crowded with people preparing her
therapy. Sydenham ordered a second purge to be prepared adding to
plantain (*Plantago major*) stinging nettles, an invaluable astringent and
anti-haemorrhagic.

Take of the Leaves of Plantain and Nettles, each a sufficient
Quantity; beat them together in a Marble Mortar and press out the
Juice, then clarifie it: Let her take six spoonfuls cold three or four
times a day, after the first purge applie the following Plaister to the
Region of the Loins.
   Take of *Diapalma*, and of the Plaister ad *Herniam*, each equal
parts, mingle them and spread them on Leather. (Sydenham, 1701)

Diapalma was a desiccating mixture of palm oil, protoxide of
lead and sulphate of zinc, which Sydenham suggests mixing with
another compound used externally to shrink hernias, perhaps in some
understanding that the shrinking of the uterus which begins in the
peri-menopause will soon put a natural end to the metrorrhagia of
menopause and should be aided rather than opposed. Thus dosed with
her red electuary, her astringent julep, her red purge and her green,
resting under her plaster, 'the Sick' was allowed a treat, which seems
to have been an intrinsic part of popular treatments for menopausal
distress.

A cooling and thickening Diet must be order'd, only it will be
convenient to allow the Sick a small draught of Claret-wine, once or

twice a day, which tho 'tis somewhat improper, by reason 'tis apt to
raise the Ebullition, yet it may be allow'd to repair the strength; ...
this is very beneficial to Women thus affected ...

The cooling diet was part of the herb women's treatment for
menopause. When Madame de Sévigné was taking the waters at Aix
in 1675, her physician Pierre Bourdelot treated her with 'melons and
ice' (vol. I, p. 150), to the horror of her friends, who were sure the
treatment would kill her. The Marquise was forty-nine; it seems likely
that the treatment was intended for the metrorrhagia of menopause.
A few months later she was complaining of joint pains:

> ... the same stiff neck was in truth a very pretty fit of rheumatism;
> it is a disorder attended with violent pain and want of rest or sleep;
> but it gives no apprehension respecting the consequences. This is
> the eighth day; a gentle dose of medicine and a sudorific will restore
> me again. I have been bled once in the foot and now abstinence and
> patience will put the finishing stroke to the disorder. (I, p. 185)

The Marquise's discomfort was actually far from over, for the 'cure'
caused her to swell alarmingly and for many weeks she complained of
'flying pains' which may be a mistranslation of 'ardor volaticus', the
Latin name for hot flushes.

Given the labours of Sydenham and Pechey, it is curious that in
1988 the official historian of menopause, Joel Wilbush, D. Phil., Fellow
of the Royal College of Obstetricians and Gynaecologists of Canada,
affirms without any sign of doubt that 'the first reference in English to
discomforts associated with the female climacteric occurs in a guide for
women published early in the 18th century.' He is referring to *A Rational
Account of the Natural Weaknesses of Women and of Secret Distempers
peculiarly Incident to Them*, of which no copy of the first edition
survives. Wilbush cites it by the title of the third and seven subsequent
editions, *The Ladies' Physical Dispensary or a Treatise of all the Weaknesses,
Indispositions and Diseases Peculiar to the Female sex from Eleven Years of
Age to Fifty or Upwards*. He quotes from a later edition of 1739:

> ... between forty and fifty years of Age, their Courses begin first
> to dodge and at last to leave them; for then they are frequently

troubled with a Severe pain in the head and Back, and about the
Loins; oftimes also with Cholick Pains, Gripes, and Looseness,
at other Times with Vapours to a Violent Degree; likewise
with feverish Heats, wandering Rheumatic Pains and general
Uneasiness. (p. 1)

Though he gives his own recipes, the anonymous physician refuses to
identify some of the ingredients, such as his 'mineral powder', because
his main intention is to sell his own specifics. His account of the brewing
of his 'uterine drops' makes quite clear that it is beyond the scope of
even the best-equipped still room and quite justifies the enormous
price of three shillings and sixpence that he is asking. The sufferer
from metrorrhagia is to be let eight ounces of blood from the arm
and purged, as recommended by Sydenham, then given 'the Cooling
Anodyne Powder', the 'Restraining Electuary' and the 'Consolidating
Apozem', in all costing fifteen shillings and sixpence, and this at a time
when most middle-aged working women would have been earning
something like one pound a month. The anonymous man-midwife
gives no rationale for his treatment; his prescriptions are derived from
no pharmacopoeia, classic or otherwise, but he sternly admonishes his
clientele to accept no imitations.

Wilbush sees in this quack-salver's advertising pamphlet the
emergence of menopause into medical literature, which he relates to
increased rates of survival of women who, once they had reached the
age of twenty, were likely to live nearly ten years longer in 1730 than
they were in 1680. In truth the anonymous author is less interested
in advancing the state of medical knowledge than in exploiting the
newly emergent semi-literate female middle class. He makes use of no
authorities and, except to vilify a rival who plagiarised his own book and
increased its saleability by making references to female masturbation,
makes no reference to his medical colleagues, if indeed he was a qualified
physician at all. He contemptuously dismisses the remedies used by
'Midwives, Nurses and other Good Women who chiefly undertake the
Cure of the Secret Indispositions of the Female Sex' (1742, Sig A2).

Isinglass boiled in milk, Turpentine Pills, Clary fried with Eggs,
Arcangell Flowers, Armenian Bole, *vulgarly call'd* Bole Armonick,
Sperma Ceti, Confection of Alkermes, Penny-royal Water, *Dr*

Stephens Water, and compound Bryony water, *commonly called*
Hysterick Water *are in a manner their whole Magazine of Remedies.*

For diagnosticians the difficulty was to decide whether the cessation
of the monthly flow represented the natural cessation of ovarian
function or the suppression of the menses. Concern that the failure
of the menstrual flow led to the development of dangerous symptoms
persisted well into the nineteenth century. Pioneering psychiatrists
John Charles Bucknill and Daniel Hack Tuke in 1858 recorded in their
influential *Manual of Psychological Medicine* that 'amenorrhoea is a
frequent cause or consequence of, or concurrent phenomenon with
mental disease; and its removal leads to recovery of sanity' (p. 436).

The observation was essentially correct; Bucknill and Tuke are unusual
in that they confess that they do not understand the connection between
amenorrhoea and mental disturbance, but clearly they thought that if
you could correct the amenorrhoea your patient would recover her sanity.
Earlier doctors were not always so conservative or so rigorous. Though
both Sydenham and the anonymous author of *A Rational Account* did
not believe that the disorders of menopause were the direct result of
the failure of the menstrual discharge to cleanse the blood of 'excrementitious humours', most other male practitioners did. They treated
distress in the early part of the climacteric by setting up or encouraging
'vicarious menstruation'. Any bloody discharge in a menopausal patient
was to be encouraged and on no account to be stopped. If no such
discharge, from a bleeding ulcer, from haemorrhoids or from the nose,
for example, was to be observed, then a vein was to be opened and the
woman cupped, or leeches were to be applied to the anus or the groin.
Better still, a continuous issue could be provoked, by opening a wound
and keeping it open with setons, threads drawn through the flesh and
left in place. Though this approach is clearly derived from classic medical
literature, which was never relevant to female healing practice, Wilbush
attributes these invasive practices to women practitioners:

> Female healers first tried to ensure a continuation of natural
> 'excretion' by emmenagogues, leeches applied to the genitalia
> or, with the help of barber surgeons, directional phlebotomies.
> When these measures failed they opened other routes of excretion,
> purgation, issues, cauteries, setons or others. (pp. 2–3)

He quotes the example of the lady in Lesage's picaresque novel *Gil Blas*, who retained her youthful beauty by means of an issue in each buttock, and forgets to add that the issues in question were regularly opened by a male surgeon, which is the point of the scabrous episode.

All of these interventions were practised in fact by male practitioners, even distinguished male practitioners. Some went so far as to push the seton needle through the neck of the womb itself. Wilbush writes:

> Though treatment was far from pleasant, women were only too
> eager to follow it. Haunted by the threat of losing their sexual
> attraction, and with it much of their status, they were ready for any
> measures which promised results. (p. 3)

He cites no authority for this observation. What the scant evidence seems to show is rather that these grim procedures remained popular with doctors for more than a hundred years, despite the protests of their patients. Queen Victoria's obstetrician Sir Charles Locock, writing of the disorders of 'the dodging time' in *The Cyclopedia of Practical Medicine*, a compilation published in 1833, makes clear his own position:

> The production of artificial discharges by means of issues,
> setons or perpetual blisters, so much in vogue formerly, is now
> no longer fashionable, from the dislike patients have to such
> remedies; but viewing what is often effected naturally, we cannot
> doubt but that their more frequent employment would be highly
> advantageous.

Perhaps because he was under the impression that the torturers of menopausal women were other women, Wilbush is very ready to identify their medical treatments as the cause of their sufferings.

> Backache and pains 'about the loins' were probably due to
> emmenagogues, for these often affected the urinary tract causing
> strangury. 'Cholick pains, Gripes and Looseness' were due to
> purgatives, Headaches and 'Uneasiness', being general complaints,
> could be either functional or iatrogenic. The same applies to the
> vapours and, to some extent, to 'Rheumatik Pains' and 'Feverish
> Heats'. The iatrogenic character of the symptoms listed therefore

constitutes strong evidence of a tradition of treatment for
climacteric stress. (p. 3)

Wilbush is untroubled by any circularity in a position which identifies
climacteric syndrome by its symptoms and then accuses the (female)
people trying to deal with them of having caused them. In fact the
symptoms were both endogenic and iatrogenic; the worst suffering was
caused not by the women so contemptuously dismissed by the men-
midwives but by the grand doctors who regularly tortured monarchs
and their children like Indians at the stake, to adapt Macaulay's phrase.
Among literate women there was a strong tradition of distrust of doctors.
The painful surgical procedures inflicted on menopausal women were
justified principally by a masculine conviction that menopause was
'l'enfer des dames', hell on women. The purpose of such propaganda was,
as it is now, to create a vast and obscenely lucrative medical speciality.

The American doctor William P. Dewees noted that for some
months prior to the cessation of the menses there is more frequent
blood loss, sometimes very heavy blood loss, interspersed by long
periods with no losses. Unlike other doctors he did not treat the
amenorrhoea of menopause. Most of his treatments were for the
flooding of menopause, which was considered by him and the more
enlightened of his contemporaries as the only dangerous aspect of the
process. The consequences of metrorrhagia are vividly described by
Dewees: the patient 'becomes pale, debilitated and nervous; ... from
the too frequent returns of this discharge, or its too great abundance
...' (p. 146)

Dewees's treatments are for the most part conservative and sensible:
'... a milk and vegetable diet, together with pure water as a drink; regular
exercise not carried to fatigue; keeping the bowels open by well selected
food, as the fruits of the season in proper quantities; the bran bread
if necessary, but not by medicine, unless absolutely required' (p. 149).
During heavy bleeding the patient was to lie down, and all motion,
even turning in bed, was forbidden. The room was to be kept cool, all
food and drink was to be cold and ice-packs were to be laid against the
woman's body. Her legs and feet, however, should not be permitted to
get cold. What seems less conservative and sensible is the dosing of the
patient with 'two or three grams of the acetate of lead, every hour or
two, guarded with a sufficient quantity of opium or laudanum' (p. 150).

To prevent 'excessive return', bloodletting and other poisons, extract of 'Cicuta' (*Cicuta virosa*, Water Hemlock) were necessary and 'all kinds of liquor, and spices should be absolutely forbidden'.

Dewees was very well aware that he had little success in controlling excessive bleeding in menopausal women, and he gives a curious and very rare glimpse of an alternative practitioner who was more successful than he. He tells us that one of his patients 'was told by some old woman that hiera picra was a certain cure for her complaint'. 'Hiera picra' was a name given to many preparations in the ancient Greek pharmacopoeiae. The name means 'holy bitters' and describes a purgative compound of aloes and cinnamon bark which was in constant use for hundreds of years. Hiera picra figures in Timothie Bright's clister for melancholy, along with Marshmallows, Hollyhocks, Pellitory of the Wall, Camomile, Hops, Melitot and other plants decocted in ale or beer with honey 'wherein Rosemarie-flowers have been steeped' (p. 262). Dewees did not scruple to express his contempt for such 'hickery-pickery' (for the name was synonymous with quackery), but to his chagrin the 'old woman' cited two cases that she had treated successfully. Dewees was honest enough to interview the ladies who 'warmly recommended' the treatment, which was half an ounce of hiera picra dissolved in a pint of gin, a wine glass to be taken at bedtime. His patient took it and was drunk all night and sick all the next day; that evening she tried again, thinking her reaction the second time might not be so bad, and suffered equally (p. 152). Dewees had pills made up in which a much smaller dose of hiera picra was mixed with oil of cloves and syrup of rhubarb, which procured the desired result.

The first whole book on the menopause was *Conseils aux Femmes de l'Epoque de l'Age de Retour* by Charles François Menville de Ponsan, which appeared in 1839, and in a second edition as *De l'Age critique chez les Femmes* in 1840. Menville de Ponsan believed that the last death throes of the womb caused the inconvenient symptoms that women experienced. The physician's job was to correct the derangement of the nerves and the digestion, which in any case was temporary; 'The critical age passed, women have the hope of a longer life than men, their thought acquires more precision, more scope and vitality' (p. 47).

Samuel Ashwell, writing a few years later, noted that women of the plethoric type 'who have been healthy prior to the change often become corpulent after its completion and are more than usually liable to attacks of apoplexy, paralysis, pulmonary obstruction and cough'. Nevertheless he did not approve of the measures taken to reduce plethora.

> I have now under my care a lady who has ceased to menstruate
> for three or four years, and who, by the adoption of a spare and
> vegetable diet and the almost daily use of purgatives throughout
> the whole time, has become gradually so exhausted, irritable and
> neuralgic that her life is a burden. (p. 200)

Ashwell's therapy for women whose menstruation had not yet ceased included purgatives, small bleedings, exercise and abstinence from 'wine, spirits and malt liquor'. So frequently do the ladies' doctors repeat the prohibition of alcohol, it seems reasonable to suspect that there was a popular tradition that encouraged women suffering menopausal distress to drink more than was usually thought proper.

> I have lately attended several cases of decided insanity consequent
> on the improper use of wine and spirits during the period of
> catamenial decline … In one … these stimulants had been
> employed in the hope that they would relieve the languor and
> depression. The affection assumed all the characters of violent
> mania; eventually however subsiding into what we feared would
> be incurable madness. Nevertheless the patient entirely recovered
> in two years: the efficient remedies being *frequent* leechings of the
> cervix uteri, moderate purgatives, nutritious diet with malt liquor
> and light wines, and extreme tranquillity in the country. (p. 202)

Gin, which is sometimes called 'mother's ruin', is assumed on that ground, and because it is flavoured with juniper berries, to have been a specific in procuring abortion. It is more likely, on linguistic and medical grounds, that the name refers to the fact that women of menopausal age were encouraged to use gin to combat 'low spirits', whereas alcohol is generally prohibited to women of breeding age. For a visible number of middle-aged women, alcohol dependency was the fairly rapid outcome.

Ashwell also implies that the theory of 'vicarious menstruation' was not yet dead and the provocation of blood loss was still being practised: he prefers less wrong-headed procedures 'as mustard hip baths and pediluvia, frictions with stimulating embrocations, and the flesh brush, the continuance of sexual intercourse, and the encouragement by any gentle means of the catamenial flow' (p. 201). His recommendation of sexual intercourse for middle-aged women is highly unusual, as we shall see.

No sooner had the menopause attracted the attention of professional gentlemen than they began competing with each other, belittling each other's theories and methods, writing books to justify (and to publicise) their own practice, and perfecting a bedside manner that would bring society ladies of a certain age flocking to their rooms. Edward John Tilt is a perfect example of the ladies' doctor. After studying at St George's Hospital in London he went on to qualify in Paris where, through the efforts of Gardanne, Menville, Moreau de la Sarthe, Brierre du Boismont and Dusourd, awareness of climacteric syndrome was much higher than in England. After travelling as the family physician with the family of Count Shuvaloff, he settled in London in 1850 and practised there as a fashionable ladies' doctor.

Tilt strongly disagreed with those of his medical contemporaries who declared that nothing significant happened in the 'seventh septenniad' of women's lives, quoting Brierre de Boismont's sample of 107 women of whom eighty suffered considerably, and his own experience of 539 women of whom he had 'only met 39 who have not suffered'. On the other hand he refused to espouse the view that the menopause was in itself dangerous. His descriptions of the climacteric in *The Change of Life in Health and Disease* published in 1857 are based upon the rare practice of listening to women themselves and are thoroughly sensible. Tilt saw the climacteric as a period of exceptional somatic stress, out of which 'arise a beautiful series of critical movements, the object of which is to endow woman with a greater degree of strength than she previously enjoyed' (p. 4). He noted that older women were far less prone to infection than younger ones and had greater endurance than women who were still subject to the demands of menstruation, pregnancy and childbirth. He saw a new role for older women as the guardians of the mothers and the arbiters of taste and manners, but their accession to it required time: 'Nature cannot work at a railway pace,' he writes. 'A habit of 32 years cannot be interrupted without periods of hesitation, trial and infirmity previous to health being regained' (p. 116).

It would never have occurred to Tilt to try to postpone or counteract the natural processes of the climacteric. A womb that is shrinking should not be stimulated; ladies who might be contemplating matrimony at this time were considered by him to be risking their physical and mental health. He quotes examples of middle-aged women treated for occluded menses, when actually they had ceased to ovulate, who were driven into melancholy and mania after a series of heavy breakthrough bleeds. Whenever Tilt encountered, in the absence of an external stimulus, increased sexual interest in a middle-aged woman he immediately suspected the cause to be pathological, and he had found diseases of the womb often enough to be confirmed in his suspicions. In the case where an external stimulus was to be found, the uterine excitation of courtship put the woman's life in danger. At no time does Tilt refer to the sexual demands of a husband. His sole concern is for the woman herself. In each case he built up a picture of the patient's entire reproductive career starting with her experiences at puberty, and he treated each one in a manner suited to her type, which he classified under one of three heads, 'plethoric', 'chlorotic' or 'nervous'.

'Visiting different medicated springs' was, according to Tilt, 'at once the most agreeable and effectual mode of restoring health at the change of life'. This was no more than orthodoxy, and popular orthodoxy at that; ladies of a certain age were a conspicuous proportion of the floating population of Bath and Tunbridge Wells long before the baths were roofed over and became places of fashionable resort. Dr Tilt liked to send his patients further afield, to Aix-en-Savoie, now better known as Aix-les-Bains, 'combining varied medicated waters with good society and a country abounding in beautiful scenery'. His patients were also encouraged to avoid sexual excitement, to take a tepid bath three times weekly and to spend several hours each day 'on the sofa'. They should eat less, take only 'one dinner' a day and avoid red meat. Dietary restrictions upon older people have a long and mostly unwritten history. Though the medical establishment may have had little understanding of or interest in the physiology of ageing, it seems likely that the carers, the women upon whom the care of older people devolved, did understand the changing dietary needs of older people.

Tilt is adamant about the inappropriateness of alcohol as a treatment for the climacteric syndrome 'by which a temporary support only can be obtained at the expense of an increase in the faintness, flushing and nervous symptoms' (p. 123). His aim is to help the organism to do what it was already trying to do and speed the accomplishing of the change. Like his predecessors, in the case of heavy bleeding in the peri-menopause he recommends bleeding by venesection or by leeching, but only for patients of the 'plethoric' type. By our standards Tilt was rather too keen on administering purgatives. The preferred sedatives for those of his patients who were 'driven to the verge of insanity by ovario-uterine excitement' were camphor, lupulin, opium and Henbane 'whether given as an extract in pills, or a topic in plaster' (p. 97). When it comes to Henbane Tilt insists on using the fresh extract, pressed out of the macerated plant, but unfortunately he gives no hint of the degree of dilution, and Henbane is highly poisonous. Camphor is obtained by distilling the aged wood of the camphor tree, *Cinnamomum camphora*, which is indigenous to China and Japan. Its medical properties had been known since Avicenna (980–1037); in the twelfth century the Abbess Hildegard of Bingen used it. In the eighteenth century 'camphire' was considered an ideal antimanic. Inhaled it relieved fainting fits and convulsions; rubbed on the skin it caused inflammation and was used as a counter-irritant; taken internally it caused vomiting, diarrhoea and sweating, and 'exhilarated' or, in larger doses, 'refrigerated' the nervous system; in larger doses still it functioned as convulsive therapy. It is not immediately obvious why Tilt should say that camphor 'was made for women with whom it always agrees, while it always disagrees with men' (p. 105), but it has been used internally as a sedative in cases of hysteria, as well as abating convulsions and epileptic fits. In Cuba it used to be used as an anaphrodisiac, which together with its use in cases of 'hysteria' seems to indicate that it was thought to act directly on the uterus.

Tilt prescribes 'lupulin' or extract of Hops (*Humulus lupulus*) because of its function as a soporific and, as he thought, anaphrodisiac. He favoured pessaries and instillation through the anus as a way of administering sedatives. Not all his chosen specifics were as respectable as the ones discussed above; he was not shy of using opium or belladonna, or Epsom salts, or sulphur 'for all the diseases of ageing'. He had also succumbed to the Swiss enthusiasm for cherry laurel water, which is prepared from the leaves of *Prunus laurocerasus* by distillation. Its function as a sedative, which would be due to the presence of cyanide derivatives, has never been demonstrated and the preparation is now considered too dangerous for use.

Generally Tilt's attitude was in complete contrast to the modern approach which treats menopausal distress as a deficiency disease. He would have thought it unethical and mischievous to dose women with hormones so that they would continue to experience or respond to sexual desire. He prescribed ambergris 'to withstand the overexciting effects of the present civilisation on the nervous system by deadening the reproductive stimulus which only lingers on to disturb health'. As he understood it, the processes of the menopause were as natural as the processes of childbirth and his job was to make both easier. If the body sweated excessively during menopause, the treatment was not to attempt to dry up or inhibit the secretion but to encourage it, principally by bathing, for the warm bath functioned as 'a giant poultice' for the whole body. He was not keen on the application of leeches to the cervix, or on the use of counter-stimulants and blistering, as favoured by Ashwell, and he returned again and again to the most popular and successful treatment of all:

> Travelling is a great strengthener of the nervous system, for it places the patient in entirely new circumstances, every one of which makes a fresh call on her attention, solicits her interests, captivates her faculties, and completely leads her from trains of thought, to which, perhaps, she had been long enchained. (p. 127)

In 1885, three years before he died of diabetes at the age of forty-seven, Dr J. Milner Fothergill published *The Diseases of Sedentary and Advanced Life: A Work for Medical and Lay Readers*, in which he spelt out his own attitudes towards 'the change of life'.

> ... females at the change of life, or the menopause, are often in feeble health. They are not infrequently stout, with flabby muscles; the heart, being a muscle, is weak; and there is an incapacity for exertion, with palpitation on effort. The nervous system is often debilitated, and self-control is impaired, and the sufferer becomes pettish or fretful, or irritable or nervous. (p. 113)

Dr Fothergill would have been incensed if anyone had taken an equally uncharitable view of his own poor health. He was in fact mountainously obese and notoriously bad-tempered.

> The bowels are apt to become irregular, while the diet becomes capricious. As to the uterine functions, the changes in them take

various directions. Sometimes a barren wife becomes a mother, like
Sarah of old, when all hope of offspring is dying out. Or a widow
or spinster, who hitherto has led a decorous life, suddenly develops
strong erotic tendencies … (pp. 113–14)

Perhaps because he was tormented by gout, Fothergill tended to see it
everywhere. Painful menstruation in the peri-menopause was probably
caused by 'latent or suppressed gout'. Moreover, he argued, 'Flatulence
is not rarely also present; and then this adds to the disturbance of the
heart, and aggravates the condition of nervousness present. Attacks of
breathlessness, or palpitation, come on at other times than upon effort.
Sometimes they are set up by flatulence; possibly at other times they are
set up by latent gout affecting the vaso-motor nerves. Or the patient
wakens up, with one or both, out of her sleep, and is gravely alarmed
…' (p. 114). The only preventative of such derangement is 'a regulated
regimen' and light food.

A generous wine may be indicated; and some stimulant be at hand
when attacks of palpitation, etc., come on. It is well to lie down
when not feeling well, so as to limit the demand upon the body
powers. Some tonic should be given, as digitalis and strychnia,
or lily of the valley or belladonna, and be combined with a
carminative, or cascarilla, or other aromatic. (p. 115)

Though the bowels must be kept open, the menopausal lady is not to
be distressed by griping and she is to drink nothing cold.

If these matters be not attended to, the lady will be very liable
to change her medical adviser, until she finds some one who
understands her condition, and her requirements. (p. 115)

Fothergill appears more concerned that he might lose a patient than
that the treatments he offers be effective (in which case he would lose
a patient). With or without the benefit of an adviser the climacteric
eventually passes:

After the perturbations of the menopause are past and over, woman
passes into a period of calm; relieved from those tumults which

mark the period of her reproductive life, and continues an almost
sexless existence; except in very rare cases, of which the illustrious
George Eliot was an unfortunate instance. (p. 115)

It is slightly shocking to discover that Dr Fothergill, in a work
published for the general reading public only four years after her death,
does not shrink from identifying George Eliot as a fatality caused by
unseasonable passion. He may indeed have been baiting his superiors,
for sixty-year-old Eliot did seek medical advice before she accepted the
marriage proposal of Johnny Cross, who was twenty years her junior. On
19 April 1880 the distinguished surgeon Sir James Paget called on her and,
after a long consultation, advised her to accept (Haight, 1969, p. 536).

The happy couple were on honeymoon in Venice, when Johnny Cross,
who never before or since showed any signs of mental derangement,
jumped from the balcony of their hotel room into the Grand Canal.
He was pulled out by gondoliers, given chloral to calm him, and
Eliot telegraphed for his brother Willie to come and help nurse him.
He recovered, and they continued on their trip through Austria and
Germany. Cross lived on until 1924 but 'the illustrious George Eliot'
died a few months later. The Venice incident was given out as an
intestinal complaint. (For further discussion of George Eliot's marriage
to Johnny Cross, see p. 333.) Though Eliot's biographer, Haight, did not
discover the truth until 1968, Fothergill takes for granted that George
Eliot did feel a sexual passion for her husband and is not in the least
reluctant to make her an example of fatal uterine excitement.

By the turn of the century women were already being dosed with
the extracts of animal glands, most of which were inert. Doctors had
become intensely aware of fibroids, which they were attempting to
extirpate by highly experimental and often quite dangerous methods,
including surgical hysterectomy, castration by X-ray, and ablation of
the endometrium by electrocautery. Though the learned gentlemen
would have rebuffed the charge that they hated and feared the womb as
much as any old medieval celibate, they inflicted outrages upon it in so
exemplary and inventive a fashion as to defy explanation. No matter how
grisly the procedure, there was never any shortage of middle-aged ladies
delighted to discover that their womb was the cause of all their woes and
prepared not only to undergo torture by uterine sound, by curette and
by electrified rod, but to pay through the nose for the privilege.

10

The Treatments – Alternative

If the traditional medical procedures of alleviating the sufferings of the menopausal woman by blasting her body with purges and vomits, inducing copious sweats, letting blood, sometimes in enormous quantities, to the point of inducing convulsions and syncope, worked at all, it seems they must have worked as aversion therapy, or maybe shock treatment. Perhaps a patient felt relief when the treatment had run its violent course simply because the assault upon her body was over. When alternative, exotic and sometimes even bizarre systems of health care were advertised, women of a certain age were among the first to offer themselves as suitable cases for treatment.

Common to many alternative treatments is the idea that the body is not a hostile entity, with an innate tendency to go painfully wrong, but a homeostatic mechanism which will cure itself of most disorders, if given a chance. Coupled with this notion there is often a corollary, that modern civilisation is hostile to the demands of the body, exposing it to toxic levels of stress, as well as a multitude of environmental poisons. The typical alternative view that 'We become ill when we violate nature's laws' is not actually tenable. The sufferer from malaria or sleeping sickness is obeying a natural law which decrees that the malarial parasite or tripanosome can survive only within his body. The diseases of ageing also follow a natural law: all that is born must die. Nevertheless most of us would accept the paired dicta of Hippocrates that the body should be aided in its self-adjustment and that the cure should not be more destructive than the disease. The most abused word in this spectrum is 'natural'.

Though life in the non-industrialised countries is shorter and more painful than life in the industrialised world, most of us would agree that industrialisation and urbanisation have consequences deleterious to health. The middle-aged woman who understands that she needs plenty of exercise if she is to minimise the risk of developing osteoporosis can do very little about it if she lives in a city where she can't take long walks in safety or without stifling in traffic fumes. If on the other hand she is a labourer in rural India she has no choice but to walk long distances with a load on her head, which will keep her skeleton healthy, at a cost. (Recent studies have shown that her poor diet results in low bone density, but the predicted fractures do not occur.) The city-dwelling woman who has no job is doomed to become a couch potato; if she has an office job, she must suffer all the inconveniences of sedentary office life and commuter travel, neither of which is what the alternative doctor would order. Given the fact that most women have no chance of fulfilling the basic conditions of alternative health care, most are best advised to try to take advantage of the only treatment the establishment can offer for climacteric syndrome and the inconveniences of ageing, namely HRT, a drastic therapy for a brutalised lifestyle.

With the onset of menopause one thing becomes clear, that is, that we must work at being healthy. We can no longer abuse the organism and get away with it. A positive commitment to health might involve the decision to move away from the city, but people who have grown up in an urban environment could find life intolerably dull or arduous if suddenly transplanted to the country. Still, there are strategies for self-purification that can profitably be undertaken without moving away from overcrowding and pollution. Among the rites of passage that the middle-aged woman can choose for herself there should be the ceremony of renouncing her addictions. Sugar and tobacco, as well as coffee, tea and alcohol, exacerbate vasomotor disturbance, so the time of hot flushing is the ideal time to give them all up. Alcohol burns off the small post-menopausal oestrogen supply and interferes with calcium metabolism; evening primrose oil, usually suggested to women as an oestrogen precursor, might be more important to menopausal women for the function signified by its botanical name, Oenothera, as a counteractive to alcohol. Coffee and salt can cause calcium to be excreted and should be banned from the middle-aged woman's regimen. Taking calcium supplements by mouth is no way to compensate for failure to eschew coffee, salt and alcohol, being more likely to cause kidney stones than to prevent bone resorption. Nevertheless commercially available food supplements recommended for post-menopausal women almost always include some version or another of calcium.

It is the most difficult thing in the world to tail off an addiction; a dramatic renunciation often works much better. The most dramatic renunciation of bad food habits is giving up food altogether, that is to say, fasting. Fasting is no more difficult than acquiring, preparing, serving and eating food, not to mention clearing up after it. Fasting might sound duller than eating, but the processes of excretion that are activated by fasting are quite dramatic, spectacular enough to take your mind off what you are not eating. Many alternative health regimes involve longer or shorter periods of fasting, intended as jolts that will cause the system to jump the rails of a noxious habit and enter upon proper self-regulation. Alternative practitioners will tell you not to fast without supervision; indeed, some will want to you fast from everything but distilled water for weeks at a time in a hospital. Linda Burfield Hazzard is thought to have starved to death more than forty of the patients who attended her sanatorium in Olalla, Washington State in the 1890s and early twentieth century. In 1912 she was convicted of manslaughter in the case of Claire Williamson who weighed only 50 pounds when she died. Hazzard was found to have forged her will and stolen all her valuables. She was sentenced to a term of from two to twenty years' imprisonment, released after two years and then, inexplicably, given a full pardon. Her death in 1938 is thought to have been caused by her trying her fasting cure upon herself.

Herbert Shelton's Health School in San Antonio, Texas, was only one of a dozen set up in the US in the 1940s where patients were confined to their rooms and obliged to rest while fasting: many of the patients had 'vainly spent years seeking cure of relief from orthodox medical sources'. These patients were 'usually women in their 50's or 60's' who saw the fasting cure 'perhaps as a final opportunity to turn the tide of deteriorating health' (Roth, p. 21). Such a regimen is every bit as punitive as the tortures devised for complaining women by conventional allopathic medicine. In 1978 49-year-old William F. Carlton checked into Shelton's Health School to be treated for his ulcerative colitis. After twenty-nine days on nothing but distilled water, he had lost more than sixty pounds and his life. He was the sixth person to die while undergoing treatment at the school. Four years later a federal court jury awarded \$872,000 in damages to his wife and children and Dr Shelton's Health School was closed.

The notion of 'fasting to save your life' has never quite gone away. According to American neuroscientist Mark Mattson, 'intermittent fasting results in increased production of brain-derived neurotrophic factor (BDNF), which increases the resistance of neurons in the brain to dysfunction and degeneration in animal models of neurodegenerative disorders; BDNF signaling may also mediate beneficial effects of intermittent fasting on glucose regulation and cardiovascular function.' It makes no odds that Herbert Shelton himself was incapacitated by an unnamed degenerative disease, probably Parkinson's, for ten years before he died.

The average middle-aged woman has quite enough common sense to decide how she will fast and for how long; if the decision is hers she is much more likely to carry it out. Many religions require the faithful not involved in childbearing or heavy labour to fast one day a week. One day a week on nothing but water will do no harm and may do good. Naturopaths recommend aiding the body in the excretion of toxins during fasting by the use of a long-handled 'skin brush' to stimulate the circulation under the skin. Another way of doing the same thing is to take a sauna bath and gently switch the skin with bundles of soft young birch twigs. In Scandinavia these are gathered in the spring and stored in the deep freeze, to be taken out a day or two before the planned sauna, when they will bud.

Many alternative therapies take time and determination to follow, and can absorb the mental energy that otherwise might be spent hankering after old addictions. Instead of longing for a sweet or chocolate or a cigarette, the woman who is looking for a change can follow one of the simplest and oldest ways of purifying the body, by drinking lots of water. Because drinking lots of our tap water could be a way not only of flushing out the kidneys and bladder but of ingesting large quantities of chlorine and nitrates, the self-purifying ritual should involve efficient filtration of tap water or finding alternative sources of H_2O. Developing a discriminating taste in water and finding the perfect water can be every bit as demanding as choosing wine; it is, moreover, a good deal cheaper. People who have grown up on chlorinated recycled water imagine that water is at best tasteless, but people who have never had piped water know the different characters of the different springs in their area, and are well able to distinguish what water comes from where. Once your palate is so refined that you can distinguish the different tastes of untreated water, you are in a fair way to have detoxified yourself.

Since the beginning of human history springs have been endowed with sacred, magic and medicinal properties. The therapeutic effects of drinking spring water with a high mineral content have been understood since the earliest times; where the water that gushed so inexplicably from the earth was unsuitable for drinking, the human animal found other ways of using it to relieve aches and pains, or to clean infections and parasites off the skin. Copper Age (4500–3500 BCE) implements have been found in sulphur baths on the island of Malta. Sea-bathing was used for similar purposes. Before entering the salt water, patients often buried themselves in the hot pebbles or sand or mud of the beach. Older women have always constituted a significant proportion of the clientele at mineral baths and seawater bathing establishments. Sixty years ago, groups of grandmothers were the only people to be seen on the beaches of Calabria and Sicily. Middle-aged women may be shy of exhibiting themselves on today's crowded beaches but swimming is one kind of exercise that the city-bound woman should take if possible.

Hydrotherapy, the system of self-medication based upon a belief in the healing properties of plain water, is one of the earliest of the alternative systems of medical care. It may consist in 'applications of hot and cold water, either externally or internally in the form of baths, packs, compresses, sprays and douches or sitz-baths (hip) in which the lower half of the body is immersed in hot or cold water, while the feet are put in water of a contrasting temperature' (Westkott, p. 140). Hydrotherapy developed in reaction to the conditions prevailing at the fashionable spas, including the spread of contagion from diseased persons, exposure to the elements, shortage of attendants, lack of privacy and offences against modesty brought about by the lack of dressing facilities and the mingling of the sexes (Donegan, 1986).

Private use of cold-water baths as a treatment was first advocated by John Floyer in *Psychrolusia, or History of Cold-Bathing*, initially published in London in 1702 and five times subsequently by 1722. Floyer's were ideas whose time had come; he was followed by the author identified as 'John Smith', who published *The Curiosities of Common Water* in 1723, with a reprint in Boston. Tobias Smollett was a follower, if we may believe his *Essay on the External Use of Water* (1752). According to John Wesley in *Primitive Physic, or an Easy and Natural Method of Curing Most Diseases*, first published anonymously in 1747, 'Cold bathing is of great advantage to health; it prevents abundance of diseases. It promotes perspiration, helps the circulation of the blood; and prevents the danger of catching cold.' The great prophet of the water-cure as a panacea, however, is Vincent Priessnitz, who developed a whole system of wetting and sweating. In 1826 he opened a water-cure centre at Gräfenberg in Silesia; there he applied a regimen which involved not only the water-cures but also plenty of fresh air and exercise and a diet of coarse, heavy food, invariably served cold. By 1840 he had accumulated a clientele of the rich and great, who were astonished at the improvement in their condition. In America hydropathy became an enduring craze that claimed a million followers (King). Now called hydrotherapy, it is unlikely to be encountered anywhere but in veterinary practice.

The next of the more venerable European alternative therapies is homeopathy, a system of treatment devised by Samuel Hahnemann in the early nineteenth century. The homeopathic approach to discomforts of ageing and the climacteric is first of all to relate the symptoms to a complete profile of the sufferer. It is assumed that symptoms are generated by the body's own response to factors operating upon it. By imitating the distorted function, the homeopathic treatment of opposing like with like makes it possible for the organism to cease its deranged operation. An inflammatory condition will be treated, for example, by an inflammatory substance. Which inflammatory substance will be decided upon the basis of the patient profile. All the remedies consist of minute traces of the active agent to be taken in granule form on an empty stomach. Before any homeopathic treatment the patient must renounce all toxins, including coffee, tea, alcohol and nicotine. A homeopathic practitioner who does not insist upon this as a condition of prescribing is wasting his patient's time and money. At first the remedy may cause the symptoms to worsen, in which case it is the right remedy. As the original symptoms retreat, the remedy should be taken in smaller and smaller quantities until it is discontinued altogether. The effectiveness of homeopathic prescribing may be no more than a combination of detoxification and the placebo effect; however, I have found it effective for treating disorders in animals, when neither needed to be taken into account.

The first person to use hypnosis in treating the sick was Franz Anton Mesmer. He was trained as a philosopher, and graduated MD from Vienna in 1766 with a treatise on the influence of heavenly bodies upon human health. He followed the English physician Richard Mead in describing the influence that the sun and moon appeared to exert as 'animal gravitation'. His first experiments consisted of placing magnets on the affected parts; when he found he could obtain the same astonishing results with his hands he coined the term 'animal magnetism' to explain the mechanism. When his colleagues in Vienna rejected him, he took his discoveries and his practice to Paris, where he elaborated his theories and his treatments. Patients sat in a darkened room, and to the strains of soft music were connected up to an enormous tub of magnetic fluid by iron branches passing through its perforated lid; the aim was to induce a trance-like state that would in turn lead to healing convulsions. When he set up a Society of Harmony to train other practitioners, the French medical establishment demanded an investigation of his claims, which dismissed the very idea of magnetic fluids in the body. None could deny the effectiveness of his treatments; eventually it was understood, though not by Mesmer, that hypnosis worked through the mind and not through bodily fluids.

Hypnosis is still used, not only for mental disorders but in the treatment of complex physical symptoms, including climacteric syndrome. The marked placebo effect in HRT trials suggests that hypnosis would have a marked effect upon the patient's subjective impression of well-being and this in turn would stimulate her internal secretions. Dr Caroline M. Shreeve, author of *Overcoming the Menopause Naturally*, published in 1987 and still in print, would recommend that the woman with sexual difficulties at menopause 'seek out a hypnotherapist' because 'Stress reactions, and anxiety, coupled with an inability to relax, lie at the heart of very many psychological disturbances, phobias and anxieties that arise in women in their forties and fifties.'

Investigation of the effectiveness of hypnosis in dealing with hot flashes has been taken up rather more recently by the team led by Gary Elkins, Professor of Psychology and Neuroscience at Baylor University in Texas. In September 2015, a review by a panel of experts commissioned by the North American Menopause Society reported that of all the alternative treatments available for the distresses of menopause, hypnosis was the only one that could be seen to be effective. One study showed that women who had hypnotherapy five times a week had a dramatic reduction in the number and severity of hot flashes (Carpenter et al.). Hypnotherapists advertising on the internet quote £70–£90 per session, which would place hypnotherapy beyond most women's means.

Autohypnosis is certainly cheaper than hypnotherapy and both Professor Elkins and Dr Shreeve give rather more importance to it. In one example Shreeve describes, a 53-year-old widow hypnotises herself by, after bathing, relaxing in a dimly lit room and concentrating on a candle-flame, counting backwards to ten, telling herself that she is going further and further into trance. When she is in a trance and can see herself in her mind's eye, she tells herself: 'I am cool and calm. My memory is getting better and better. I feel happy, serene and relaxed' and she believes herself. The key it seems is relaxation, which may be achieved not only by hypnosis or autohypnosis but by 'autogenic training', in which the subject is taught first how to stretch all her muscles, and then let them go limp, until she is completely floppy and concentrating on the physical process of breathing, when she is to visualise individual parts of her body and tell herself how they feel, so that she experiences them that way. In 2003 an issue of *Women's Health Issues* was given over to 'mind control of menopause', and familiarity with the techniques is increasing. MP3s and CDs available online for self-hypnosis include a 'A Menopausal Relief Set' of four for $49.94.

Other ways of exerting mind over matter include yoga, meditation transcendental and otherwise, and biofeedback. One thing is common to all of them: if they are to work the woman herself must make a positive commitment to them. The methods simply systematise the woman's own attempt to take control of the situation and herself: all are different ways of doing the same thing, examples, not of right and wrong therapies, effective and ineffective, but of the different strokes natural to different folks. Women who are unable to 'discipline themselves' in the matter of alcohol, nicotine, caffeine or food abuse find it easy once they have made an investment of time and mental energy in a system of self-regulation. Instead of saying no to a host of compulsive behaviours, they are saying yes to a new idea of self. They are born again without religion. Traditionally, of course, women past their childbearing were born again within religion; they fasted and meditated and prayed to something outside themselves, but when they did it wholeheartedly the result in terms of tranquillity and detachment was probably similar.

Therapies which require the woman to submit to another person's control, allow herself to be put into trance, or needles to pierce her flesh, or pressure to be placed upon her feet, her ear lobes, her acupuncture points, or her joints to be manipulated or her body to be anointed with aromatic oils, will not perform the function of persuading her that the locus of control is within herself which, psychologists tell us, is essential to well-being. The climacteric is the time of taking control; part of the shock of the climacteric is the cold-water effect of discovering that one has no choice but to do so. Having professional alternative therapists work upon one's body can be very pleasant; the uncaressed woman may well feel invigorated after her skin has been stroked and gently pummelled. If the treatment has cost a good deal of money the woman has an interest in making it work. If the woman has no money she will not be able to afford hours of massage or acupuncture or psychotherapy, no matter how much she would like it.

Lately there has been a push to promote acupuncture as a treatment for hot flashes. A study led by Dr Nancy Avis at the Wake Forest Baptist Medical Center in the US recruited women who had an average of four hot flashes or night sweats a night and divided them into two groups, one of which received twenty acupuncture treatments over six months and the other 'no acupuncture or any other alternative remedies'. Nearly half of the acupuncture group reported a 47 per cent drop in the frequency of flashes within eight weeks, 4 per cent thought themselves cured completely, but more than a third reported an improvement of less than 10 per cent. In Britain the initial acupuncture treatment will cost between £50 and £70 and subsequent treatments between £35 and £50 each.

The best way to approach the climacteric is to be in shape. At this time of life food needs are declining sharply. The menopausal woman should cut down her total food intake, and avoid protein and cholesterol. Discomfort at night can be eased to some extent by common-sense measures like eating less at the evening meal. A spoonful of honey at bedtime can help to raise night blood-sugar levels and avoid waking in fright.

It is probably inevitable that alternative treatments of menopause distress overlap with strategies for mitigating the effects of ageing. Most modern rejuvenation therapy was devised by men for men. One of the advantages of eternal youth, after all, is that it enables the successful senior male to enjoy all the young females who fall to his lot. Historically, many of the seekers after eternal youth were convinced that they could steal youth from another living creature by destroying it and absorbing some part of its living body. Stories abound of despots who had young virgins killed in order that they might stay young by drinking or bathing in their blood. Others merely inhaled the breath of young girls or sucked milk from their breasts.

Murder and cannibalism are not within the range of privileges allotted to civilised man; the later purveyors of eternal youth plundered non-human species. Rajahs afflicted with torpor and general debility ate the testicles of tigers. From 1889 when Professor Charles Brown-Séquard, who was seventy-two years old, injected himself with an extract of animal testes and proclaimed himself rejuvenated, the emphasis has been upon virility. Brown-Séquard was followed by Arnold Lorant, author of *Old Age Deferred*. Serge Voronoff transplanted hundreds of glands from the testicles of chimpanzees, popularly known as 'monkey glands', into the scrota of human males. Alexis Carrel believed that 'man' wore out prematurely because of insecurity, overwork and an inappropriate nutrition. Ilya Metchnikoff believed that ageing was caused by the ravages of intestinal bacteria and recommended daily ingestion of yoghurt to neutralise them, encouraged perhaps by the extraordinary longevity of Georgian peasants who eat yoghurt every day. Alexander Bogomolets, who is believed to have injected Stalin with his elixir, antireticulocytotoxic serum, in attempt to prolong his effective life, held that:

> A man of sixty or seventy is still young. He has then lived only half of his natural life. Old age can be treated just as any other illness because what we are accustomed to regard as old age is actually an abnormal, premature phenomenon. (Hannon, p. 50)

The most successful elixir of youth was the saline solution of fresh cells from the organs of lamb foetuses which was injected into degenerating tissues in what was known as Niehans's cellular therapy. A 1990 article in *In Health* magazine described Paul Niehans as a 'public relations genius' and stated that the Clinique La Prairie, which he had founded in Clarens-Montreux, Switzerland, had attracted 65,000 patients. The average age of Niehans's patients was forty-five. In his view men began to age at sixty when glandular secretions began to fail; women's biological age was determined by menopause ten years or more earlier.

Niehans treated thousands of powerful men and a few women, among them Gloria Swanson, Queen Victoria Eugenia of Spain, Marlene Dietrich, the Gish Sisters, Hedda Hopper and Ann Miller. Current advertising by the clinic states that 'a six-night Weight Management Approach programme costs £13,330; the six-night Revitalization programme is £20,560.' Patients are advised to return every two years for a top-up.

In London Niehans's disciple Peter M. Stephan offered rejuvenating injections of animal cells at £200 a course. He advised that a woman should have her first injections at about thirty, and further injections every five years. 'I don't promise she won't age,' he said, 'but she will age well and comparatively slowly … She will most likely look anything from ten to fifteen years younger than she is all her life' (Hannon, p. 106). Accepters of what Stephan called Therapeutic Immunology could expect memory to improve, tiredness to vanish, skin, hair and nails to improve, muscles to refirm, lines to fade and face to sag less and less. In *New Life for Old* (1980) David Abbott included case histories such as that of Patient B, who first approached Stephan when she was forty-five. He diagnosed 'total exhaustion' and treated her with extracts of various animal tissues, after which she provided a testimonial stating: 'I live an 18 hour day to the full and have my health, vitality and looks that reflect both' (pp. 126–7). Abbott was convinced that Therapeutic Immunology was about to be adopted on a national scale. Stephan stood at the crossroads; he awaited only the indoctrination of all the GPs and the education of secondary school students in the necessary ancillary techniques to sweep aside all other systems of medication and confer upon mankind 'the secret of eternal youth'.

Having discovered the miraculous properties of Viagra, Big Pharma is now competing to find something to combat lack of interest in sex in women, which has a new name, Female Sexual Dysfunction or FSD. The compound most recently hailed as the 'female Viagra' is flibanserin, originally developed as an antidepressant, and now sold as a specific for 'hypoactive sexual desire disorder' or HSDD, and sold under the trade name Addyi but, whereas Viagra can be used effectively for men of all ages, flibanserin is considered suitable only for pre-menopausal women, who are probably not the ones who need it. Its effects must be considered less than spectacular. The women in the clinical trials reported only a half to a single added sexually satisfying event in a given month compared to those taking the placebo. Besides flibanserin has some unpleasant side-effects, such as dizziness, nausea, fatigue, fainting, insomnia and worrying drops in blood pressure when combined with alcohol. FDA clinical reviewers voted to refuse approval for the drug but were overruled by senior administrators on the grounds that there was an unmet need in the case of 'female sexual interest/arousal disorder' (FSIAD), which seems as bizarre a misinterpretation of feminist priorities as could be imagined.

Combinations of esterified oestrogens and methyltestosterone marketed under the names Covaryx, Essian, Estratest, Menogen and Syntest, which unlike flibanserin are designed for post-menopausal women, could be expected to enhance sex drive. Unfortunately in women who still have wombs they need to be opposed with progestogens, which may diminish their effectiveness. Online reviews report that Covaryx and Estratest are effective in restoring lost sex drive in hysterectomised women, but difficulties in acquiring the medications and changes in the law regarding their availability have resulted in completely avoidable confusion and disappointment, as well as more serious symptoms associated with withdrawal.

Royal jelly is another of the elixirs of youth. Though it was proved by the AMA to contain no more than vitamins of the B group, and US shipments of royal jelly were impounded in 1962, it is still to be found, and at a high price, on the shelves of health-food shops. Individuals can be found who 'swear by it'. When Dr Ana Aslan, who combatted ageing with H3 or 'Gerovital', which was simply procaine hydrochloride, visited England in 1959 this therapy too was discredited, though Dr Aslan had patients who swore that they felt much younger and healthier than before they took her elixir. When the first hormone replacers began their careers they were anxious to dissociate themselves from the pedlars of rejuvenation, but the planeloads of women who arrived from all over the world at the Atlanta clinic of Robert M. Greenblatt in the early Seventies came with the same suggestibility that worked so well for Stephan, Aslan and the royal jelly industry.

The term 'aromatherapy' was invented by René Maurice Gattefosse in 1928; the techniques were further developed by Dr Jean Valnet, who used essential oils from plants first to treat severe burns and battle injuries and then in psychiatric practice, and founded the Société Française de

Phytothérapie et d'Aromathérapie. Like virtually all alternative medical systems, aromatherapy claims to treat the whole person, rather than an afflicted part; illness is seen as an imbalance of the energies in the body which can be rebalanced by the absorption of selected volatile oils distilled from plants, either through direct application to the skin, by massage or hot and cold compresses, in creams, lotions or aromatic waters, or as baths. Nevertheless, *Aromatherapy: An A–Z* by Patricia Davis, Principal of the London School of Aromatherapy and one of the founders of the International Federation of Aromatherapists, does not at all illustrate the idea that the absorption of the volatile elements in the oil of plants acts upon the whole organism. The patient is divided up into parts and encouraged to medicate herself using methods familiar from Queen Philippa's herbal; indeed, Davis claims that aromatherapy has been in use for 4,000 years. Human beings have deliberately inhaled pleasant and unpleasant scents for longer than that and have been sensible of effects varying from nausea to drowsiness. Under 'Menopause' Davis describes a treatment which is not so much aromatherapeutic as conservative, involving the old favourite essential oils of geranium, rose, bergamot, clary sage, jasmine, lavender, neroli, sandalwood and ylang-ylang.

Davis claims that attar of roses 'has a powerful effect upon the uterus', 'cleansing, purifying, regulating and tonic', invaluable for women 'who have menstrual irregularities or are tense, depressed and sad' (p. 290). The best attar is Bulgarian or French, being obtained by the enfleurage method in which rose petals are laid on fat spread on sheets of glass which are stacked in wooden frames so that the oil is gently squeezed out into the fat. Each day the petals are renewed until the fat can absorb no more. Then the fat is shaken in alcohol to separate out the essential oil. It is tempting to consider whether the efficacy of attar of roses is not directly related to its costliness, which acts as an objective indicator of the user's worth to herself and others, not least the aromatherapist who is charging her for all this tender loving care. An easier way to extract oil from one's own roses is to spread the petals on muslin impregnated with refined olive oil, laid on glass and stacked, changing the petals each day. After three weeks you should be able to press out or distil a usable body oil. Any roses of the gallica, damascena or centifolia group can be used.

By geranium, Davis means *Pelargonium odoratissimum*, which is sometimes used in men's perfumes and has no medical application outside aromatherapy. Davis claims that Culpeper describes this plant as under the dominion of Venus, which she takes to mean that it has some special affinity to the female organs of generation. In fact, Culpeper does not describe *Pelargonium odoratissimum* at all. He describes two other members of the geranium family, Herb Robert and Cranesbill, neither of which has or had any application in female problems.

Of the antidepressant oils, most have no medical application outside aromatherapy. Bergamot has no connection with the plant English gardeners call by that name (*Monarda didyma*), being instead the cold-pressed oil of the rind of *Citrus bergamia* from Sicily. Clary Sage is *Salvia sclarea*, which has been used to scent wine for hundreds of years. Elsewhere Davis claims that oil of jasmine is 'a valuable uterotonic', an effect not noticed anywhere but in the literature of aromatherapy. Neroli is the oil of Seville oranges, and has presumably a similarly uplifting effect to bergamot. Ylang-ylang is the oil of *Cananga odorata*, an Asian tree.

Davis also informs us that: 'Fennel is a plant which contains plant oestrogens, so fennel tea is a valuable drink' (p. 223). This is a confusion to be found so often that it is important to refute it. Many plants contain what are now more often called phyto-oestrogens, but though they may be ingested in various ways, they are not usually bio-available as the equivalent of endogenous oestrogen. Indeed they may function as oestrogen antagonists. The list of plants that contain them is huge; it includes as well as Fennel, and its relatives Fenugreek, Anise and licorice root, soy, linseed, oats, barley, beans, lentils, hops, wheatberries, alfalfa, apples, carrots, pomegranates, Red Clover and goodness knows what else. Their usefulness in menopause is still under review; there is certainly no evidence that drinking tea made from fennel has any effect at all (Lethaby et al.). Black Cohosh does contain a phyto-oestrogen, but is found to be inert. However, it is often the case that traditional remedies undergoing clinical assessment are prepared using inappropriate methods. Their action is often synergistic in ways that cannot be duplicated in the laboratory. Under 'phytoestrogenic foods that will keep your hormones happy', Canadian inspirational speaker Rosalie Moscoe lists 'soy (in moderation), pomegranates and flaxseeds'. Other websites list pages of exhortation to increase soy intake, as well as pages of evidence that vaccination causes autism and Zika virus is a medical hoax.

It is obvious that aromas do exert powerful immediate effects on living organisms, whether to attract or repel them. Nasal receptors communicate rapidly and forcefully with the brain. In the 1960s, when Ivan Popov, the medical adventurer who first introduced placenta and embryo extracts into cosmetics, was working for the French scent manufacturer Anton Chiris, he drew up a chart of 400 aromatics, assigning to them eight basic characters: fresh, stimulant, exaltant, erogenous, heavy, narcotic, tranquillising, anti-erogenous. When Patrick McGrady interviewed him for his book *The Youth Doctors* in 1968, Popov was sure that 'if anything is going to revolutionize the field of rejuvenation in the next few years ... it's going to be aromatics (especially stimulant and tranquilizing aromatics). Alone, they have incredible properties. Used in conjunction with other treatments, they often possess a powerful synergism, greatly accelerating and augmenting the regular beneficial effects. Moreover, their application is utterly simple' (McGrady, p. 179).

Popov was also interested in reflexotherapy.

Reflexotherapy has to do with simply smelling the aromatics. Through action of certain extremities of the central nervous system they can have a direct effect on the brain. It is now being studied in the Paris Medical School. (p. 179)

Rather than reflexotherapy, Patricia Davis chooses twenty years later to discuss reflexology, in which pressure is applied manually or with a special vibrating device to selected points on the feet in order to produce reactions in the rest of the body (Davis, P., p. 284). A spot under the instep is associated with the adrenal glands; and the uterus is reflected in two, one just behind the heel and another six inches or so higher on the leg. According to Patsy Westcott and Letarsia Black (1987, p. 154), foot massage is particularly useful in problems of menopause.

The idea that volatile substances acting on the extremely sensitive nose might affect the brain, and enter the bloodstream by inhalation and through the skin, is not in itself improbable. The idea that the foot is connected by mysterious sympathies to every organ in the body is more difficult to credit, especially when we are also told by the acupuncturists that the organs are connected by meridians conducting energy through the length of the body, or the ear or the hand. The justifications of treating one part of the body by inflicting pain on another sound no more convincing than the notion of counter-irritation that justified some of the most painful therapies of the eighteenth century. When we find electric currents being passed through acupuncture needles in order to stimulate the flow of endorphins, we might call to mind all the other attempts to affect disease processes in the body by sending electric currents through selected parts of it. The notion that there are energy conduits which may become blocked resurfaces in many guises, as chakras, meridians or sen lines.

In the twenty-first century most of the costly substances dispensed by apothecaries for the treatment of menopausal women over the centuries have disappeared, only to be replaced by an extraordinary array of newer alternative remedies sourced from the farthest corners of the world. Ginseng, known though not used in the West since the seventeenth century, is now the most widely used medicinal in the world. The botanical name of ginseng, Panax, comes from the same Greek root as the word 'panacea', meaning universal remedy. The Chinese name transliterated as ginseng comes from words meaning 'shaped like a man', referring to the root, which has a thick trunk with limb-like lesser roots attached. In one Finnish study doctors found that ginseng 'helped dry vagina, hot flushes, sweats, tension, anxiety and palpitations', according to 'established reporter on women's health issues' Patsy Westcott, whose *Alternative Health Care for Women* devotes a mere two and a half pages out of more than 170 to the menopause. There are in fact various varieties of ginseng: *Panax pseudoginseng*, which is native to damp, cool woodland in Manchuria and Korea, *Panax quinquefolium* or American ginseng, *Panax fruticosum*, used as a food and a medicine in some parts of Polynesia, and Siberian ginseng, *Eleutherococcus senticosus*. The most important of these is *Panax pseudoginseng*, which comes in various commercial grades, the most valuable being Red Korean ginseng. Centuries of collecting mean that ginseng is rarely found in the wild in China and Korea, where commercial cultivation of the root, which takes nine years to mature, is undertaken on an increasing scale and carefully controlled by the government. The virtues so long extolled by Oriental pharmacists have now been recognised by Western pharmacognosy, which has coined a new word, 'adaptogen', to explain the combination of tranquillising and energising functions of ginseng.

Ginseng root contains 'volatile oils, comprising sapogenin and panacen (stimulating the central nervous system); a saponin, panaxin; panax acid; ginsenin (with hypoglycaemic activity); a glycoside, panaquilon (acting as a vasoconstrictive stimulant); ginsennosides; phytosterols; hormones; vitamins B1 and B2; mucilage; several other substances; all combining to produce a complex total effect' (Stuart). As their names indicate, most of these constituents are found only in ginseng. As an adaptogen ginseng is particularly indicated as a therapy in times of exceptional somatic stress, and therefore in the peri-menopause. The difficulty for the woman treating herself with ginseng is to understand how much she needs to take and in what form. The drug is available in a bewildering variety of expensive commercial preparations, all of which make different and conflicting claims for the effectiveness and suitability of their own mode of administration. For women who are feeling agitated rather than listless, ginseng is not the drug of choice.

The entire Chinese pharmacopoeia has been ransacked for remedies for menopausal distress; the Chinese herbs mentioned in hundreds of preparations include *Angelica gigas, Bupleurum falcatum, Camellia sinensis, Cnidium monnieri, Curculigo orchioides, Cynanchum wilfordii, Ginkgo biloba, Magnolia officinalis, Paeonia lactiflora, Phlomis umbrosa* and *Rehmannia glutinosa*. As Chinese prescribing is personalised, and herbs are viewed as working synergistically with each other and with the patient's own biochemistry, the addition of most of these (here identified by their Western binomial names) to a heterogeneous assembly of all kinds of ingredients from all over the world is pointless. Since the discrediting of HRT, 'natural' remedies for the ills of menopause have proliferated. There are now hundreds of 'natural' alternative remedies. As most of them are marketed as dietary supplements rather than drugs they have never been tested for efficacy.

Angelica sinensis, or Dong Quai, is another adaptogen, sometimes called 'female ginseng', and as such is recommended for those women who have 'pale and dull complexion, dry skin and eyes, blurry vision, ridges in their nail beds, frail body and rapid heart beat'. Preparations of the root are used for period pain, PMS and menopausal symptoms, to purify blood, and treat hypertension, infertility, joint pain, ulcers, anaemia, constipation, allergies, loss of skin pigmentation and psoriasis. It is also to be found in preparations applied to the penis to prevent premature ejaculation. Donna Gates, ageless 'expert in candida, adrenal fatigue, autism, autoimmune diseases, weight loss and anti-aging', founder of the website *Body Ecology*, decided that fermenting the root 'would make it more powerful and provide the healthy, immune-boosting benefits of healthy microflora'. The result of the fermentation process is an 'immune boosting probiotic liquid'. As might be suspected from the wide range of vague ailments that Dong Quai is considered useful in treating, it cannot reliably be shown to be effective in any.

The ingredient in herbal remedies for menopause ailments most extensively studied is Black Cohosh (*Actaea* or *Cimicifuga racemosa*), native to eastern north America. This would have been used there and nowhere else until the modern era, but now we find it marketed worldwide as, for example, Femular, 'a natural medicine manufactured in Switzerland'. Online promotions claim that 'Femular has been shown to relieve a range of menopausal symptoms. Femular has been shown to have a 50% reduction in menopausal symptom severity and a 60% reduction in hot flushes/night sweats.' Womenlivingnaturally.com tells us that 'structurally Black Cohosh resembles estradiol' that even so it has no oestrogenic activity and actually protects against cancer of the endometrium, ovaries and breast. Yet, even though Black Cohosh is the best-researched herbal medicine on the market, it cannot be shown to be much more effective than placebo. It has also been linked with an increased risk of liver damage and breast cancer. In one case a 47-year-old woman used Black Cohosh for only three weeks before suffering liver failure. No other cause of liver disease was identified (Whiting et al.). The American website Livertox, which provides 'clinical and research information on drug-induced liver injury', sums up the current state of ignorance thus: 'Black cohosh does not appear to be inherently hepatotoxic, and the clinical features of cases suggest that the liver injury is an idiosyncratic reaction which may be immunologically mediated. The specific component of black cohosh responsible for the hepatic injury is not known. As with many HDS (herbal dietary supplement) products, unknown adulterants or herbals mislabeled as black cohosh may be the actual cause of hepatic injury.'

Another American native, *Sanguinaria canadensis* or bloodroot, is favoured by homeopathic practitioners, as is *Strychnos ignatii* from the Philippines. Another, *Chamaelirium luteum* or False Unicorn Root, often still listed as '*Helonias dioica*', contains steroidal saponins that are converted through digestion to the sapogenin diosgenin; this plant has been so diligently harvested over so many years that it is now considered threatened in the wild and is being grown commercially. Unfortunately, the conditions required for successful commercial growing of medicinals as extensive monocrops under glass militate against the plants developing their active constituents.

The lists of ingredients for these herbal potpourris are sometimes bewildering, blinding the reader not so much with science as with nonsense. Zalestra, to name but one of more than 200 examples, consists of unspecified amounts of 'green tea, guggul, octopalean, maca root powder, jojoba meal extract, indole-3-carbinol, borage oil powder, mega soy extract, manganese, black cohosh, DHEA, vitex fruit extract, bioperine, gelatin, cellulose, and magnesium stearate'. According to NHS Choices green tea (*Camellia sinensis*) 'contains B vitamins, folate (naturally occurring folic acid), manganese, potassium, magnesium, caffeine and other antioxidants, notably catechins' and 'is alleged to boost weight loss, reduce cholesterol, combat cardiovascular disease, and prevent cancer and Alzheimer's disease'. There is no conclusive evidence for any of these claims.

Guggul is an Indian shrub (*Commiphora wightii*), for so long harvested in the wild in Gujarat and Rajasthan that it is now on the IUCN Red List as critically endangered. It is now commercially grown in India. Its active ingredients, known as guggulsterones, are marketed as enhancing thyroid activity and lowering cholesterol, though in the dosages available over the counter neither function has been demonstrated. The Creative Compounds website tells us that octopalean is 'a new ingredient from Creative Compounds. The active ingredient, octopamine (also known as norsynephrine), is a stimulant-free, naturally occurring amine that is closely related to norepinephrine'. According to the vendors, octopalean 'stimulates beta-3 adrenoceptors like ephedrine and has been shown to increase metabolism, stimulate lipolysis and promote insulin sensitivity'.

Maca (*Lepidium meyenii*) is an adaptogen from Peru; as one online site has it 'Maca root contains many chemicals, including fatty acids and amino acids. However, there isn't enough information to know how maca might work'. Or if. Another site warns us that only 'Royal Macha' will do, because cheaper versions don't work. Credibility is not enhanced when we find Maca being promoted online as 'a very potent aphrodisiac'.

Jojoba oil is recommended as a perineal lubricant for menopausal women, but what jojoba meal extract can do for them must remain a mystery. Indole-3-carbinol (I3C) is derived from the breakdown of glucobrassicin, a compound found in cruciferous vegetables like sprouts; its risks and benefits are still largely unquantified but it has no obvious role in post-menopausal therapy. The botanical binomial for borage, *Borago officinalis*, makes clear that it has always been considered a medicinal herb, but only a single wobbly study connects it with controlling hot flashes.

'Mega soy extract' is available as just that, and its purveyors tell us that: 'Once [*sic*] study showed that soy isoflavones promote and [*sic*] anabolic effect on bone tissue in post-menopausal women by binding to the estrogen receptor sites in the bone' – a statement which even the person who copied it onto the Mega Soy website couldn't understand. There is little more than a remote possibility that some post-menopausal women might be deficient in manganese, and significant risk is associated with overexposure to manganese, so it is not generally included as a therapy for menopausal ills.

It is surprising to find Black Cohosh so far down the cast list. DHEA is dehydroepiandrosterone, used by some in the belief that it can slow down the ageing process; as far as the US National Institute on Aging and the US National Center for Complementary and Alternative Medicine have been able to determine, there is no ground for this belief, while long-term use of DHEA may do harm. 'Vitex fruit extract' is supposedly derived from *Vitex agnus-castus*. Bioperine is a concentrated extract of black pepper said to enhance the bioavailability and the benefits of the other ingredients. Magnesium stearate is a flow agent used in the manufacture of tablets; it is potentially toxic and may negatively affect the absorption of the active ingredients.

As this example demonstrates, purveyors of the menopause remedies offered as dietary supplements are now making up preparations composed of heterogeneous mixtures of ingredients from all over the world. Beside the usual suspects Dong quai, Soy, Wild Yam Root, Black Cohosh, et al., Menoquil, one of the leading menopause remedies, contains the pro-erectile herb *Cnidium monnieri* from China. A principal marketing mechanism for preparations like Menoquil is a promise of money back if the product is returned within a period; judging by the complaints aired on the web this is often more difficult than might be imagined.

Most of the firms involved are small operations, set up specifically to exploit the particular wonder herb and capable of little in the way of customer service.

The role of soy in the management of menopause is difficult to quantify. Commentators are either vehemently for or as vehemently against. Some insist that soy should be used as in whole foods rather than as a dietary supplement; others argue that the effective agents are soy isoflavones rather than soy. According to the website of the late John R. Lee, which offers saliva tests to establish hormonal status and sells Lee's hormone-balancing cream at a mere $21.95 for a two-ounce tube, attempts to judge the efficacy of soy have failed.

In one comprehensive study from the Bowman Gray School of Medicine in North Carolina, researchers looked at the effects of soy phytoestrogens on women aged 45 to 55 with menopausal symptoms. This study was big news because the women who took a phytoestrogen-rich soy supplement reported a 50 percent decrease in the severity of their hot flashes. What most news stories didn't mention, however, is that the placebo group reported a 35 percent reduction. Furthermore, this study showed small reductions in the *severity* of hot flashes, but none in their *frequency*.

In October 2010 a closed workshop on soy and soy isoflavones was convened in Chicago by the North American Menopause Society. Evidence was heard about 'the prevalence of use of soy and soy isoflavones; the molecular, cellular, and physiologic effects of isoflavones; and the effects of soy and soy isoflavones on menopausal symptoms, breast and endometrial cancer, atherosclerosis, bone loss, and cognition'. In almost all categories the results were inconclusive or outright contradictory and the conclusions were that more research needed to be undertaken. The authors of the report, which was published in *Menopause*, the journal of the North American Menopause Association, in 2011, blamed much of the discrepancy on small sample sizes and inconsistent methodology.

The website of Andrew Weil MD lists among 'natural treatments' 'soy foods': 'The isoflavones in soy foods help balance hormone levels and have some estrogenic activity'. Soy isoflavones are said to exert mild oestrogenic activity for about half of the study populations, and nothing for the other half. Isoflavones are polyphenolic compounds produced in fabaceous plants, with soya, otherwise known as Lima Beans (*Glycine max*), as the leading contender. Because some isoflavones, such as genistein and daidzein, exert mild oestrogenic effects they are called phyto-oestrogens. Structurally similar to oestrogen, soy isoflavones have the capacity to bind to empty oestrogen receptors and relieve hormonally based symptoms of menopause such as hot flashes. It is this ability to inhibit hormone reception that may be the mechanism by which some phyto-oestrogens seem to prevent hormone-dependent cancers.

Despite the fact that soy isoflavones have a chemical structure that is very similar to the hormone oestrogen, small variations in that structure can produce physiological effects that are very different. Both isoflavones and oestrogen bind to and activate oestrogen receptors in cells. Oestrogen will bind to either of the two kinds of receptors in human cells, but isoflavones bind more readily to one than the other. Thus the two types of receptors can produce different, sometimes completely opposite, effects. Isoflavones may have oestrogen-like effects or anti-oestrogenic effects, or no effects at all. For this reason, isoflavones are considered to be selective oestrogen receptor modulators (SERMS). Research into the potential health benefits of isoflavones, particularly as safe alternatives to oestrogen, continues and potential adverse functions are gradually being identified: not only can isoflavones disrupt the delicate balance of hormones; they can also act as goitrogens, suppressing thyroid function. One school of thought holds that the isoflavones in soy need to be fermented, as is the case in a wide range of foods eaten in China, Korea, Vietnam, Japan, India and Indonesia, of which the best-known, after soy sauce, are miso, natto, tempeh and fermented tofu.

In 2001, at age fifty-four, American entertainer Bette Midler claimed to have overcome the discomforts of menopause by the use of 'a soy and primrose oil thing'. The source of 'primrose oil' is not a primrose, but the American native *Oenothera biennis*, Evening Primrose. Online practitioner Ann Louise Gittleman, who put together the combined dietary supplement marketed to peri-menopausal women under the name 'The Essential Woman', claims that 'in study after study, women have found evening primrose oil to be outstanding for irritability, mood changes, headaches, anxiety, and PMS and perimenopausal discomforts such as fluid retention and breast tenderness.'

The last of the 'natural treatments' listed by Dr Weil is one or other of evening primrose oil or blackcurrant oil on the grounds that both 'are sources of gamma-linolenic acid (GLA), an essential fatty acid that can help influence prostaglandin synthesis and help moderate menopausal symptoms'. What the menopausal woman is to make of a statement like this is anybody's guess. The role of 'prostaglandin synthesis' in menopause has yet to be determined; prostaglandins are known to stimulate and inhibit bone resorption and formation, although after twenty-five years of study we still do not know how to balance these contrasting capacities in the menopausal woman. Something that 'can help influence' cannot be shown to have any effect at all.

'Visionary pioneer' Dr Christiane Northrup recommends perhaps the most exotic of the exotic specifics for the treatment of menopause, namely Kwao Krua Kao, native to northern and north-eastern Thailand and Myanmar, which was given the name *Pueraria mirifica* by botanists K. Suvatabandhu and H. K. Airy Shaw in 1953. It seems that the plant is properly *Pueraria candollei* var. or subspecies *mirifica*; the confusion seems to have resulted from the appearance on the market of inactive preparations offered at the same high prices as those that appear to be the real thing, but the whole spectrum is fogged. The FDA, who have permitted the sale of *Pueraria mirifica* preparations in the US as dietary supplements, describe *Pueraria mirifica* as 'used by Thai women in and around Thailand for the relief of vasomotor symptoms (hot flashes and night sweats) associated with menopause. As part of the current practice of botanical medicine in Thailand, menopausal women are encouraged to consume the roots of *Pueraria mirifica* in powder form orally once a day before bedtime to alleviate hot flashes and night sweating.' The active constituent is a phyto-oestrogen called miroestrol, which is said to increase sex drive, make breasts bigger, firmer and perkier, fight osteoporosis, delay ageing, improve memory, and to be more potent than oestrogen. In the US the dried powder of the roots is principally taken by both men and women desirous of enlarging their breasts. If the results alleged in online websites are to be believed, the product would seem to be too active to be taken for an extended period; no scientific analysis of its mode of action, certainly no double-blind trials, have been carried out. From 27 December 2016 Dr Northrup has been selling via the website of A-ma-ta, a company she set up for the purpose, an 'exclusive patented extract' of *Pueraria mirifica* which she calls Puresterol at $29.95 for sixty capsules (a month's supply).

The main ingredient in Femestra, 'an all-natural formula that helps women combat the symptoms of menopause', is a kind of rice bran from Japan; the active agent is gamma oryzanol or ferulic acid, which was first investigated as a treatment for menopausal symptoms in the 1960s with inconclusive results. Though Canadian chiropractor and naturopath James Meschino can be seen and heard to explain its mode of operation in online videos, the consensus appears to be that the effectiveness of gamma oryzanol in controlling hot flashes cannot be reliably demonstrated.

In the case of 'Passion Revive Herbal Remedy', recommended for people of both sexes suffering loss of interest in sex in mid- and later life, the list of active agents includes *Mucuna pruriens*, Ashwagandha, Catuaba, *Curculigo orchioides*, *Rehmannia glutinosa*, *Muira puama*, Mulberry, Shilajit, and *Schisandra chinensis*. *Mucuna pruriens* or 'Velvet Bean' is touted as an aphrodisiac; apparently male rats given the substance mounted the females ten times more than the control group and had shorter post-ejaculatory intervals of inactivity. The Sanskrit name 'Ashwagandha' literally means 'the smell of a horse'. Preparations of the root of this plant (*Withania somnifera*), the Indian ginseng, are said to enhance sexual potency in both men and women. 'Catuaba' is the name given to a number of herbal preparations using the bark of various Brazilian trees, chief amongst them *Trichilia catigua* and *Erythroxylum vaccinifolium*; the name means 'what gives strength to the Indian'. Catuaba is principally used to enhance sexual function in men. In the Chinese pharmacopoeia the rhizome of *Curculigo orchioides* is used for erectile dysfunction in men and for post-menopausal osteoporosis. *Rehmannia glutinosa*, the Chinese Foxglove, is thought to counteract the loss of bone density. *Muira puama* is another aphrodisiac said to improve sexual desire and up the frequency of sexual intercourse in women with a low sex drive. It is derived from the bark of two Brazilian trees, *Ptychopetalum olacoides* and *P. uncinatum*.

There were always health-care providers who thought that, if menopause was not a disease, it was not to be treated by pills or potions. As the apothecaries mixed new and ever more expensive nostra, other practitioners, aware of the scale of the placebo response, were trying different approaches. One online adviser recommends masturbation, claiming that 'paddling the pink canoe can help with menopausal symptoms by preventing vaginal narrowing, helping to promote lubrication, and facilitating desire.'

The woman seeking a remedy for what ails her will find in the old herbals many treatments for insomnia, flushing, nervousness, rumbling guts, lethargy, depression, bloating, and the like. There is no reason why she should not try her own combinations and her own modes of administration, bearing in mind that herbal substances are anything but harmless. *Agnus castus*, for example, is also called wild pepper, and can scorch the throat if taken in infusion. Nightshade (*Solanum dulcamara*), used for treating night sweats, and Henbane are too poisonous for internal use in any form, though hyoscine hydrobromide or scopolamine is used in remedies for travel sickness and excessive salivation, and hyoscine butylbromide as buscopan is used for irritable bowel syndrome. Oil of Henbane or a poultice of fresh leaves is valuable in treating joint pain; women wanting to try Henbane for menopausal distress might like to experiment with external plasters, or Andrew Boorde's 'dormitary', which I take to be an impregnated compress of fresh extract. Otherwise minute quantities of Henbane tincture are still used in homeopathic prescribing.

An easy and pleasant way for a woman to avail herself of the relaxing effects of the volatile oil contained in the female strobilus of Hops is to collect the Hops from the hedgerows in autumn, dry the seedheads (not in sunlight) and stuff a small pillow with them, so that during spells of insomnia she can rest her cheek upon it and inhale the soothing scent without having to leave her bed or disturb others. Such a sleep cushion should consist of an inner butter-muslin bag of herbs and a pillow-case of fine lawn, which can be easily laundered. The ladies of Queen Elizabeth's bedchamber strewed it with Meadowsweet (*Filipendula ulmaria*) by her order; an alternative to green stains on the carpet could be a few sprigs of this fresh herb or any other of the fragrant soporifics in a variant of the sleep cushion. Another way to use herbal sedatives is to add a few drops of the essential oil to a bedtime bath and inhale the active constituents that way.

Most dried herbs sold in commerce are not only old and valueless, but can be contaminated by the presence of other material and may not correspond at all to the label. The usual quality controls do not apply to herbal preparations, often marketed as dietary supplements, which can be costly. Preparations of fresh material are not only more reliable, but are usually very much more effective and should be used in much smaller quantities. Juice expressed from the fresh plant ferments very quickly and may become dangerous, while refrigeration may destroy its effectiveness. All the traditional remedies are slow-working and need time to exercise their effect. When collecting fresh material it is important to consider whether it is affected by herbicides or other poisons. In some circumstances, for example if they are grown in greenhouses, overfed and overwatered, herbs may have grown lax and weak and lack the properties they develop in the right cultural conditions.

The naturopathy of old wives cannot be approached like the modern standardised commercial pharmacopoeia. It is pointless to set off to the health food shop to buy remedies that have in the past been associated with various kinds of distress, imagining that they can be taken like aspirin. Ideally the sufferer should collect her own plant material, carefully following any indication she can find of the part of the plant that was traditionally used, the time it should be collected, and the way it should be treated. Fresh plant material can be prepared in infusion or decoction, macerated and steeped in oil or white wine, or carefully dried away from sunlight. Some valuable plants, like Rocket and Watercress, which both contain calcium, should be eaten raw; others are only useful dried. There are two good ways to get to know how plants behave and what they are likely to be good for; one is to study them in their natural habitat, the other is to grow them. Walking or working among living plants is very much the best way of absorbing their active constituents, which rub off on skin and arise from bruised leaves. If you are scrambling across a mountainside with a swag of fresh herb on your back, you are absorbing its volatile elements into a well-oxygenated bloodstream in ways that cannot be duplicated on the therapist's couch or in your bathroom.

The efficiency of absorption of therapeutic substances into the bloodstream by the nasal route has probably not received sufficient attention. Plant oestrogens are known to exert a powerful influence upon animal behaviour; the oestrus of many species is triggered by the presence of plant oestrogens in pasture in springtime, probably not by ingestion but by inhalation. Human beings seem to be like other species in this respect. Most people feel exhilarated in springtime whether the sun is shining or not. Some women have noticed that even if they are having a majority of anovulatory cycles they will ovulate in spring. Our receptors for phytosterols, if they do act upon the human organism, are most likely in the nose or the upper respiratory tract. We are unlikely to be able to devise a mode of administration of any derivative of phytosterols which does not offer the same problems of overdosing and inappropriate biological pathways that we find in our use of equine steroids.

Millions of women between the ages of forty-five and fifty-five discover gardening. Other people imagine that this is because they have nothing else to do. In fact there is always something else to do, as every woman who gardens knows. The time spent in the garden is time stolen from some other less rewarding task. Gardening cannot be recommended as good exercise, because too much time is spent virtually motionless and in awkward positions, while muscles chill and bones seize up, and feet get colder and colder, even if they are not wet. Though lower back pain and gardening go together, gardeners feel very much better for gardening, back pain and all. The effect is so like the 'mental tonic' effect alleged for HRT that we may be justified in suspecting that there are volatile oestrogens in living plants that do not survive in treated plant material.

When she was fifty-seven, sophisticated, intensely gregarious Lady Mary Wortley Montagu astonished her friends and family by turning gardener. She wrote to her daughter from her villa at Gottolengo near Brescia in 1748:

> I am realy as fond of my Garden as a young Author of his first
> play when it has been well receiv'd by the Town, and can no more
> forbear teizing my Acquaintance for their aprobation ... Gardening
> is certainly the next amusement to Reading ... (Montagu, II,
> pp. 407–8)

With the letter she sent her daughter a little plan showing her plot divided by covered walks and her dining arbour with a cupola above it. She may not have known it, but her wobbly drawing is on exactly the same plan as the *hortus conclusus* which is how the Garden of Eden was shown in medieval iconography. A garden is a kinetic work of art, not an object but a process, open-ended, biodegradable, nurturant, like all women's artistry. A garden is the best alternative therapy.

11

Misery

The misery of the climacteric comes from without and from within. It is less sharply painful than grief and differs from grief in that no mourning will appease it or express it. Misery is the dull pain or dreariness that cannot find relief in tears; there is no loftiness or nobility in it. The external cause of misery is to be found in the attitudes of others. The internal source is the awareness of the stigma, which persists despite the classic response, the denial that one is a menopausal woman or, worse, an old woman. One strategy for dealing with stigma is to assert and reassert that you do belong to the stigmatised class, confident that you're so unlike the stereotype that the stigma can be clearly seen to be nothing but bigotry, but it doesn't always work.

To call someone, anyone, 'old' is to insult him or her. It will take a great deal longer to teach the world that 'old is beautiful' than it took to teach people not to use the word 'black' as pejorative. 'Old' is familiar, shabby, belittling. When 'old' is paired with 'woman' it becomes an insult for either sex. When Joseph Addison mounted an attack upon what he called 'old Women's Fables' in 1711 in the twelfth number of his new magazine the *Spectator*, he took as his text a quotation from the Roman satirist Persius: *veteres avias tibi de pulmone revello*. We must, he argued 'pull the old woman out of our Hearts …'

Helen Walmsley-Johnson, fifty-eight years old, writing in the *Guardian* on 8 October 2014, wondered whether it was 'insulting to be called an old lady? As a woman inhabiting that strange hinterland between youth-erly and older-ly, I find I am more relaxed now about thinking of myself as "old". "Old" in itself (and to me certainly) is not a pejorative term; "old" means familiar and comforting, wise and steady. It's only when someone adds something nasty to it such as "dried-up old [insert four-letter word of your choice]" that it becomes an insult.' Somehow Ms Walmsley-Johnson managed to overlook the invariably unflattering term 'old bag'. An old bag can be familiar and comforting, wise and steady, but not if it's you.

Fifty-two-year-old Marina Benjamin, Senior Editor at *Aeon* Magazine 'knew that middle age was dowdy and maudlin and complaining, that our hormones ride rollercoasters; that we thrill to adulterous affairs; that in midlife we lose parents and sometimes friends and feel as if our identities are dissolving – it's why we cry over empty nests, fret over our truncated futures, suffer breakdowns and breakups and mourn our disappearing youth' (the *Telegraph*, 11 June 2016). In another column we learn that in autumn 2013 aged forty-eight she had a subtotal hysterectomy with ovaries and Fallopian tubes all removed. When she turned fifty she wrote a much-admired book called *The Middlepause*.

> Spurred by her own brutal propulsion into menopause, Marina Benjamin weighs the losses, joys and opportunities of our middle years, taking inspiration from literature and philosophical example. She uncovers the secret misogynistic history of HRT, and tells us why a dose of Jung is better than a trip to the gym. Attending to ageing parents, the shock of bereavement, parenting a teenager, and her own health woes, she emerges into a new definition of herself as daughter, mother, citizen and woman.

Good for her. However on 11 June 2016 an edited extract from *The Middlepause* sounded a different note.

> Outside in the square as I write this, it happens to be spring, and the cherry trees are starting to bud. With a sorry heave of my chest, I recognise that I have no part of it any more because the time of my life that was ruled by such cycles, that was attuned to the moon and the tides as to the moods of the seasons, is over. Spring in particular is no longer for me. I am not just out of sync with nature's rhythms: I've got no rhythms. (the *Telegraph*, 11 June 2016)

It is simply not true that post-menopausal women have no rhythms. The moon still shines in at the window on some nights and not others, the animals still mate in due season, the oestrogens still fly up from the pasture grasses. That feeling of irrelevance, of out-of-stepness, is misery.

In 1785 William Hayley dedicated *A Philosophical, Historical and Moral Essay on Old Maids … in Three Volumes* to the 'Poet … Philosopher and … Old Maid' Elizabeth Carter, without her permission. He assumed that everybody, including 68-year-old Miss Carter, would agree that old maids were universally afflicted with 'curiosity, credulity, affectation, envy and ill-nature', only partly counteracted by their potential for 'ingenuity, patience and charity'. Miss Carter illustrated his case by failing to accept the dedication with the 'polite good humour' that he stipulated. She was offended; there was no way the expression 'old maid' could be anything but derogatory. 'Old' plus a female noun, 'old woman', 'old girl', 'old cow', 'old bitch', is always insulting. The insult lies in the combination of the age with the sex; to be called 'old man', 'old boy' or even 'old dog' is not in the least insulting.

We are not here concerned with male anophobia as much as with the anophobia of women themselves, which so complicates their own ageing. It is understandable, but not therefore forgivable, that young women, whose oppression is often dealt out to them by older women, should react against them with bitterness and ridicule. Schoolteachers, overseers, manageresses, mothers-in-law, social workers, health visitors, all are likely to be older women whom the younger woman perceives as interfering in her life, criticising her, disapproving of her. It is a permanent aspect of all kinds of oppression among human groups that the oppressed are forced to act out institutionalised oppression and exert pressure on those immediately beneath them in the power structure. The sales manageress who herself was never allowed to sit down never allows a younger saleswoman to sit down, although (because) her own legs and feet are screaming from the pain of such abuse over the years. The younger saleswoman damns her in her heart and aloud. A cruel system is then seen to be personified in the old bitch who notices how long a saleswoman stays off the floor when she goes to the toilet, but not how pale and tired she is from trying to keep up with the demands of husband and family. The odd thing of course is that a man could behave in exactly the same way and it would not be so bitterly resented.

Female writers, regardless of their own grey hairs, were quick to root the old woman out of their hearts, and to write as intolerantly of older women as any man. If we scan the works of George Eliot for fifty-year-old female characters, for example, we find very few. There is Adam Bede's mother, Lisbeth, 'an anxious, spare yet vigorous old woman' (p. 54), although probably not yet fifty, who does nothing but whine and wail. Eliot gives vent to her own rejection of her own ageing in the construction of this character; her identification with a perpetual daughter is repellently clear in the writing as she rejects Lisbeth as 'The long-lost mother, whose face we begin to see in the glass as our own wrinkles come, [who] once fretted our young souls with her anxious humours and irrational persistence' (p. 56). An older woman's concerns are not concerns but 'humours', and her pressing of her case is not persistence but 'irrational persistence'. All old women are hags; all old hags are batty old hags. Needless to say, Eliot is not interested in Lisbeth, and does not dwell upon the change in her life and character that ensues when her alcoholic husband tumbles into a stream and drowns. One day, perhaps, someone will write a novel called 'The Deliverance of Lisbeth Bede'.

Part of the misery of the menopause is the suspicion that one might be going crazy, that one's identity is dissolving, in Marina Benjamin's phrase. At the time when George Eliot was writing, most medical practitioners believed that menopause caused derangement. In his *Practical Treatise of the Diseases of Women* (1844) Samuel Ashwell declared that of the disorders of the menopause, the commonest was 'functional derangement of the brain and nervous system'. The mental aberrations included 'timidity, a dread of serious disease, irritability of temper, a disposition to seclusion, impaired appetite or broken sleep, with physical weakness and inquietude ... Hysteria, of marked intensity, not infrequently exists, and with two patients formerly under my care, a stranger, seeing the extent of mental aberration, might, without careful investigation, have concluded that they really were insane.' Happily, Ashwell thought they were not, otherwise they might have joined the throngs of women walled up in madhouses, their temporary aberration forever complicated by institutional psychosis.

The first psychiatrists included among the psychoses something they called involutional melancholia, which afflicted women of climacteric age and men ten years older.

The onset is gradual, with a slow build up of hypochondriasis, pessimism and irritability, finally flowering into a full-blown depressive syndrome. The most prominent features are motor agitation and restlessness, a pervading affect of anxiety and apprehension, an exaggerated hypochondriasis (sometimes with bizarre delusions), and occasional paranoid ideation which infrequently dominates. These distinguishing symptoms may be thought of as superimposed on a basic depressive substrate with insomnia, anorexia and weight loss and feelings of guilt and worthlessness. (Rosenthal, p. 23)

The syndrome was first identified in 1907 in the fifth edition of Kraepelin's *Psychiatrie*; he recommended bed rest, diet and prevention of suicide. Depression in older patients of both sexes is nowadays unlikely to be attributed merely to the processes of ageing, but it is so common and so difficult to treat that researchers have had no option but to return to it time and again. In the 1920s enthusiastic investigators reported 'excellent treatment results' with whole ovary and corpus luteum extracts – the same substances that in later years were shown to be inert (Rosenthal, p. 24). In the 1930s oestrogen was found to work wonders with involutional melancholia, but these results were difficult to repeat and the treatment was as often derided. In 1944 electroconvulsive therapy – shock treatment – was used successfully on women whose melancholy failed to respond to oestrogen. The groups of women studied were all small, there was no double-blind and many of the guinea pigs had been institutionalised for years.

In 1951, John C. Donovan of the University of Rochester set about identifying a climacteric syndrome by regularly interviewing 110 patients referred to him. He found that more than half of them had many current symptoms that could not be explained by their menopausal status, or had symptoms that varied from visit to visit, or had a past history of similar complaints, or were highly suggestible. After the other cases had been further worked up, they too tended to resolve into the same three categories; if they demanded treatment, Donovan often gave them saline injections, pretending that they were hormone, and the patients all claimed to feel better as a result. Donovan was irresistibly led 'to speculation that if a woman has been able to withstand the stress of living without prominently resorting to symptom formation and if the menopause has no catastrophic emotional meaning for her, she will experience the menopause without undue difficulty' (p. 1287). In 1979 involutional melancholia was deleted from the *Diagnostic and Statistical Manual of Mental Disorders*, for it had been proved to the compilers' satisfaction that women of all ages suffered depression with no significant peak in the climacteric (Weissman, 1979).

Nevertheless, women continue to complain of mental disturbance during the peri-menopause. John Studd, the British Master in Menopause, told the *Daily Mail* in 2015 (26 January), 'I see five new patients a day at my clinic complaining of anxiety, depression, tearfulness, mood swings, anger or panic attacks.' A bevy of women told journalist Hannah Ebelthite that 'it was like someone had inhabited my body' or 'I had no idea I might hit my mid-forties and feel like I was losing my mind' or 'I felt fuzzy in the head, like I was tipsy …'

The 'Menopause Health Hub' of the A[lfred] Vogel website states that 'women going through the menopause are four times likelier to suffer from depression than women who are younger than forty-five'. No source is given for the statement. Depression is here described as 'a mental disorder that can lead to further complications and requires the attention of doctors'. The account of clinical depression given here describes it as 'a feeling of extreme sadness lasting for more than two weeks, with no specific cause that can be identified, and which interferes with everyday life. Depression can be accompanied by suicidal thoughts. If you are continually feeling worthless and are having changes in your sleeping and eating patterns, these may also be indicators of depression.' Interestingly we are also told that it needs to be 'diagnosed and treated by a doctor' and it is important for the woman to discuss all her symptoms 'with him'.

Dr Sarah Jarvis is both a doctor and female. Her list of identifying factors for depression goes like this:

Little interest or pleasure in doing things
Feeling low or hopeless
Changes in sleep (not just caused by hot flushes and sweats)
Changes in appetite
Feeling that you have let others down or are a failure
Problems concentrating
Being so sluggish or nervy that others have noticed
At worst, thoughts that you'd be better off dead.

Dr Jarvis is now in her fifties and may be considered to know whereof she speaks. A contributor to a menopause chatroom can be found snarling:

> My doc is still in her 20s. What the hell does she know? SSRIs caused me such horrible digestive problems I am now dealing with that on top of everything. Quit the pills but the problem remains. Thanks a lot. Tried talk therapy. I agree, blah blah blah. I too am old, fat, and cranky plus my looks are gone AND am treated like a problem by the world. 'Get out of the way old lady, life is for the young.' Want to start using a cane so I can accidently trip up these arrogant neophytes. Oh. Tired of being invisible too.

When I read out this lament to a younger woman she said, 'She's just a horrible person' and refused to sympathise.

It is no consolation to find that depression at menopause is pretty much like any other depression. In some ways it is helpful to think that a physical process can be blamed for mental phenomena, especially when that process is understood to have a beginning, a middle and an end. If a woman is allowed to think that she is tearful, irrational or aggressive because she is having a bad menopause, she can escape part of the burden of guilt that attaches to such misbehaviour. She 'has not been quite herself' as the expression goes, and she can therefore return to a self unsullied by her temporary aberration. Once the idea gains ground that the sleepless, exhausted, touchy middle-aged woman is so because she is a 'bad coper', she can be pardoned for regarding a future of failing to cope with ever-increasing problems without the least enthusiasm.

Though involutional melancholia proved to be a phantom of theorisation founded on anecdote, the basic assumption that psychological upheaval was characteristic of the climacteric refused to die, particularly for those who accepted the Freudian account of the process. In 1924, forty-year-old Helene Deutsch addressed a meeting of psychoanalysts at Würzburg on the subject of the climacteric. The paper she gave is the basis of the last chapter in *Psychoanalysis of the Sexual Functions of Women*, published in German by Freud's publishing house in Vienna in 1925. Deutsch's account of the climacteric goes like this:

> Woman's last traumatic experience as a sexual being, the menopause, is under the aegis of an incurable narcissist wound.

In complete parallel to the physical process, this represents a
retrogressive phase in the history of the libido, a regression to
abandoned infantile libidinal positions.

The presupposition, that menopause marks the end of a woman as a
'sexual being', is deterministic to the point of being chilling. It also
appears to be wrong; women past menopause are still sexual beings, but
Deutsch elaborates her distorted vision.

At the menopause everything that was granted the female being
at puberty is taken back. Simultaneously with the processes of
genital retrogression, the beautifying activity of internal glandular
secretions ceases, and the secondary sexual characteristics come
under the aegis of the loss of femininity.
    The libido, now without the possibility of cathexis and with a
diminished capacity for sublimation, has to go into reverse and
seek out earlier positions, *i.e.* set out on the path that is familiar
to us from the formation of neurotic symptoms. (Deutsch,
1984, p. 56)

None of Deutsch's argument is susceptible to proof, nor is any of it
logically necessary. It represents a masculine view, of course, being very
little more than the systematic application of Freudian theory to an
event about which Freud never theorised. The 'complete withdrawal
of the libido from the genitals' cannot be shown to be the inevitable
consequence of the involution of the uterus or the cessation of ovarian
function; the assertion demonstrates a degree of biological determinism
that would seem to imply that all adult females who had never had
congress with the penis had to be insane. Deutsch places the beginning
of the climacterium at age thirty, when

Though still capable of conception, the woman already feels the
threatened devaluation of the genitals as an organ of reproduction,
and on top of this there are the external frustrations to which that
function is exposed (social difficulties, etc.) ... the genitals fight
to regain their position. It has often been suggested that a purely
hormonal process lies behind the pre-climacteric increase in libido
... (p. 57)

– if only a pre-climacteric increase in libido had been actually
demonstrated, which it had not. According to Deutsch clitoral
masturbation is mobilised again, as the ageing female regresses toward
her pre-genital condition, and she becomes sexually rapacious.

> The impulse is provided by the progressive devaluation of the vagina
> in its significance as the organ of reproduction as well as failure
> in the outside world resulting from the greater difficulty of object
> finding, after which an increased libidinal hunger persists in the
> narcissistic need to be desired and loved. The tragi-comic result
> is that the older and less attractive she becomes, the greater is her
> desire to be loved. Under the pressure of failure the vagina gives up
> the struggle ... (pp. 57–8)

Given the element of disguised autobiography in this article, it is not
irrelevant to ask oneself how much the stereotype of the 'dangerous age'
had to do with explaining and containing Deutsch's sexual aberrations
in her thirties. It might make more sense to relate a marked increase in
sexual interest in women in their late thirties, supposing any such change
had ever been observed in any but Deutsch herself, to completed family
size and/or the removal or otherwise of fears of pregnancy. According
to Deutsch, in the pre-menopause women who have hitherto coped
with frigidity now break down; masculinised women 'fall ill over the
femininity complex at menopause'; clitorally centred women suffer
castration anxieties. The incest prohibition breaks down and the pre-
menopausal woman begins to fantasise about repeating the Oedipal
situation with her son; Deutsch cites three cases in illustration for, as
we all know, what drives the attraction of older adults to younger ones
and vice versa is the ubiquitous Oedipus complex.

> The reversion of the libido to objects that are subject to the incest
> prohibition that now sets in as well as the inversion of the psychical
> life by unconscious fantasies lead to a characteristic personality
> change as well as numerous organic symptoms that generally have
> the quality of conversion formations. (p. 59)

It would be interesting to know if Deutsch recognised the
'characteristic personality change' when it started happening to her for,

as we have seen, few women who have actually experienced menopause agree that anything drastic or permanent has happened. Far be it from me to suggest that to proceed from an assumed physical process, described by Deutsch as if it were the defeat of the warring genitals, to psychic manifestations and then back to physical manifestations, which are then denied any connection with bodily events, is arbitrary or preposterous. Climacteric distress, according to Deutsch, is caused by unavoidable frustration: the adolescent's 'too early' is neatly balanced by the premenopausal woman's 'too late'.

> The typical irritability of the unsatisfied, their liability to depression, numerous equivalents of anxiety (giddiness, palpitations, high pulse rates etc.) closely resemble the numerous complaints that appear at puberty ... Of the numerous organic symptoms such as headaches, neuralgia, vasomotor disturbances, heart sensations, digestive troubles etc., a large number must be regarded as conversion symptoms ...
>
> The psycho-neurotic events that take place in the phases of the early climacteric ... come under the heading of hysteria. Later pathological developments come under the pre-genital, that is to say the post-genital heading, i.e. they are obsessional, melancholic, paranoid. (pp. 59–60)

It is worth turning to the entry on the menopause by E. Borner in the *American Cyclopaedia of Obstetrics, and Gynaecology* (1887) to hear the voice of common sense:

> The phenomena of this period are so various and changeable, that he must certainly have had a wide experience who has observed and learned to estimate them all. So ill-defined are the boundaries between the physiological and the pathological in this field of study, that it is highly desirable in the interests of our patients of the other sex, that the greatest possible light should be thrown upon this question.

A hundred and twenty years down the track huge amounts of work have been done, but so far the result of so much light is only deeper shadows.

It must be understood that Deutsch was not writing about the significance of menopause in the general population, but of the mechanisms behind symptom formation in the climacteric, but her account does suggest that women will only cope successfully with the menopause if they can maintain 'male-oriented relations to life' or continue 'psychical motherhood in relation to the outside world', that is, they must either have careers or continue nurturing. Though Deutsch would not have held with the notion of an involutional melancholia as such, she recommended 'an analysis begun just before the menopause' as a precaution against eventual symptom formation. Neither the putative analysts nor the putative patients responded with enthusiasm.

As a Freudian Deutsch was obliged to concentrate on the individual as the source of her own woes. If she had looked at how women treat each other she might have noticed that younger women feel and express hostility towards older women at every stage of life; 'old' is part of practically every insult spoken or thought by a younger woman towards an elder. In the mind of a twelve-year-old a silly bitch is a silly old bitch even when she is not yet thirty. Youth in women is prized by men and, therefore, by women themselves; a younger woman is prompted by a thousand cultural goads into thinking of herself as a newer and therefore better model. There is in our throwaway culture no suspicion that an individual might improve with age and accumulate desirable characteristics.

The tradition of ridiculing older women seems neither to surprise nor to infuriate them. They watch without complaining as television commercials show them to be too stupid to understand the instructions on a detergent packet and too bigoted to see that new chemicals might make it possible to wash soiled clothes in cold water. In 2016, an ad selling dining chairs showed an older woman at Christmas dinner sitting on a kind of improvised seating so low that it left her barely able to see what was on the table. The disparagement was subtler than usual; few people would have noticed the subliminal message that it was only to be expected that grandma would get the worst seat. A TV ad for Heinz ketchup shows a grannie in a pinny producing food for a brat who will not eat it until grandad gives him a bottle of ketchup; when the grannie puckers up for her goodnight kiss, with hideous close-up – grandad brings the ketchup, signifying that it's so good it could even help you stomach grandma's kiss. A supremely nasty ad for Ripolin paints shows a dilapidated painted wall as the wasted breasts of an older woman. The movie *Madagascar* features a character called Nana who is vengeful and violent, 'one seriously mean old lady', capable of beating up a lion as a 'bad kitty'. Very funny, if you're not an old lady.

A recent TV commercial for Tostito potato crisps shows the Tostito repair team removing not just inferior chips from a party venue but also an 'unwanted relative'. According to the Huffington Post, 'one of the crew members, dressed in blue uniform and yellow safety helmet, is shown pushing a hand truck on which an immobilized elderly woman is strapped and wrapped in moving blankets, like a piece of discarded furniture. A disclaimer subtly runs across the bottom of the screen: "Not responsible for damaged relatives." To make it worse, it appears that the woman is smiling innocently, which could only be the case if she were cognitively impaired in some way.' This element has not found its way into the advertising campaign by accident. The ad is contrived to harvest deep-seated intolerance for older people, especially women.

The creation and imposition of these stereotypes of older women involve the cooperation of women themselves. While there are still very few women writing television commercials or working as art and campaign directors in the agencies, there is no lack of actresses prepared to caricature themselves and their mothers. From 1987 to 1994, J. Walter Thompson employed a Jewish actress in her forties, Maureen Lipman, to caricature a 55-year-old Jewish woman, Beattie Bellman, who was adept at creating confusion on the telephone. The campaign was funny but, like lots of British humour, it was also sexist, racist and ageist. Such a campaign relies for its acceptability on the fact that no one cares about older women, not even older women themselves. Lipman regarded Beattie as her masterpiece; the account of the first two years that she co-authored with Richard Phillips admonished readers: 'You've seen the ads … now read the book – then phone your mother.' The discarded relative in the Tostito ad could well have been a mother. Elisa Gabrielli and 77-year-old Marion Ross were more than happy to voice Nana, the 'abusive old lady' and 'ninja-nanny' in the *Madagascar* movies for Dreamworks Animation.

In twenty-first-century society rejection of the mother is almost a condition of entry into adulthood. What answer can there be to the mother who confides to a web blog … 'being a single mother, doing my best and raising two adult boys who are now successful men, husbands, and fathers, I feel a deep sadness. I am not included, and always made to feel like I have done them a horrible wrong in some way. I can't do anything right. I am starting to wonder what's wrong with me. Yet their father and I divorced when they were small, he rarely saw them, paid little support, lives 3,000 miles away and they welcome him into their homes. I wish I could let it go. It makes me feel so small. Like I am a failure.'

Under the rubric 'Mother damned-est', the website 'Psychology Today' reassured readers that 'in a sense difficult mothers are the norm. Our need for a mother's attention, appreciation, and understanding is great; our expectations are high. We tend to be critical of responses that are not precisely what we hope for. Her shortcomings – the endless reminders to be careful; her compulsive checking-up whether you have your keys as you head out the door, when you forgot them only once, two years ago; her inability to read an instruction manual – irritate and embarrass us, because we retain our idealization of the powerful nurturer of infancy.'

The importance of advertising in our culture can hardly be exaggerated. Market research investigates attitudes and responses in order to establish the imagery that will be effective in presenting products as desirable or indispensable for their target audience. That imagery is based in prejudice and relies on prejudice for its subtext. Advertising cannot but reinforce the prejudices existing in the community. Only the subtlest and most intelligent, and hence the least effective, advertising can buck the system. With the ageing of the population a new rich market exists for new services and new products, retirement homes, pension plans, fiscal services of all kinds, health products, treatments, tourism and so forth; the problem is how to sell them. Old faces, old bodies sell nothing, if only for the reason that most people perceive themselves as essentially younger than they are. A car advertised as specially suitable for a senior citizen would not be bought by senior citizens, none of whom want to be stereotyped in that way. No old person wants to go on a tour that has only old people on it. A TV ad for Volkswagen shows young men buying a used Golf from one ancient careful lady driver with flashbacks of her popping wheelies and making handbrake turns. It is important to register the fact that all such positive views show white-haired grandmothers rather than middle-aged women. In the winter of 2015 much was made of a passing fad amongst designers for models over the age of seventy to front their campaigns. That was daring; putting their expensive creations on fifty-year-olds would have been simply stupid.

The advertising industry though aimed at women is run by men. As recently as 2010, women working in the advertising industry set up the '3% Conference' in response to the fact that only 3 per cent of creative directors were women. Women make around 75 per cent of all purchasing decisions but only 11 per cent of advertising creative executives are female. Protests against the sexualisation of women in advertising in all media are made every day, but nobody, not even the few powerful female executives in the industry who are themselves middle-aged, points out that women over thirty have no place in the advertising world.

The gender bias in the industry is probably why it remains stubbornly resistant to the fact that middle-aged women have more spending power than younger ones. Instead of finding middle-aged women selling products to other middle-aged women we are astonished to find, at all hours of the day, well before the watershed, women of a certain age targeted in ads that are downright humiliating. They are there to typify sufferers from 'sensitive' or 'overactive bladder', of which as many as one woman in three is said to be a victim. Middle-aged women, otherwise absent from our screens, are shown daring to laugh and run and even dance because their urine leakages are now under control, skilfully absorbed by products laughably labelled 'Always Discreet' and the like. Some global companies have made efforts to address gender bias and stereotyping in the campaigns they use to sell products to the female public. In July 2016, household goods company Unilever said it would 'unstereotype' its adverts after research suggested that only 2 per cent of ads showed intelligent women. Odds are than none of the 2 per cent were over the age of thirty-five. Unless of course the subject was incontinence pads.

Fifty-year-old women laugh along with everyone else when male comedians guy whiskery-chinned shrieking old bags in ridiculous hats, their bums stuck out in a nanny's stoop and their feet bulging with bunions. Men seem unable to resist dressing up as women on the slightest pretext, and when they do they and everyone around them seem to find them irresistibly funny. Any white comedian who blacked his face would nowadays be considered deadly unfunny, as would any gentile who put on a big nose to impersonate a Jew. The cross-dressing travesties devised by both straight actors and comedians are often no less grotesque and contemptuous than these examples, but women are constrained to laugh at them, if they are not to be accused of having no sense of humour. When Les Dawson or Benny Hill or Dick Emery created female characters, there was nothing tender or empathetic about them, especially if they were over thirty. The endless female characters created by Eric Idle, Michael Palin, Terry Jones, John Cleese and Graham Chapman in *Monty Python's Flying Circus* were hardly less repulsive, being more in the way of a public schoolboy's eye view of matron than a recognition of a middle-aged woman as a human being. Middle-aged women can be funny, but when they are it is automatically assumed that it was inadvertent. Their own jokes are, as it were, on them. Unfortunately all too often female comics are indeed the butts of their own comedy. Jo Brand, fifty-eight years old, told an interviewer (*Guardian* 15 May 2016) that the first question she had been asked in a Q&A which she had recently done for charity was 'What's it like to be hated?' Every middle-aged woman could answer that question.

In 2013 *Mrs Brown's Boys* was found to have the highest audience appreciation rating of any British comedy, though critics unanimously condemned it as the worst TV comedy ever made and 'about as funny as a colonoscopy'. Mrs Brown is played as a foul-mouthed middle-aged woman by 57-year-old Brendan O'Carroll. Bizarrely, the community that announced itself offended was not the female majority but the transgender minority. Their contention that '*Mrs Brown's Boys* demonstrates that as long as the majority laugh, the minority are screwed' was countered by Rebecca Ellis: 'actually it is a tradition that gets its laughs ultimately by mocking women' ('Mrs Brown's Boys and gender-bending comedy', Funnywomen 27.2.2013). So secure is *Mrs Brown's Boys*' position as the 'best British sitcom of the twenty-first century' that two special episodes were aired for family viewing on Christmas Day 2016.

Middle-aged women do not see how much of the hatred of Mrs Thatcher derived from the fact that she was fifty-three when she became prime minister, or how much the high-principled rhetoric of the opposition parties made use of knee-jerk animus against the aged female. So far there has been no speculation about the menopausal status of Britain's second female prime minister, sixty-year-old Theresa May, whereas Mrs Thatcher's possibly mythical patchet was famous.

In the popular TV series *Acorn Antiques*, conceived as a parody of the ITV soap opera *Crossroads*, which ran from 1985 to 1987, Julie Walters, then thirty-five, created the 'decrepit cleaner' Mrs Overall. As Laura Thompson wrote in the *Telegraph* in 2012 (19 June): 'Although Acorn Antiques was brimful of glorious jokes, it was the tentative emergence of Walters on to the set – old-lady legs stumbling into cardboard walls, hair-netted head and widow's hump just visible above a tray laden with 'home-made macaroons' – that tipped the whole thing into hysteria.' When Walters, described as Britain's best-loved actress and a national treasure, was given a lifetime award by Bafta in 2013 she is said to have been happy for Mrs Overall, who was largely her invention, to be her enduring legacy. According to a series of statements she made in the Twentyteens about her menopause, when 'she would sometimes endure as many as 15 hot flushes in a night', she weathered a prolonged and difficult peri-menopause, and yet she evinces no embarrassment if anyone should remind her that one of the most often quoted jokes from *Acorn Antiques* is about poor Mrs Overall. Miss Babs says: 'Mrs Overall can't have gotten far. That's one of the blessings of osteoporosis.' Walters was also happy to play Bren's elderly sick, 'self-centred', 'delusional' and eventually dying mother Petula Gordino in *Dinnerladies*.

The British viewing public never tired of the 'monstrous snob' Hyacinth Bucket in *Keeping Up Appearances*, created by Roy Clarke, who claimed in an interview with the *Mirror* (26.2.2016), 'I knew Hyacinths who kept their husbands confined to the kitchen. Hyacinth Bucket was the least invented of all my characters; I took her largely from life.' The woman who aligns herself with old women and objects, on behalf of old women, to the casual abuse of old women will be told that she is not old. Present company is excluded so that old women in general can be vilified and mocked.

Simone de Beauvoir wrote *Force of Circumstance* between June 1960, when she was fifty-two, and March 1963. At thirty-nine she had had a rather unsatisfactory affair; at forty-four, when she was already obsessed by the spectre of advancing age, 26-year-old Claude Lanzmann telephoned and asked her to go to the movies with him. De Beauvoir

was so pathetically grateful for this attention that when she replaced the
receiver she burst into tears. Within weeks he had moved in with her.

> Lanzmann's presence beside me freed me from my age. First, it did
> away with my anxiety attacks. Two or three times he caught me
> going through one, and he was so alarmed to see me thus shaken
> that a command was established in every bone and nerve of my
> body never to yield to them; I found the idea of dragging him
> already into the horrors of declining age revolting. (De Beauvoir,
> 1965, p. 297)

In fact de Beauvoir had suffered from panic attacks all her adult life,
but in *Force of Circumstance* she relates them specifically to ageing. In
The Second Sex de Beauvoir prefigured her own condition:

> Long before the eventual mutilation, woman is haunted by the
> horror of growing old ... she has gambled much more heavily than
> the man on the sexual values she possesses; to hold her husband
> and assure herself of his protection, it is necessary for her to be
> attractive, to please ... What is to become of her when she no
> longer has any hold on him? This is what she anxiously asks herself,
> as she helplessly looks on at the degeneration of this fleshy object
> that she identifies with herself. (pp. 587-8)

Like Helene Deutsch, de Beauvoir tends to see her subjective
experience as universal. When she wrote *The Second Sex* she was only
forty-one yet she was already vividly aware of the signs of her bodily
ageing. It seems unlikely that all her love affairs would have ended because
her body was ageing, rather than because of growing incompatibility
or boredom or dislike. (She chooses not to discuss her relationships
with younger women, or why it was that she handed so many of the
women she had sexual relationships with over to Sartre.) What seems
more likely is that de Beauvoir interpreted male loss of interest itself as
evidence of ageing, and internalised the value judgement that she had
foisted on to her lover/lovers. It is not intrinsically improbable that her
lovers felt both unable to reassure her, given the intensity of her anxiety,
and unequal to the demands her anxiety made upon their failing sexual
prowess. Helene Deutsch would have explained de Beauvoir's phobia as

what happens when a successfully masculinised identity is undone by the femininity complex of the pre-menopause, and predicted that an Oedipal affair with a much younger man was on the cards.

By 1959 de Beauvoir and Lanzmann were moving apart.

When I had first known him I was not yet ripe for old age; he hid its approach from me. Now I had found it already established inside me. (p. 480)

She was in fact barely fifty-one years old.

De Beauvoir does not show any signs of realisation that her view of her age was wildly distorted. She certainly seems not to consider the possibility that living in propinquity with a much younger man is not likely to assist with adjustment to one's own ageing. By mid-1959 Lanzmann had moved out; in 1963 he married his first wife. De Beauvoir meanwhile had settled into a shallow but interminable depression:

I no longer have much desire to go travelling over this earth emptied of its marvels; there is nothing to expect if one does not expect everything ... To grow old is to set limits on oneself, to shrink ... I have lived stretched out towards the future, and now I am recapitulating, looking back over the past ... once my worktable is left behind, time past closes its ranks behind me ... suddenly I collide again with my age. (pp. 670–1)

There is not much point in preserving people to live to be full of years if they are to spend the reclaimed time in futile repining. Simone de Beauvoir is, she tells us repeatedly, an intellectual; notwithstanding, she faces the future as unprovided as any empty-headed beauty queen.

Old age. From a distance you take it to be an institution; but they are all young, these people who suddenly find that they are old. One day I said to myself: 'I'm forty!' By the time I recovered from the shock of that discovery I had reached fifty. The stupor that seized me then has not left me yet ...

Often in my sleep I dream that in a dream I'm fifty-four, I wake and find I'm only thirty. 'What a terrible nightmare I had!' says the young woman who thinks she's awake ... (p. 672)

De Beauvoir regards this obsession – she says herself the nightmare recurs 'often' – as no more than reasonable. She is excessively revolted by her own appearance:

> Before the mirror I often stop, flabbergasted at the sight of this incredible thing that serves me as a face. I understand la Castiglione who had every mirror smashed … When I was able to look at my face without displeasure I gave it no thought, it could look after itself … I loathe my appearance now: the eyebrows slipping down towards the eyes, the bags underneath, the excessive fullness of the cheeks, and that air of sadness round the mouth that wrinkles always bring … when I look, I see my face as it was, attacked by the pox of time for which there is no cure. (pp. 672–3)

This despondency seems to be specifically related to menopause. The conviction that her death has already begun, because it 'haunts' her sleep, is quite irrational. De Beauvoir could have died at any time, and did not in fact die for another twenty years. Though we might imagine that our death comes on stealthily, we have no way of knowing if it is thundering towards us or is still forty years away. Characterising ageing as dying is the kind of category mistake that a woman as well instructed as de Beauvoir should blush to make. It is ironic that she is unashamed to present herself as a nightmare-ridden narcissistic phobic, but ashamed to offer an explanation in terms of a menopausal syndrome. On the one hand she had everything that any middle-aged woman could ask – health, work, independence, fame and friends; on the other, she had never been a beauty. Perhaps her desolation is the outcome of the impoverishment of existential philosophy itself: she can find no joy in the idea that she is drifting away from an earth whose injustice and misery disgust her. It is as if she has no interior landscape.

> One after another, thread by thread, they have been worn through, the bonds that hold me to this earth, and they are giving way now, or soon will.
>   Yes, the moment has come to say: Never again! It is not I who am saying goodbye to all those things I once enjoyed, it is they who are leaving me; the mountain paths disdain my feet. Never again shall I collapse, drunk with fatigue, into the smell of hay. (p. 657)

Why ever not? we must ask. There is no lack of fatigue, no lack of hay. There may be no truth in the idea of involutional melancholia, but there does seem to be something radically wrong with 54-year-old Simone de Beauvoir, who suffered for years from anxiety attacks and then gratuitously identifies an anxiety attack as one of the 'horrors of declining age'. If one were to coin a word to describe her state it would be 'anophobia', irrational fear of the old woman. It would seem to be deeply rooted in fear of the mother and rejection of the mothering role, and in the kind of insecurity that requires the winning of male attention as a condition of self-approbation. Her condition is not so different from that of the old concubine in Aphra Behn's *Oroonoko* who confesses that 'certainly, nothing is more afflicting to a decay'd Beauty, than to behold in itself declining Charms, that were once ador'd; and to find those Caresses paid to new Beauties, to which once she laid Claim; to hear them whisper, as she passes by, that once was a delicate Woman' (Summers, V, p. 147).

De Beauvoir's self-defeating mental processes, her vivid awareness of death, her nightmares and obsessions, are the misery of the climacteric. Like the sweats and the pins and needles, they will recede, but if this brief agony has reminded us of our weaknesses and inadequacies, it should have left us sadder, wiser and more merciful than before. We can no longer permit ourselves to say as de Beauvoir does that 'my species is two-thirds composed of worms, too weak ever to rebel, who drag their way from birth to death through a perpetual dusk of despair' (1965, p. 654). The healthy, wealthy, literate woman who lives to menopause only to find herself brought low, struggling to get from one day to the next, knows that life is all but too hard for all of us, and hardest for the poor and hungry, who nevertheless create as much joy and beauty as richer women do, and more. The woman who can write that two-thirds of her species are nothing but worms seems to have lost her bearings; her disillusion seems to have reached toxic levels.

> Nothing will have taken place, I can still see the edge of hazel trees
> flurried by the wind and the promises with which I fed my beating
> heart while I stood gazing at the gold-mine at my feet: a whole
> life to live. The promises have all been kept. And yet, turning an
> incredulous gaze towards that young and credulous girl, I realize
> with stupor how much I was gypped. (p. 658)

So wrote Simone de Beauvoir in 1963 when she was just fifty-five. Her heart was (of course) still beating. No one had diddled her; she deluded and diddled herself. Her disappointment with her life is endogenous; it arises in her. We have to assume that Simone de Beauvoir's attitude to the actual cessation of the menses was entirely negative, if for no better reason than that she refuses to mention it.

Thirty years later we are told that researchers have charted a gradual change in attitude towards menopause from negative to more positive, which is considered a good and helpful phenomenon. In so far as women's anxiety about menopause may be lessened by the inculcation of less negative notions perhaps it is, but if the nett effect is to lessen the already scant sympathy that others feel for the woman struggling with menopause, the change in attitudes can only be a bad thing. Studies of attitude to menopause are misleading, however. In 1963, psychologists Bernice Neugarten and Ruth Kraines of the University of Chicago devised an ATM (attitudes toward menopause) test, which they administered to four groups of women: women in their twenties, between thirty and forty-four, from forty-five to fifty-five and from fifty-six to sixty-five. Attitudes were divided into seven categories: negative affect, post-menopausal recovery, extent of continuity, control of symptoms, psychological change, unpredictability and sexuality. More than half the women in their twenties and the women actually traversing the climacterium thought that menopause was an unpleasant experience. Two-thirds of the women over forty-five thought that women felt better when the menopause was over, in sharp contrast to younger women, of whom only 19 per cent in their twenties and 27 per cent of the others agreed. Likewise, under the heading of continuity, three-quarters or more of the older women tended to think that menopause did not change a woman in any way, but only half the women in their twenties. If a woman is the sum of her changes it is puzzling to know what they can have made of the question about continuity; older people are not the same as younger people. Life would be very dreary and rather pointless if they were; the question seems to test ego strength rather than 'continuity'. Under 'control of symptoms' was registered the attitude that women who had problems at menopause were those who expected them, and, surprisingly, three-quarters of the older women agreed. When under 'psychological change' we find the example 'women often get self-centred at the menopause', we must wonder how far these notions were prompted; in any event, only half or fewer of the women under fifty-five agreed, and only a third of the older women (Neugarten and Kraines 1965, Neugarten et al., 1968).

A constant feature of attitudes to menopause is the resentment of the young. Virtually all the studies of attitudes to menopause show that they are more negative among the young (Eisner and Kelly, 1980; Dege and Gretzinger, 1982) than among the middle-aged themselves. The loaded description of menopausal women as 'more self-centred' in the Neugarten and Kraines sample might have been substituted by 'less self-sacrificing', 'more preoccupied', 'less accessible', 'less predictable' or 'less biddable'. Mothers and wives are, in my experience, seldom self-centred to begin with, especially by comparison with both their husbands and their children. The perception of a less obliging female as more self-centred seems to carry part of the resentment felt by family members if the mothering function ceases to be the focus of a woman's life.

When it comes to having a 'positive image' of the menopause, the mind begins to boggle. It is hard to feel positive about vasomotor disturbance, painful intercourse and ageing; if saying that you reckon you can handle it is regarded as the expression of a positive attitude, the notion of positivity that is being invoked would seem to be paler than pallid. The truth seems to be that the question itself instructs the 'coping' response; women who appear to be coping best may in fact not be facing the situation at all. They may be sparing their partners and family members from facing it too. Though such gallant behaviour will be perceived as positive, it is actually anything but. Researchers might ask about a woman's attitude to the loss of her reproductive function and be told that it makes no odds at all. If family size was completed years before, even fifteen or twenty years before, and contraception has been a problem ever since, it would be strange that any woman should regret the cessation of ovarian function. If the same woman were to be asked how confident she felt in her power to attract male attention whether in bed with her partner or in the forecourt of the petrol station, the answer might be very different. Though she sees men of her age having no difficulty at all in attracting the attention of women, and holding it, and flirting as much as they ever did, she knows that she has become invisible, and is now expected to be inaudible. She has a choice, to become the kind of stentorian bully who can be heard apostrophising saleswomen from the other side of the department store, or to fade out of sight and hearing. The combination of ageism and sexism in our society is what makes menopause utterly negative; asking the woman herself whether she shares the negativity is to challenge her own self-esteem, and to call forth the classic response to stigma.

The menopausal woman herself is not likely to be heartened at the conclusion of a survey by the International Health Foundation (Akzo) that Subjective Adaptation (satisfaction with daily life, health, physical appearance and daily tasks and view of the future), Role Identity (dependency on others, identification with traditional female, maternal and sexual roles), Family Relations and Wider Social Relations all deteriorate with age, some with a dip at menopause, some not. John G. Greene is quick to notice that in discussion the authors of the report of the IHF survey frequently use the term 'menopausal crisis' despite their own findings, and he rejects their final conclusion, namely that 'it is clear that for many women the menopause is a period of disorientation, physical problems and psychological imbalance' (p. 49). The confusion here is one we have encountered throughout discussion of menopause, that the processes of ageing cannot be intelligibly distinguished from those of menopause. Greene's opinion remains that 'the impact of the menopause per se on most of the psychological and social characteristics of middle aged women in this survey appears to be relatively benign, certainly in comparison with that of chronological age' (p. 79).

In the early 1970s Greene was asked to see patients with possible psychological symptoms from Dr David Hart's Menopause Clinic at Stobhill Hospital in Glasgow – the first menopause clinic in Europe – and this resulted in the seminal paper 'A factor analytic study of climacteric symptoms' which was published in 1976 in the *Journal of Psychosomatic Research*. In 1998 he published the pivotal article for menopause research, 'Constructing a Standard Climacteric Scale', which was intended to provide uniform criteria that would guarantee comparability of measurement all over the world. Women presenting for assessment in research programmes using the scale had to fill out a twenty-five-item questionnaire. Greene's scale was widely used, for example, in Holland (Barentsen et al.), Australia (Travers et al.) Ecuador (Sierra et al.) Hong Kong (Chen et al.) Bangalore (Chattha et al.), and in Uttarakhand, northern India, where 'most of the women rated menopause as a positive change in life' (Kapur et al.).

In 1975 Scottish psychiatrist Barbara Ballinger of Royal Dundee Liff Hospital undertook a survey of all the women between the ages of forty and fifty-five listed in six general practices in Dundee in order to find out how many of them were suffering any kind of latent or manifest psychiatric illness. As well as a questionnaire about their menstrual cycle and family situation the women were all sent the General Hospital Questionnaire, which lists sixty symptoms and asks respondents to mark which ones they have; a score of eleven identifies a suitable case for treatment. No fewer than 30 per cent of the 539 women who responded were identified as probably psychiatric cases; among women between forty-five and forty-nine the figure was as high as 40 per cent. The case seemed to be proven. In fact it was not, for hot flushes are included on the symptom list, and six items relate to disturbed sleep, which in menopausal women can be caused by vasomotor disturbance. Neither should have been included as a psychological symptom. Ballinger's publications (1975, 1976, 1977) are all based on this study, which, though its flaws have been stringently analysed by John G. Greene (1984, pp. 55–6, 80–81, etc.), is itself the authority for dozens of articles on the psychotropic effects of HRT.

It is only to be expected that in discussion of depression in women in their fifties, allopathic medicine would place all the emphasis on a possible biochemical basis for it. Though we find, as Mansel Aylward found in 1973, that menopausal women are low in indoleamines, and in particular tryptophan, we ought perhaps to consider the possibility that these substances are not secreted in sufficient quantity because patients are depressed. Low levels of tryptophan are as likely to be a symptom as a cause. The organism may react to grim and painful conditions by failing to secrete the chemical of joy and serenity. Administration of oestrogens may free bound tryptophan, but given the pronounced placebo effect noticed in all double-blind trials of oestrogens, it is impossible to conclude from that that oestrogen will 'cure' the misery of middle-aged women. It seems equally possible that the display of genuine interest in the middle-aged woman and the expression of concern for her state of mind and health will raise her spirits, and the objective sign of raised spirits will be higher levels of tryptophan. It would seem from the marked placebo effect noticed in studies of menopause that with menopausal women a very little help and support goes a long way.

Those of us who see that women's lives predispose them to anxiety and depression can see pretty clearly that not only menopause but also ageing can cause both to intensify in midlife. Sofia Andreyevna Tolstoy was married at eighteen; her husband, the great novelist, was thirty-eight. Sofia Andreyevna loved him with the kind of mature, genitally centred passion that Deutsch would have regarded as appropriate; he responded to her intensity and then hated himself for it, not least because he made her pregnant thirteen times. Sofia Andreyevna learned the full extent of his contempt for her when she read his diaries, in which he claimed that he had to get away from her, that a wife like her would drive anyone mad. One of the torments of her life was that her husband showed the diaries to other people. Though he called her his ordeal, he continued to use her body when he felt the need, until the last year of his long life. After these episodes of compulsive sex, he would treat her with contempt even colder than before. She never gave up her struggle for his love, but he never granted what she yearned for: tenderness, intimacy and respect. The verdict of history is that she was a paranoid, hysterical nightmare who tormented the great man beyond endurance. As he lay dying, she was prevented from being by his side in case she should upset him.

A woman whose ego is under such pitiless onslaught can hardly be expected to deal calmly and quietly with her change of life. By the time of her fiftieth winter on earth, in 1895, Countess Tolstoy was in a sorry state. Her last-born child, Ivan, was her joy and consolation, but he was frail and often ill. Tolstoy never took her place by Ivan's bedside for a moment. To her worry and exhaustion was added the stress of the climacteric. She confided to her diary:

Something is broken inside me – I ache inside and cannot control myself. (12 January)

My body has stopped – my body and soul have come to a halt. (14 January)

I am exhausted by Vanechka's illness and my own situation. I feel weak, and breathless from the slightest exertion. (16–17 January)

I have never learned to do anything properly! ... It's fine, 6 below freezing, a moonlit night. But I am still depressed and my soul is asleep. (19 January)

I am in poor health, constantly bothered by asthma and palpitations. If I walk fast my pulse shoots up in five minutes from 64 to 120. (1 February)

I am passing through yet another painful period ... it is so terrible, so difficult, and so clear to me now that my life is going into a decline. I have no desire to live and thoughts of suicide pursue me ever more relentlessly. Save me lord, from such a sin. Today I again tried to leave home ... (21 February)

Demented by 'the old grief of having loved him so much' when Tolstoy had never loved her, she had run off in the snow in her nightclothes and slippers.

He has killed my very soul. I am already dead ... Having tortured my soul, he then called in the doctors to examine me ... so the neurologist prescribed bromide and the specialist in internal diseases prescribed Vichy water and drops. Then the gynaecologist Snegirev was called in, referred cynically to my 'critical time of life' and prescribed his particular medicine. I haven't taken any of it.

On 23 February little Ivan died. Sofia Andreyevna wrote in her diary, 'My God, and I am still alive!' For two years her diary lay untouched. By the time she took up her pen again her condition had changed. She had ceased to menstruate and accepted that she was in the 'critical time of female life'.

... today I left the room in which I have slept for 35 years and moved into Masha's old room. I have started to want more privacy, besides it was stiflingly hot in the bedroom and I am drenched in sweat all day as it is. (3 July 1897)

However much my children criticise me, I can never be again as I was. I am worn out, my passionate maternal feelings are exhausted ... I feel happier with outsiders, I need new, more peaceful and straightforward relationships with people now ... (23 July)

Needless to say, Tolstoy was bitterly jealous of his subject wife's attempts to find in other relationships the esteem that he withheld. Simone de Beauvoir sees the storminess of their relationship as merely the psychopathology of age; according to her, Sofia Andreyevna had 'always hated' sleeping with Tolstoy, for whose contradictory attitudes towards his own sexuality de Beauvoir seems to have considerable sympathy. She notes quite neutrally that Tolstoy 'slept with' his wife on his seventieth birthday (p. 398), with no sign of awareness of how the old man's cold and selfish lust devastated Sofia Andreyevna. (A better account of the sexual economy of the Tolstoy household can be found in Andrea Dworkin's book, *Intercourse*.)

In her book *Life Change* (1988) Barbara Evans is principally concerned to make a distinction between the endocrinological and the psychological causes of climacteric depression. As she has seen HRT relieve the symptoms she goes for the endocrinological version, even though the doses used in one of the few trials of oestrogen in cases of depression were up to ten times higher than those used for vaginal atrophy and vasomotor disturbance. Interestingly endocrinologist Edward L. Klaiber, who ran this American experiment, came to the conclusion that severely depressed women had actually become resistant to oestrogen. We could reverse the order of biofeedback in the case of mood-regulating hormones as well and argue that angry women will not tolerate their own tryptophan, rather than assuming that they are angry because they do not have enough of it. In 2002 Klaiber brought out his popular book *Hormones and the Mind*, in which he 'draws upon recent advances in the emerging field of psychoneuroendocrinology to show how certain hormone "cocktails" tailored to each person's particular biochemical profile can work as an effective remedy against depression, moodiness, irritability, memory loss, and sexual dysfunction by restoring the proper hormonal balance to the mind and body'. The book is not addressed to 'each person'; it is subtitled 'A woman's guide to enhancing mood, vitality and sexual vitality'. Klaiber's 'unique system of individualised hormone modulation' is presumably accessible at a price from his medical practice in Worcester, Massachusetts. One delighted patient bears witness online:

> He sat with me for well over an hour, asking detailed questions about my health and family history. He knew after talking to me that my hormone levels would be low, and drew blood. Two weeks later when I received the results, which were appallingly out of whack, I was overwhelmed and relieved and very, very grateful that

fate had sent me to him. I had always *known* in my gut that there
had to be a real, biological reason for my poor energy levels and
persistent depression … now, finally, a doctor had (rather easily)
documented WHY.

Needless to say, Klaiber's personalised cocktails use 'bioidentical'
hormones; according to another witness he also prescribes Prozac,
Paxil, SSRIs and Zoloft, which is a shame, when it seems that when he
was younger he was on to something different and better.

It does not do to argue in a world where a woman's only friend and
counsellor is her doctor that there may be causes for women's misery
that are not endogenous. The doctor must treat the patient as a closed-
loop system, because the sociocultural wheels that grind her cannot be
moved by medical prescription. The doctor, who cannot operate upon
the body politic, can only attempt to adjust the patient to it.

If the misery of menopause is associated with ageing rather than
menopause itself, the inference must be that it will not go away, but
will steadily, quietly and inexorably worsen. Likewise it seems that loss
of interest in sex is not menopause-related but age-related. However,
the state of current understanding is not such that we need to believe
either proposition. A good deal of the misery of older women is
actually a concomitant of menopause, and does fade when the stress
of the climacteric is past. In 1798 when Elizabeth Inchbald was forty-
five she was well and busy rehearsing her play *Lovers' Vows* in London.
She declared herself 'Happy but for a suspicion amounting almost to
a certainty of a rapid appearance of age in my face'. A year later she
described herself as 'extremely happy but for the still nearer approach
of age'. Two years later, in 1801, when she was mourning the death of
her 'best friend in the world', Perdita Robinson, she made one of the
very few references in literature to the menopause as 'the suspicion of
never more being as a young woman again', adding that she was 'very
happy but for my years'. The next year she declares herself 'very happy
but for ill health, ill looks, etc.' But by 1803, despite leaving her London
home for ever and fearing an invasion of the French, she could describe
herself as simply 'very happy'.

Even so, there is an ineluctable social dimension to the dreariness
that enwraps some post-menopausal women. Margaret Powell, in *The
Treasure Upstairs*, tells us that when she was a door-to-door canvasser

she met many women who were pathetically grateful for someone to talk to.

> One middle-aged and quite well-to-do widow assured me that
> she always filled in every form sent to her by the council or the
> government, 'because,' she said, 'for a brief while it gives me
> the feeling that I'm alive and my existence is noted somewhere.
> Otherwise every day is so much like another that I could be in a
> dream and not in the real world at all.' (p. 104)

When the only person a woman has a right to talk to is her doctor, and only the doctor is obliged to listen, we cannot be surprised that so many women seek consultations, thus putting themselves in mortal danger, for the doctor must prescribe, and nothing a doctor can prescribe will make an empty life worth living. Overprescription of tranquillisers threatens the health of women of all ages, including women in the climacteric. Overprescription of tranquillisers is the price we pay for pretending that misery is disease and not an appropriate response to oppressive circumstances. Though there is no psychopathology that arises from the cessation of ovulation and the involution of the uterus, there is a psychopathology that threatens the older woman's mental health. It is a complex of sexism and ageism further complicated by greed, intolerance, impatience and callousness. Giving women medicines to help them to deal with it is another case of medicating one person for another's illness.

12

Grief

One of the subtlest changes during the fifth climacteric is the encroachment on the consciousness of the idea of death and – even less acceptable to most people – the idea of one's own death. Quite suddenly and without warning or deliberation, after fifty years of feeling immortal, we begin to see an end to our journey on earth. Rachel Brooks Gleason, a woman doctor who with her husband ran a hydropathic establishment called the Elmira Water Cure in the 1880s, used to tell her patients that 'the menopause tells us that we are looking toward the sunset. But is there not a brighter morning in that land where there is no night, where no one is sick, none is sad and all are satisfied?' (p. 217). History does not record whether her patients found this observation cheering, or whether they fled howling.

Dr Gleason was not terribly sympathetic to women's anxieties; she admitted to wishing that her more anxious patients suffered in reality from the infirmities that they imagined that they suffered from, so that she could send them home to die. Nowadays a therapist who allowed, let alone encouraged, menopausal women to spend any time trying to understand death would be accused of dereliction of duty. The middle-aged woman's new consciousness of the finiteness of the individual life, which involves an awareness of the limitations on what can be accomplished in a single life, is another of her guilty secrets. In consumer society everything may be talked about, the most intimate anatomical and personal matters may be discussed in any company, but not death.

In 1969 Iris Murdoch wrote a strange and interesting novel called *Bruno's Dream*. At its centre is Bruno, an old man who is bedridden, waiting for death. He is a curious figure, with a huge head and withered limbs, who might be thought to resemble one of the spiders that have fascinated him all his life. A spider is not only capable of living for months without nourishment, with only the thinnest flicker of vital force that will nevertheless suffice to launch it into killing mode if prey should come within its reach; in dreams the spider prefigures the womb, and Bruno's is a dream. Though in treating this odd old man whose head is 'a mass of crumpled flesh' as a figure of the womb in process of involution there is a considerable risk of appearing solemnly absurd, and Iris Murdoch would have been the first person gently to ridicule any such reading, the novel makes a good deal of sense if we pursue the analogy. Bruno continues to die throughout. His fortune resides in a collection of stamps which is eventually lost. It would be too much perhaps to insinuate that the stamps are like the undeveloped ova, blueprints for something of immense value that can never be built. They are lost, of course, in a flood.

Around Bruno's deathbed revolves a cast of characters who dovetail like a Chinese puzzle: Danby Odell, the womaniser, who married Bruno's daughter Gwen, who died when she dived into a river, the same river that will flood in the novel, to rescue a child; Miles Greensleave, Bruno's son, who married Parvati (goddess of plenty), who died (pregnant) in a plane crash, and then Diana (goddess of chastity), and Diana's sister, Lisa, the unfulfilled spinster, ex-Poor Clare, actually in love with her sister's husband, together with the low-life trio of Adelaide the Maid, Nigel the Hippy and his twin brother Will, the unreflecting male animal. Bruno himself had betrayed his intense wife Janie with a prostitute called Maureen, whom he had to give up when his wife discovered the affair when she came across them both in a fitting-room in Harrods. Bruno wants to reconcile himself with his son, Miles, but the meeting causes only greater bitterness. It also brings Danby into contact with Miles's wife, Diana. Diana, the calm, the beautiful, the orchestratress of existence, is menopausal, 'nearly fifty' as she says.

> She had spent so many years waiting for children and only lately
> had consciously told herself that the wait was over. She had
> occupied so many years – how had she occupied them? … She still

counted herself fortunate. Though lately, perhaps prophetically, collected quietly in the kitchen at night, she had found herself looking a little with new eyes, had felt a vague need for change, had sensed even the possibility of boredom. (pp. 90–1)

This is the view from inside of the menopausal woman's bad behaviour, and it is not so very bad after all. Diana begins a flirt with Danby, meaning to hold off physical intimacy, but needing the excitement and the confidence that the flirtation gives her. She wants the romance and courtship signified by old-time dance music.

I am middle-aged, thought Diana, looking around the ballroom at the dreamy couples who were so far from young. I belong with these people … Had Diana now reached an age where there had to be, at last, one novelty after another? (p. 93)

Two crushing blows knock Diana out of the game once for all. Her new suitor has barely declared himself before he falls intensely in love with her younger sister, Lisa, and then Diana's husband finds that he is in love with Lisa too. Diana is stripped of everything she has lived for. It is as if she has realised that her lovers are all in love with herself when young, and she is moving inexorably away from them to a realm where they cannot follow.

Because 'April is the cruellest month' the novel is obsessed with barrenness amid the fresh lushness of early spring, the season of narcissi and anemones. Danby courts Lisa, who to other eyes than his is simply 'a gaunt untidy middle-aged schoolmistress', in Brompton Cemetery. Actually she is the angel of death, and the cemetery is a mass of tiny graves like the follicles of the failing ovary.

Behind her were the graves of children, tiny pathetic stones half lost in the meadowy vegetation. The silent sleepers made a dome of quietness. (p. 146)

Bruno is a dome, inside a dome, the cage of his bed, a sarcophagus that contains a barely living body. Though it is risky to assume that a writer is not in control of her material, the return of these elements within *Bruno's Dream* suggests something not quite worked out, indeed, something not quite confronted. The contrasting women of the novel are like aspects of the same woman before, after and during her changes, one mourning her never-born children and one her lover and one her youth.

Adelaide the Maid is Danby's housekeeper, and his mistress.

Adelaide, though putting on weight and no longer very young, was really quite beautiful … She was heavy about the hips and stomach but her shoulders and breasts were classical. She had a round face and a naturally rosy complexion and a great deal of long hair of a rich brown colour. (Her hair was dyed, only Danby had never realized this.) (p. 20)

Adelaide's reaction to losing Danby to Diana seems accurately pre-menopausal, although she is too young to be described that way.

She had that heavy graceless fat feeling which she identified as the feeling of growing old, the feeling of no return. She had made some sort of life-mistake which meant that everything would grow worse and never better. Was there no action which she could perform which, like the magic ritual in the fairy tale, would reverse it all and suddenly reveal her hidden identity? But she had no hidden identity. (p. 133)

Adelaide is a kind of living proof of those researches that show that uneducated blue-collar women suffer more at menopause than women who have options not connected with sexual and reproductive function. Adelaide cannot cope with Danby's loss of interest. She deliberately does dreadful things, smashing fragile china, stealing a valuable stamp, destroying a camera, and then painfully regrets them. She is rescued by Will's constancy; they marry despite everything, though the bride is fearfully flushed and hot and tearful. Adelaide alone proves fruitful. Her husband becomes a knighted actor, and her tall twin sons, Benedick and Mercutio, a Russian expert and a mathematician, respectively. Adelaide's happy ending is Murdoch at her most perverse. It is told out of sync, before we reach the real ending which must be Bruno's death. In Adelaide's case Eros wins and Thanatos is held at bay, but it is Thanatos we are really concerned with. The consignment of Adelaide to life is perfunctory.

Diana knows about her husband's love for Lisa as soon as he does. She tells him 'things will never be the same again, never, never, never' (p. 174); the whole book cries out that 'the most precious thing is gone, lost forever'. What is lost was not truly valued until it was lost. The bitter pangs of regret that rack the pages are typical of menopausal mourning, but Murdoch does not allow herself to dwell upon the mental state of any single character. We move in and out of the mental states of all the characters in what seems to be an omniscient fashion but, though we see the tears shining on Diana's cheek as she lies rigid in bed alongside her husband, we do not feel them. The experience is held at bay. The book speaks to itself in riddles. Lisa gives Miles up, sentencing him to 'real death', and declares her intention of going to India.

> If only they had gone away, thought Diana, I could have survived. Of course it would have been terrible. She tried to imagine the house suddenly empty, deprived of that dear familiar animal presence. They had lived together for so long like animals in a hutch. But all she could feel was the hollow misery of her irrevocably transformed marriage, 'Things will never be the same again, never.' But if they had gone, she thought, then all the energy, all the pride, all the sense of self would have been on the side of survival ... Every way I lose. She has taken him from me, she has destroyed our married love, and I have no new life, only the dead form of the old life ... My pain and my bitterness are sealed up inside me forever. I have no source of energy, no growth of being, to enable me to live this hateful role ... I am humbled by this to the point of annihilation ... (p. 33)

At this point Diana does not know that Danby too loves her sister. She is told it by Nigel, the *deus ex machina* who, when she asks 'What about me?', instructs her: 'That is what they all cry. Relax. Let them walk on you. Send anger and hate away. Love them and let them walk on you. Love Miles, love Danby, love Lisa, love Bruno, love Nigel' (p. 239).

The doctrine is a hard one, but it is the only one that can help a suffering woman to cope with the eclipse of her womb. Diana must extract her ego from the business of loving; she must rise above the narcissism that is luring her to the quintessentially narcissistic act of self-murder. Nigel takes the sleeping pills out of her handbag and returns them to the place she pinched them from. The black tide of the river rises; Adelaide and Bruno both fall into the water and the stamps are lost. Somehow everyone survives and the story resumes the next spring, in Brompton Cemetery again, where Diana and Miles are walking 'like an old couple'. Suddenly Lisa reappears and offers herself to Danby because she wants all the things she has always denied herself, 'warmth and love, affection, laughter, happiness'. The angel of death is humanised and takes what is on offer, although it is only second-best. Diana meanwhile has to contemplate the slow demise of Bruno and grows to love him.

> And now, she thought, I have done the most foolish thing of all, in becoming so attached to someone who is dying. Is not this the most pointless of loves? Like loving death itself ... He could give her nothing in return except pain. And it seemed to her as the days went by and Bruno became weaker and less rational, that she had come to participate in his death, that she was experiencing it too. Diana felt herself growing older and one day when she looked in the glass she saw that she resembled somebody. She resembled Lisa as Lisa used to be. Then she began to notice that everything was looking different. The smarting bitterness was gone. Instead there was a more august and terrible pain than she had ever known before. As she sat day after day holding Bruno's gaunt blotched hand in her own she puzzled over the pain and what it was and where it was, whether in her or in Bruno. (p. 309)

The mourning is not easy, nor is it soon over.

> The pain increased until Diana did not even know whether it was pain any more, and she wondered if she would be utterly changed by it or whether she would return to her ordinary being and forget what it had been like in those last days with Bruno. She felt that if she could only remember it she would be changed. But in what way? And what was there to remember? What was there that seemed so important, something she could understand now and which she so much feared to lose? She could not wish to suffer like this throughout the rest of her life. (p. 310)

But eventually her grieving has accomplished its work, and run its
course.

> Let love like a huge vault open out overhead. The helplessness of
> human stuff in the grip of death was something which Diana felt
> in her own body. She lived the reality of death and felt herself made
> nothing by it and denuded of desire. Yet love still existed and it was
> the only thing that existed.
>
> The old spotted hand that was holding on to hers relaxed gently
> at last. (pp. 310–11)

A novel is perhaps not the best way to confront the anguish of the
middle-aged woman, but it is one way to tease out the elements of the
conundrum without appearing to beg for diagnosis, treatment and cure.
For many of our female poets grief was a medium in which they
worked all their lives, but even in such cases the grief of the climacteric is
distinct, tougher, more grinding, for it is grief that cannot ask or expect
to be assuaged. Elizabeth Barrett chose invalidism and reclusiveness
until her virgin fastness was invaded by Robert Browning. Their love
story is commonly perceived to be without blemish; in fact a degree of
ennui and irritation seems to have crept in long before Elizabeth's death
at the age of fifty-five. In the volume of poems published the year after
her death, there is one that strikes the note of climacteric grief. It is to
Robert Browning's credit that he did not attempt to expunge it from
the Barrett Browning canon, for it specifically denies the myth that
Robert and Elizabeth lived happily ever after.

> You see we're tired, my heart and I.
>   We dealt with books, we trusted men,
>   And in our own blood drenched the pen,
> As if such colours could not fly.
>   We walked too straight for fortune's end,
>   We loved too true to keep a friend;
> At last we're tired, my heart and I.
>
> How tired we feel, my heart and I!
>   We seem of no use in the world;
>   Our fancies hang, grey and uncurled

About men's eyes indifferently.
    Our voice which thrilled you so, will let
    You sleep; our tears are only wet:
What do we here, my heart and I? ...   (p. 566)

Understandably, such poems do not make a poet's reputation. The celebration of middle-aged dreariness does not have the glamour of blighted love or premature disillusion, but to the middle-aged woman herself it is a comfort, if a cool one, to know that other women have stood on the same bleak promontory and wondered if there was any point in surviving the crossing. Elizabeth seems in fact to have given up, for her health declined rapidly in this period; within a few months of penning these lines she was dead.

Christina Rossetti, who deliberately chose the life of a celibate semi-recluse in preference to the kind of middle-class marriage that was offered to her, who loved in secret and writhed in lifelong frustration, expressed the bereavement of the climacteric in typically encoded form in the poem given by its editor, Rossetti's brother, William, the title 'A Life's Parallels'.

Never on this side of the grave again,
    On this side of the river,
On this side of the garner of the grain,
        Never.

Ever while time flows on and on and on,
    That narrow noiseless river,
Ever while corn bows heavy-headed, wan,
        Ever.

Never despairing, often fainting, rueing,
    But looking back, ah never!
Faint yet pursuing, faint yet still pursuing
        Ever.   (Vol. 2, p. 105)

Rossetti William was uncomfortable with this kind of writing, which he found harsh and unfeminine. He would have been even more uncomfortable if he had paused to consider the imagery of the ungathered ears of corn and the silent channel beside. Rossetti often thought of herself as a spiritual athlete; the imagery of life as an uphill climb reaches its apogee in another poem of the same period, 'Resurgam'.

From depth to height, from height to loftier height,
    The climber sets his foot and sets his face,
    Tracks lingering sunbeams to their halting-place,
And counts the last pulsations of the light.
Strenuous thro' day and unsurprised by night
    He runs a race with Time and wins the race,
    Emptied and stripped of all save only Grace,
Will, Love, a threefold panoply of might.
Darkness descends for light he toiled to seek:
    He stumbles on the darkened mountain-head,
      Left breathless in the unbreathable thin air,
    Made freeman of the living and the dead:–
He wots not he has topped the topmost peak,
      But the returning sun will find him there.   (Vol. 2, p.171)

Now that more and more women are publishing poetry, and more and more of that poetry deals with women's reality rather than parodying the preoccupations of men, we can perhaps expect better insights into the emotional world of the ageing woman than were available to us before. In 1978 the distinguished American poet Linda Pastan published a book of poems called by the name of the last poem in the collection, *The Five Stages of Grief*. On the jacket May Sarton is quoted as saying: 'Nothing is here for effect. There is no self-pity, but in this new book she has reached down to a deep layer and is letting the darkness in.'

What distinguishes the older woman's grief is precisely this absence of self-pity. Her lament is not about herself, nor is it complaint. It is sterner than either and more austere, repellently so perhaps to the young, who repeatedly fail to understand its 'still, sad music'. The epigraph to the book (from Shakespeare's *Richard II*) could be lettered on the T-shirt of every woman who is looking her destiny in the eye:

You may my glories and my state depose,
But not my griefs. Still am I king of those.

The five stages of grief are Denial, Anger, Bargaining, Depression and Acceptance. Perhaps menopause comes as such a shock to so many women because they have been denying their advancing age for so long. The complaint, that it has come too soon, is heard by many doctors. Emily Dickinson encapsulates this experience in eight lines:

> Consulting summer's clock,
> But half the hours remain.
> I ascertain it with a shock –
> I shall not look again.
> The second half of joy
> Is shorter than the first.
> The truth I do not dare to know
> I muffle with a jest.

(p. 697)

Denial is over, of course, as soon as a woman registers the truth that she has been denying. Linda Pastan may only have realised that the first group of poems fitted into a denial group when she had passed that stage herself.

> In this season of salt
> leaves drop away
> revealing the structure
> of the trees.
> Good bones,
> as my father would say
> drawing the hair from my face.
> I'd pull impatiently away.
> Today we visit my father's grave.
> My mother housekeeps, with trowel
> among the stones,
> already at home here.
> Impatient, even at forty
> I hurry her home.
> We carry our childhoods
> In our arms.

(Pastan, 1978, p. 3)

This small poem is full of ironies; the home that the daughter hurries
her mother to is also the grave, impatient even (still? already?) at forty,
denying the place where her mother actually lives, refusing to see where
she herself is heading, and yet the poem knows. The exploration moves
quietly on through the sequence, while unfamiliar darkness gathers
around familiar imagery:

> At the edge of the grass
> Our deaths wait like domestic animals.
> They have been there all along, patient and loving.
> We must hurry or we may miss them in the swelling dark.

The imagery of bereavement is complicated by themes of adultery,
of the departure of a lover/husband, and by the poet's fear of the end
of her creativity; the painfulness of the underlying theme of the death
of the womb is almost too deep for utterance, though there is no other
way of reading a poem like 'Egg'.

> In this kingdom
> the sun never sets;
> under the pale oval
> of the sky
> there seems no way in
> or out,
> and though there is a sea here
> there is no tide.
> For the egg itself
> is a moon
> glowing faintly
> in the galaxy of the barn,
> safe but for the spoon's
> ominous thunder,
> the first delicate crack
> of lightning. (p. 5)

In the angry phase of her grief, the poet cries out against those who
reject her, by dying, by their unthinking superiority, by adultery ('all
men are babies, my mother said'), by leaving her. In the last poem

in this section, 'Exeunt Omnes', she takes the only way out (having shrunk from suicide) by detaching herself from the life that does not satisfy her, in which she has failed, being no more than an 'average' mother/wife, to satisfy the ones she loved.

> Let everything happen
> off-stage
> Leave me
> with the scenery:
> with the stream which this morning
> is all surfaces;
> the hills which alter
> no more than their colours;
> with the old passion
> of the seasons
> changing.
> Let the only dialogue
> be between hawk and crow in their innocent
> murderous play.
> Go away
> all of you.

(p. 22)

Detachment is not so easily accomplished. In the next stage in realising grief the poet's struggle to cling to the life that is rejecting her continues, but the young are appearing more and more as an alien race. The pain of bereavement breaks open at the old site; the companion insists on leaving, having no need to feel as she does, indeed dreading the sharing of her feeling.

> Don't leave now.
> We have almost
> survived
> our lives.

(p. 28)

The failed negotiation leads to 'Depression'.

You tell me nature is no mirror
yet in the broken surface
of the lake I find
jagged pieces of my face.
Ask nature what love is.
Silence is answer enough.

(p. 37)

All the poems in this section are bleak; the familiar imagery of the beloved country is replaced by hotel rooms and 'the city'; her mother's voice on the telephone crackles 'like a brush-fire soon to be put out'. Life is a test that she has failed.

I studied
so long
for my life
that this morning when I waken
to it as if for the first time
someone is already walking
down the aisle
collecting the papers.

(p. 42)

This is the authentic regret of the climacterium, with its special feeling that if only one had been allowed a reprieve one would have done better. The notion that life is out of one's control, the decisions affecting one's whole existence have been made and acted on behind one's back, dominates the most unbearable phase of the sea-change. When we have identified the delusion, we are already on the way to refuting it.

I studied
so long
for my life,
and all the time
morning had been parked
outside my window,
one wheel of the sun

resting against the curb.
Can so much light
be simply
to read by?
I open the curtain
to see,
just as the test
is over.

(p. 43)

The test is over; the results are unimportant. Study has ended and the living is about to begin. The programmed life of response to the expectations and demands of others has ended. But for the moment the woman is blinded by the harshness of the light and can hear only the cawing of the crows. She can find no joy yet in her own observations in '25th High School Reunion':

We come to hear the endings
of all the stories
in our anthology
of false starts:
how the girl who seemed
as hard as nails
was hammered
into shape;
how the athletes ran
out of races;
how under the skin
our skulls rise
to the surface
like rocks in the bed
of a drying stream.
Look! We have all
turned into
ourselves.

(p. 45)

We have arrived at the point of 'Acceptance' but this time the poet does not find herself walking towards the sun and away from night, as

Kate does in her dreams in *The Summer Before the Dark*. Her agony is not yet over; her grief is a circular staircase and she is back where she started, ready to deny, rage, and bargain all over again.

The middle-aged woman will not find it easy to get her mourning done. Our culture demands a smiling face; it is bad enough to know oneself for an old trout, without having to add the epithet 'miserable'. We have no tolerance for female images that are solemn, thoughtful or severe. The menopausal woman finds that she is obliged to buck up, to pull herself together. If she wants to sit and think and cry a little or a lot, she is made to feel that these are bad wishes, and may not be indulged because such behaviour makes other people feel bad. Yet such feelings are not only just and proper, but necessary. Though Freud might be surprised to find his theory of mourning applied to the eclipse of the womb, because he did not understand the forms in which the womb received the investment of emotional energy, it applies nonetheless. Freud's generic mourner was male, which goes to show that he was as uninterested in older women as they were in themselves. (I have taken the liberty of changing the sex of the mourner.)

> Mourning occurs under the influence of reality-testing; for the
> latter function demands categorically from the bereaved person that
> [s]he should separate h[er]self from the object since it no longer
> exists. Mourning is entrusted with the task of carrying out this
> retreat from the object in all those situations in which it was the
> recipient of a high degree of cathexis. That this separation should be
> painful fits in with what we have just said, in view of the high and
> unsatisfiable cathexis of longing which is concentrated on the object
> by the bereaved person during the reproduction of the situations in
> which [s]he must undo the ties that bind h[er] to it. (Freud, p. 333)

The death of the womb straddles Freud's two categories of physical pain and mourning, and bears all the narcissistic weight that physical pain does, with the same propensity for 'emptying the ego'. The mourner can ignore her condition only at her peril; somehow or another the loss must be acted out. The form that the acting out takes will depend not only on the personality of the mourner but upon her circumstances. Many of the older descriptions of climacteric syndrome noticed that it involved a desire for solitude, a desire that solicitous persons felt obliged to deny. Even when mourning was considered proper and carried out in public, people who assumed that women's emotions exist in order to provoke responses in other people could see no value in a woman's unwitnessed tears.

One exception is the author of *What Every Woman of Forty-five Ought to Know*, published in the United States in 1902. Emma F. Drake was a woman doctor who likened the climacteric to 'early fall housecleaning', which is perfectly manageable unless demanding guests arrive. Though she fell for the lurid descriptions of mental and physical derangements associated with menopause, she still advised her readers to 'be quiet and patient and all will be well' (p. 67). She was prepared to suggest radical strategies that would permit the menopausal woman to get her grieving done. To women panicking that their youth is gone, she recommends taking time out to face just how far away it is.

> Run away from yourself and your surroundings for a while and forget
> for a little the every-day cares. Hunt up some old friend, the more
> closely associated with faraway times the better, and get away to her
> where you can talk over unmolested all the girlhood days. (pp. 92–3)

She encourages women to examine the life that has hitherto been unexamined, assuming, probably correctly, that all the woman's time has been monopolised by others. Long before anyone had identified a 'me generation' she was advising women to take time for themselves. She counselled a sea voyage, 'with a friend who will not tire, or be putting you in mind constantly of things you have left behind'.

> If you are in the city and cannot get away from home, buy a tent
> and set it up in the yard and sleep with nothing but canvas between
> you and the sky … Get away from home as often as you can. It will
> do the family good to miss you … Never mind what social functions
> are demanding your time, get away from them all … (p. 94)

The purpose of getting away is to reflect, to mourn and to let go. Dr Drake teaches her patients, besides the necessity of taking stock, techniques of relaxation, of letting go.

> Learn to be a child again, and go back to your childhood days, to
> remember the recesses and the restfulness. Swing your hammock
> under the trees. (p. 110)

One of the more acceptable reasons that used to be given for menopausal mourning was 'the empty nest', the house that the children have grown up and left. Though missing the children and mourning their leaving home was a perfectly healthy response, the condition came close to being given disease status, with some commentators referring to an empty nest syndrome. As more and more mothers worked outside the home, the impact of this life change became less marked. Recent studies have tended to place less emphasis on parental mourning, and not simply because in these days of crushing student debt, children cannot afford to leave home. Those not in education are finding it more and more difficult to find jobs, and they too are likely to continue living in the parental home. Children whose marriages fail, leaving them with the financial burden of maintenance, may be forced to return to their childhood homes and become part of the 'boomerang generation'. US census data from 2008 showed that as many as 20 million 18- to 34-year-olds (34 per cent of that age group) were living at home with their parents. A decade earlier, only 15 per cent of men and 8 per cent of women in that age range did so. However the grief of the ageing mother is not solely a response to the physical absence of children; Dr Drake understood that mothers miss their babies long before the young persons they have grown into have flown the coop.

Your darlings are not yours quite the same as they were before, and you mourn without meaning to do so ... (p. 117)

Once involved in the inner drama of the climacteric the ageing woman should retreat into her own spiritual world and come to terms with herself. She should not be jollied out of it, or bullied or ridiculed. To be patient she must be allowed to be quiet. Dr Drake quotes the scripture in reference to the grief of single women at menopause, likening them to 'Rachel weeping for her children' and refusing to 'be comforted, because they are not'. All mothers weep for their children's childhood, for the disappearance of those magical small people, who understood so well how to give love and how to take it. It is at least as sad for a woman to know that the love affair with her babies will never come again as never to have known it, especially now that a grandmother's physical hunger for her grandchildren is a thing of no importance.

Our culture has very little tolerance of grief. We are forbidden to mourn even the death of those nearest and dearest. A woman whose child dies is not allowed to sit with other women crying and keening, much less required to do nothing else for a certain prescribed time. A woman whose parent dies is not allowed to veil her head and withdraw from human intercourse in order to understand what has happened to her. What should be a time of recapitulation, of constructing an overview of a long and protean relationship, is expected to pass at the same ragtime pace as the rest of our lives, which are seen as a continuum. The most heartening thing that writers can find to say about the menopause is that there need be 'no change', as if human life was anything but change. The refusal to recognise change is what causes maladjustment. Sorrow is not itself evidence of maladjustment but of the adjustment process itself.

In 1984, Inner City Books, a publishing company set up to promote the application and practical understanding of the work of Carl Gustav Jung, produced a very unusual and important book by the Jungian analyst Ann Mankowitz. *Change of Life: A Psychological Study of Dreams and the Menopause* dealt with the case of 'Rachel', who was fifty-one and had 'just had her final menstruation'. Her marriage had endured, her children were grown up; her husband's parents and her father had died several years before, her mother a year before. Rachel was not complaining of particular difficulties; she simply wanted to understand how to approach the second half of her life, but together she and Mankowitz discovered that there was unfinished business that had to be got out of the way before she could be reborn as herself. Out of Rachel's dreams came evidence of profound desolation and loss.

The first dream was the image of the house in the country, where she had lived when her children were small, as a burnt-out ruin, which struck in the dream with the kind of physical shock that endures long after waking. The second was a scene inside the burnt-out house where an unburnt woman lay upon an unburnt bed, but she was dead. The next was the barn of the burnt-out house, full of dust and ashes where four wisps hung from four ropes and the dreamer recognised them as babies burnt in the fire and turned away, unable to bring herself to look more closely. At this dream Rachel baulked and it was some weeks before she could return to the dream of the dead babies.

When she first described them as looking mummified her eyes filled
with tears and the connection with Mummy, which the children
always called her, and which she called her own mother, became
clear. The number four at first puzzled her, until she remembered
her miscarriage; then she realised that these wisps represented not
just her live children but all the fruit of her womb ... (pp. 55–6)

Once she had confronted the meaning of her dream symbols, Rachel
went through several emotional stages, of shock, of revulsion, and then
of the anguish of maternal deprivation. She became angry with the
analysis, seeing it as the cause of her feelings of grief and hopelessness,
rather than submerged grief and hopelessness as the causes of the
recourse to analysis.

For a few sessions she mourned her 'dead children', her dead hopes.
She talked about the little creatures in the barn and wept over
them; she remembered in detail her births and pregnancies and her
miscarriage; she reminisced over her children as infants and toddlers
and had nightly dreams of babies. She savored the deep nostalgia
that surrounded the whole generative process from beginning to
end ... Then she said farewell to it all. It was gone forever. When
this mourning was over she reported that she felt purged of what
seemed now to be irrational grief, and she felt ready for what might
come next. (p. 58)

Margaret Christie Brown, contributing to an International
Symposium in 1975, ended by saying

I should like finally to make a point that the menopause is a time of
loss and women should not fall into the trap of feeling guilty about
their sadness or of putting doctors into the position that they must
produce a panacea so that no distress is felt at all ... a process of
gradual letting go ... is one of the purposes of mourning.

Brown does not tell us what it is that the menopausal woman is
mourning. Some would say that it is the passing of her beauty; others
that it is the children that she did not have; others that it is the children
she had who died; others that it is the children she had who grew up.

Elizabeth Barrett Browning, in a late poem called 'Little Mattie', gently chided the bereaved mother for her desperate grief, teasing her because her child in heaven could no longer be a baby.

> There's the sting of't. That, I think,
>   Hurts the most a thousandfold!
> To feel sudden, at a wink,
>   Some dear child we used to scold,
> Praise, love both ways, kiss and tease,
>   Teach and tumble as our own,
> All its curls about our knees,
>   Rise up suddenly full-grown.
> Who could wonder such a sight
>   Made a mother mad outright! (p. 557)

On the other hand the grief could be a kind of penitence for having survived the role of lover–mother, for having failed quite to annihilate oneself in altruism. At menopause an old denied self reappears like a ghost, and may indeed reproach us for having delivered our lives over to the control of others who may now appear uncaring and unappreciative. The furious reproach, that one has given 'the best years of one's life' to this or that or these or those, is mostly self-reproach. The people we upbraid will tell us that they did not require or demand the sacrifice; at menopause we are charged by ourselves with having thrown the best years of our lives away. Images of waste, of squandering, and even of charade crowd our dreams waking and sleeping. We have done our best to fulfil the conflicting demands of the female condition and after thirty-five years we have been dishonourably discharged.

The personal has survived the impersonal role of lover–mother and it is not too late, but the grief of the climacteric causes temporary blindness. The end of the old life feels like death. It is a kind of death, from which we will be reborn, but first we must mourn the passing of the other self. Her exequies should include a celebration of her contribution, but in an anti-matrist society a eulogy of the mother is unlikely to be forthcoming.

The middle-aged woman's new thoughtfulness about death may lead her back to the church of her childhood or to her lawyer's office to make a will. If it does, she is unlikely to discuss the matter with anyone other than her priest and her lawyer. Though we might not agree with Prospero in *The Tempest*, who decided that after his daughter was married he would make every third thought a thought about his death, we ought to accept the fact that death is a part of life, and one that can be handled well or badly. The way we handle it will be as much an expression of our personality as anything else we have ever done, unless of course it is taken out of our hands, unless we die not knowing that the great moment is at hand. The older woman knows the truth of the advice that the Duke gives Claudio in *Measure for Measure*, but she should not say so:

> Be absolute for death; either death or life
> Shall thereby be the sweeter. (III.i.5–6)

In the twenty-first century the woman who admits that she sees the climacteric as the entry into the antechamber of death is in grave danger of psychiatric interference. Such weird insights are better kept to oneself. If she admits that death is on her mind, it will be understood that something is wrong with her. She is not allowed to be sad, or sorrowful or melancholy; these conditions are translated into others that signify disturbance or illness. She will be described as despondent or depressed. Thinking about death is considered to be itself a morbid symptom; if its presence is suspected, some brain-deadening treatment will be ordered. If thinking about death is associated with insomnia, severe psychological disturbance will be suspected and more drastic intervention justified. Given this intolerance for grief, it is not surprising that women themselves convert their censored feelings into symptoms. To be sad is wrong; to be sick is not your fault.

Sooner or later death must be thought about. We must get used to the idea at some stage. The climacteric is a time of mourning, whether deaths in the immediate circle of family and friends occur at that time or not. The menopausal woman should be allowed her quiet time and her melancholy. There is work to be done, setting the psychic house in order, organising the basis of a new life, with a new focus and new concerns. It often falls to the lot of menopausal women, who do not themselves feel well and capable, to attend to the needs of a querulous parent or, worse, to see them through a protracted end. How often have you seen the fifty-year-old woman guiding the seventy-five-year-old around the hospital, the supermarket, the theatre foyer? You will not often see a grandchild performing this labour of love; the middle-aged women are the only ones free to do it, and the whole responsibility tends to fall on them.

It is a bitter irony that most of the caring for aged parents has to be undertaken by their menopausal daughters, who may be least able to cope with the anxiety and depression and the bone-deep tiredness that such care can involve. Perhaps in that great storm of emotions the passing of menstruation is a mere bagatelle. Then again, perhaps day-to-day dealing with the ending of life makes the climacteric worse, by underlining the theme of loss, endless irreplaceable loss. To the weight of depression is added the weight of exhaustion and grief. The world suddenly seems all loss and death; the irreversible law of entropy becomes so obvious to the middle-aged daughter who day after day watches her mother struggling with confusion and pain that it seems a law of futility.

There can be no cure for this pain, only the compassion of people with enough imagination to see how vast the sorrow of the middle-aged woman can be. The younger generation soon makes clear that it does not want to be troubled by the details of grandmamma's plight; indeed, the middle-aged woman knows that screening the grim truth is part of her duty towards them. She carries the whole weight in her heart and moves dry-eyed from day to day doing what has to be done.

There was a time when mourning was not forbidden but compulsory, and in many traditional or 'backward' countries it is so still. When my Tuscan friend Angiolina lost her mother, she was in the throes of a climacteric so painful that she had bouts of what appeared to be mental derangement; for the first time in our twenty-year association she stole from me. Sometimes she was disoriented and confused. Her mother's decline was slow and difficult, and Angiolina fretted that she was far away in the house of her daughter-in-law, who did not know how she liked to have her hair braided or how much she longed to see the wild blue hyacinths on our hills where she was born. When Angiolina's mother died, her body was brought home to our small cemetery. Every day for as long as they lasted Angiolina gathered the hyacinths and took them there. Every day she would sit for hours by the grave, talking to her mother. Nobody interfered with her; nobody tried to cheer her up. Instead, neighbours did her household tasks while she gave herself up completely to her grief. She put her bright-coloured headscarfs away and wore a black one. She saved up all her spare money and paid for masses to be said for the repose of her mother's soul.

In those weeks when Angiolina came up to work, we would sit together and sew, and she would talk to me. Her mind was running on her childhood, on her mother's struggle to protect her children from their father's severity, on the way her mother hoarded her egg money so that the children could have small treats, on her mother's suffering when the Nazis shot her eldest son dead in front of her. Normally Angiolina was unreflective; she could not read or write and she had no way of keeping a record. Under the stimulus of her grief for her mother, her memory accomplished extraordinary feats of recall. She would tell me every detail of those far-off days, the way the wind blew, whether the trees were in leaf or in bud, how good the harvest had been, what road she had taken with her goats. She told me how her father threw her out when she refused to give up the poor boy who had courted her for sixteen years. On their wedding night they had no covering to their bed, but Angiolina's mother risked a beating from her husband to creep up the hill by night bringing them the brand-new blanket that was their only wedding present, a luxury in those grim years of the *miseria*.

Angiolina's love for her mother was a passion that had never found its full expression during her mother's life; now that her mother was dead, Angiolina needed to talk to her. I would hear her in the vegetable garden, earnestly talking away as if her mother were there beside her, explaining, protesting, wheedling. Sometimes she would sit and rock for a few moments with her apron held to her eyes. Then, when her grieving was done, she laid by her black kerchief. She still goes to her mother's grave every Sunday before Mass. And she still says when the dark blue hyacinths begin to open on their purple stems, '*alla povera mamma piacevano tanto*' and we both love them the more on that account. In mourning her mother so wholeheartedly Angiolina brought her life under a measure of imaginative control. When her mourning was over her menopausal distress had vanished with it.

The time is long gone when Anglo-Saxons gave vent to their grief. Friends do not hasten to your house when you have suffered a bereavement, in order to sit by the body with you, and weep with you. Grief became first a private thing, veiled and silent, then a secret thing, and then a shameful thing. Sadness, though it is possibly the most rational and explicable state of mind, has become odd and inappropriate. If we were allowed to wear mourning we would discover as I discovered in Sicily that people are quick to offer sympathy, and under the gentle pressure of compassion to recall their own bereavements. The Sicilians would ask me for whom I mourned, when he died, what he was like. Each time I told them my heart felt eased of some of its burden of regret for the things unsaid and the things undone, the roads not taken.

Not only does grief demand expression, the expression of grief brings relief. Some of the finest poetry in our language has been written in the throes of mourning. It might do the grieving woman's heart more good to read it and find release in tears than to dose herself with tranquillisers in an attempt to ignore her justified pain. Failure to mourn makes light of loss, and undervalues the one lost. An unmourned death is made meaningless. Meaninglessness causes despair and despair kills the soul. The ageing woman cannot afford to compromise the life of her soul; her continuing ability to feel is an index of her vitality. As Karen Blixen said, quoting William Faulkner, 'between grief and nothing I choose grief.'

13

Sex and the Single Crone

Women of all ages have a right to sex. For lesbians this appears to be reasonably straightforward; you fancy someone, you tell her so and she at least entertains the idea. For heterosexual women of middle age the situation is very different. Even the richest, the most successful, the fittest and most beautiful, must proceed with caution.

On 12 April 2015 at the Coachella Festival in California, 28-year-old Canadian rapper Drake was singing his song 'Madonna' when the 56-year-old lady herself appeared in thigh-high boots and a multicoloured mac and began dancing around him, singing her new song 'Human Nature'. At that point Drake was sitting in a chair facing the audience; as she passed behind him Madonna yanked his head back, opened her mouth wide and clamped it on Drake's mouth for a full three seconds. When she released him, the audience could see, as she behind him could not, that he looked nauseated. Indeed, he leaned forward and clapped his hand over his mouth as if to stop himself from vomiting. Among the sexist and ageist comments that jammed the Twitterfeed was one from JamesJames Brown: 'Drake looks like a little 6 year old kid who's been forcibly kissed by his auntie with a moustache.' Most reactions, whether from men or women, registered revulsion at the mere thought of 'tonsil tennis with a pensioner'. Madonna may very well have been guilty of a sexual assault but, though there were a few voices who called her behaviour 'rapey', no one suggested that Drake could have filed a suit against her. So powerful is Miss Ciccone that Drake later went public to explain that it was not she or the kiss but her lipstick that was 'gnarly'. Mere days before this event, 21-year-old Justin Bieber confided

on the Ellen DeGeneres Show that he was up for a one-night stand with
Madonna, an offer that was less flattering than he may have imagined.

For the Single Crone sex remains a blood sport. She may have the
right to it, in theory, but seeking it is likely to expose her to all kinds of
risk, some of it potentially lethal. In her last book, *The Treasure Upstairs*,
published in 1970, Margaret Powell, the charlady turned best-selling
author, described the common case of a sixty-year-old woman in love
with a man in his thirties. She tells how, when she took her employer
Thora Ellis out to a pub in Hove, they made the acquaintance of some
young Canadians:

> … Miss Ellis – or Thora – was entranced by her Pete. I didn't at
> that time realize how much she'd been taken in by him. When we
> left together at closing time she talked about him all the way back
> to her home: what an interesting life he'd had, what good manners
> he'd got …

Powell goes on:

> What I didn't know was that she'd given this Pete her address and
> invited him round to the flat. So I was very annoyed when, on the
> following morning, he called at eleven o'clock, and I had to make
> coffee for three instead of two. This was the start of regular visits.
> He felt that he'd got her where he wanted her … he captivated her
> so quickly that no warnings from me would have had any effect.
> I knew she was giving him money. One day he came in wearing a
> new watch, and on another he'd a gold cigarette case. It annoyed
> me how a woman of her age could be so deluded. Surely she should
> have known that a young man of thirty-five couldn't have fallen in
> love with even an attractive woman of over sixty, let alone a plain
> one with a hairy old mole. Eventually I did try telling her that he
> was just after her money, but she wouldn't listen to me. 'He's like a
> son to me,' she kept repeating. 'A right bastard son you'll find him
> to be,' I flung at her in my exasperation …
>
> Then things got worse. This Pete moved into the flat, sleeping
> in the spare room, and he used the place as if it belonged to him.
> He now quite openly asked Miss Ellis for money, even in front of

me, and I could tell it wouldn't be long before he had me out of the place ... (pp. 131–2)

Powell wrote to Miss Ellis's lawyer brother, who threw the opportunist lodger out of the flat and took his sister home with him to Manchester ...

It was this that made me feel so awful about having written to him. I had, as it were, turned the calendar back forty years. She was again keeping house, just exchanging a martinet of a father for a martinet of a brother ... When I said goodbye to her, she didn't reproach me. I think she felt that the moment of happiness she had had made everything worthwhile. She'd had her taste of what, to her at any rate, was romantic love ... (p. 133)

For some women belief in and longing for romantic love never die. Tippi Hedren at eighty-six is still spry and able-bodied, and as slim, fragile and dazzlingly blond as ever. She lives on the Shambala Reserve that she set up in Acton, California, with seventy animals, including tigers and leopards. In September 2008 she told the *Sunday Times*, 'I'm waiting for someone to sweep me off my feet', by whom she did not mean the Grim Reaper. Her daughter Melanie Griffith, who was divorced from Antonio Banderas in 2014, is single, appears to have undergone recent cosmetic surgery but does not admit to it, but does admit to looking for romance. Tippi's granddaughter Dakota Johnson as the female lead in the film of *Fifty Shades of Grey* probably figures that she has had enough 'romance' for the time being at least.

In 1983 Elizabeth Taylor was fifty-three years old, hugely rich, and single after the collapse of her sixth marriage. She was also being treated at the Betty Ford Center at Rancho Mirage California for alcoholism and drug addiction. There she met 31-year-old Larry Fortensky, a construction worker who was there after a conviction for drunk driving. Before the seven weeks of the treatment had come to an end she was in love. Though Miss Taylor told *People Weekly* that she did not intend to marry Fortensky, explaining: 'I think I've outgrown that. In today's society you don't need to be married. You don't need to tidy up. Not at my age any way.' Even so, in 1991 she did marry him in a lavish ceremony at Michael Jackson's Neverland Ranch. They separated in 1996, but remained friends. When Taylor died in 2011, she left Fortensky $800,000.

In 1983 Joan Collins was at the peak of her fame. After two years playing Alexis in *Dynasty*, she had won a Golden Globe award and featured in a twelve-page photo layout in *Playboy*. She was also single, after her divorce from Ron Kass. By a friend's swimming pool she met Swedish one-time popstar Peter Holm. She was fifty; he was thirty-six. He later claimed that he won her heart by having sex with her three times a day. By September he had moved in with her. One of his many girlfriends would later tell the media that Holm's only interest in Collins was her money. She would also quote him as saying 'that he had hated having sex with Joan because she was old and wrinkled', that he had had to think of other women while making love to her, and that he was constantly unfaithful. Another girlfriend, whom Holm set up in an apartment with Collins's money, said Holm told her Joan was 'an old lady' and that he had to arouse himself by watching pornographic films before having sex with her. Against the advice of her friends, Collins eventually married Holm, but his treatment of her deteriorated so rapidly after the event that she sued for divorce in December 1986.

It is the more extraordinary then that within a few years she would make a rather similar mistake again.

She is not easily drawn on the subject of her close friend art-dealer Robin Hurlstone. But after three-and-a-half pretty secret years, 57-year-old Joan Collins has just openly acknowledged their special companionship and disclosed Robin's best qualities. It's 'to Robin' she dedicates her second book, 'for his patience and support. With all my love'.

Patience and support are not what younger women might thank a lover for; the cynical reader might be pardoned for suspecting that Joan and Robin, a never-married old Etonian in his early thirties, were indeed just good friends, or even that Hurlstone was what is known in the business as a walker, supplying the 'harmony, compatibility and friendship' that the star said were the most important aspects of a loving relationship. Unfortunately the tabloid press a few days later ran a story about Collins's attempt to buy a portrait of Mr Hurlstone from his close friend the Marquess of Bristol, who had originally commissioned it. According to gossip columnist Nigel Dempster, when Collins named her price, she was told by the nobleman that it would suffice only to buy pictures of rather a different kind, depicting both Mr Hurlstone and the Marquess in attitudes that she would not find particularly attractive.

Despite Hurlstone's membership of what Collins calls 'the gay monde', his contempt for her family and his unwillingness to spend time with her children, the relationship lasted for thirteen years. When he was dumped for Percy Gibson, Hurlstone was indignant not to have been paid off with a substantial gift. The old school network seems to have come to his rescue; he was last seen as Herr Schneider in *The Grand Budapest Hotel*, which was co-written by his old schoolfriend Hugo Guinness.

Gina Lollobrigida was fifty-seven in 1984 when she met 23-year-old Javier Rigau y Rafols at a party in Monte Carlo. She was then single; her marriage to Milko Skofic had ended in divorce in 1971; she had been briefly engaged to an American real estate heir before the divorce, and had had an affair with Christiaan Barnard, the pioneer of heart-transplant surgery, after it. Still ravishingly beautiful, by her own admission she had always been spoiled by men and had many admirers. She should have been able to resist the juvenile charms of Rigau y Rafols. It was not until October 2006 that their engagement was announced, only to be called off a few weeks later. In 2013 Lollobrigida began legal action against her ex-fiancé, alleging that Rigau y Rafols had staged a fake marriage in Barcelona with a 72-year-old woman impersonating her, so that he could claim her $35 million estate after her death. That case is ongoing at the time of writing, with Lollobrigida alleging that she and Rigau y Rafols never had sexual relations and him alleging that she made coarse and specific propositions at the outset. Lollobrigida also claims that 'A while ago he convinced me to give him my power of attorney. He needed it for some legal affairs. But instead I fear that he took advantage of the fact that I don't understand Spanish ... Who knows what he had me sign.' The whole business is a sad and squalid ending to a distinguished career as an award-winning actress, a photojournalist, holder of the Légion d'Honneur, a generous contributor to stem cell research, representative of UNICEF and 'the most beautiful woman in the world'.

For many years there was a belief current among gentlemen of a certain milieu that menopause often brings a surge in women's sexual urges. Its origins are lost in the annals of prejudice. In the *Spectator* No. 89, Joseph Addison, counselling women against 'the folly of Demurrage' or refusing proposals from eligible gentlemen, warned them darkly about the craziness that lay in wait:

> There is a third Consideration which I would likewise recommend
> to a Demurrer, and that is the great Danger of her falling in Love
> when she is about Three-score, if she cannot satisfy her Doubts and
> Scruples before that Time. There is a kind of latter Spring which gets
> into the Blood of an Old Woman, and turns her into a very odd sort
> of an Animal. I would therefore have the Demurrer consider what a
> strange Figure she will make, if she chances to get over all Difficulties
> and comes to a final resolution in that unseasonable Part of her Life.

The belief that menopause can turn virtuous women into sex maniacs persists. Professor d'Alba, writing in answer to readers' letters in the Italian magazine *Cronaca Vera* in April 1990, told a reader whose wife had been seduced by his African lodger that he was to blame for leaving her alone in the house with the young man. According to the 'professor', women approaching 'the tunnel of the menopause', as he called it, are often troubled with uncontrollable sexual desire, and are therefore particularly susceptible.

Ann Mankowitz feels that, though she can cite no examples, she can say with impunity:

> In fact, the pain and anger brought on by a woman's awareness of
> the decline of her feminine power in middle age can even increase
> her apparent sexual desire, sometimes to the point of frenzied
> promiscuity. (p. 5)

Tore Hallström, principal author of the Göteborg study of the sexuality of women in middle age, which began in 1968 and ran for ten years, and had as its object 'to demonstrate any possible effects of the climacteric on mental health and sexual behaviour', dismisses this notion as a myth.

Even in up-to-date texts the old concept of a specific increase of
the sexual drive in the climacteric is mentioned (e.g. Helen Kaplan,
1974 [in] *The New Sex Therapy*). The present investigation, however,
gives no support to the opinion that sexual interest tends to flare
up at the climacteric. Those women who report increasing sexual
interest or capacity for orgasm are few in number at these ages and
become steadily fewer with rising age ... (p. 166)

The study then cites its own table, which gives 16 per cent of
respondents reporting increased interest at age thirty-eight, 12 per cent
at forty-six, 4 per cent at fifty and 2 per cent at fifty-four. The numbers
reporting increased capacity for orgasm were higher; 21 per cent at
thirty-eight, 18 per cent at forty-six, 13 per cent at fifty and 6 per cent at
fifty-four. These are significant numbers even in so small a sample, and
do provide evidence that the sexually aggressive menopausal female is to
be found with sufficient frequency for most men to have encountered
one. The problem of course is to decide what the increased interest is
being compared with, and whether any of the respondents at fifty had
already experienced increased interest at thirty-eight and forty-six, and
were being asked to calculate an increase over an increase. Nevertheless
Hallström reports confidently: 'The idea of an increased sexual drive
in these years is based on mere anecdotal evidence and must now be
regarded as a myth' (p. 166).

As far as Hallström is concerned, if everybody doesn't have it,
nobody has it. The truth is that many women, especially those with
high circulating levels of testosterone, will feel increased clitoral
sensitivity during the climacteric, and a disturbing level of genital
tension, occurring regardless of the presence or absence of a partner
and often irreconcilable with the presence of a partner used to a
different pattern of response. Women using testosterone to alleviate the
discomforts of menopause may find the ensuing genital irritation and
diffuse sensations of arousal so unmanageable and disconcerting as to
necessitate the cessation of the treatment. Middle-aged women, having
perforce cast off the narcissism of younger women, are quite likely to be
more direct in their sexual advances and to make quite clear what it is
they are after, especially if, for the first time in their lives, what they are
seeking is not love but a fuck. If this is the case, it will be the first time

in their lives that they have understood the male pattern of arousal and the male search for release.

The Göteborg study had as its object 'to demonstrate any possible effects of the climacteric on mental health and sexual behaviour'. What the connection might have been between the two was possibly obvious to Dr Hallström. Of the total random sample of 899 Göteborg women, only 800 were interviewed. The study concerned itself only with 'married women and unmarried women cohabiting with a man'; no questions were asked about female sexuality, except as it was expressed in heterosexual intercourse. There was no mention of masturbation whatsoever, though the best way to assess 'capacity for orgasm' is by asking about masturbation rather than the pattern of response to a (very possibly perfunctory) male partner.

At the conclusion of the Göteborg study forty-five out of a hundred Swedish marriages were ending in divorce. Divorced women living with their children must have made up a significant proportion of the population of Göteborg. There would have been some widows, and there were the 6 per cent or so of women never married, who, we are told, do not make up a deviant or residual group of people left behind, but are part of the community, and usually a distinguished part of it, for the never-married female is typically a high achiever in the highest social class. None of the numerous members of these classes of women has sexuality worth studying, it would appear. In selecting their random sample of cohabiting women, the designers of the study must have ignored a sample almost as large as the one it 'randomly' selected. The value of the study as an indicator of changes in women's sexuality at menopause is little if anything.

The sexuality of older people has always been a subject of ridicule. Revulsion at the demanding of conjugal rights by old men is a staple of European comedy. Usually the wife of the old man is a young woman repelled by the deathly touch of old age and afire for contact with flesh as taut and warm as her own, but similar revulsion could be felt by any woman, regardless of her age. It is quite impossible to 'interiorise' the objective fact of one's age, and hardly more possible to gear one's sexual response to individuals of the right age group. Simone de Beauvoir sees that women are less aware of physical appearance in sexual partners than men are, but does not understand that this is only so in the dialectic of unliberated sex. Women who must be parasitic on men if they and their children are to survive will respond to the evidence of power and wealth, rather than beauty. Women who are financially independent may choose something more delectable; women who are rich can have their pick of very handsome, very much younger men, of the kind who will be only too happy to live off them.

The men who see women only as dependants and treat them as perpetual children do not feel the need to add physical attraction to the services they are prepared to perform. They tend to take little care of their looks and fitness. Most shave when they get out of bed rather than before they get into it. One of the surprising things that can happen to the older woman who achieves her own independence and a degree of authority is that she decide to seek sensual pleasure before it is too late. Her own sensuality leads her in the same direction as men are led, towards youth and beauty. She cannot, however, take her pick of beautiful youth with the same impudence as a man and the relationship is fraught with hazard for both parties. The tragedy of the marriage of May and December has been a theme of European literature since it began, but December in this case is always a man. The marriage of female December and male May has always seemed comic. It is generally assumed that youth is sexually attractive and age is not. From one point of view this is simply objective fact. Young people give off the pheromones that attract sexual interest. Older people don't. While it is understood that men respond to the appeal of young bodies, it is assumed that women are unmoved by it. Paedophilia, the sexual love of children, is understood to be a male attribute. Most women will reject a boy in favour of a man. This was not always the case; Eros is depicted as a youth, and boys have been seen as proper objects for the love of both sexes. This is the older woman, Venus, wooing the boy, Adonis, in Shakespeare's poem *Venus and Adonis*:

'Thrice fairer than myself,' thus she began,
'The field's chief flower, sweet above compare;
Stain to all nymphs, more lovely than a man,
More white and red than doves or roses are ...'

Venus is unlike the heroines of romanticism in that she feels sexual desire and is sexually aggressive. Shakespeare guys her aggressiveness in the poem, but he is equally mocking of the youth's cold rejection of the queen of love. In the libertine culture a very young man was expected to be taught the arts of love by an older woman; one of the routes to preferment for a young nobleman lay through the bed of a powerful woman; he was expected to use his juvenile charms in his own interest much as we now would expect young women to do. This is Aphra Behn's description of the male love object, in this case in the form of a young friar in *The Fair Jilt*, published in 1688:

> ... he wanted no one Grace that could form him for Love,
> he appear'd all that is adorable to the Fair Sex, nor could the
> mis-shapen Habit hide from her the lovely Shape it endeavour'd to
> cover, nor those delicate Hands ... (Summers, V, p. 78)

Such young men were desirable precisely because of their effeminacy, their slenderness, their silky curls, the pink and white of their hairless cheeks. Both men and women were presumed to desire this kind of beauty which, though it lies in a realm beyond gender, did not exclude sex. The exaggerated potency of young men was a part of their attractiveness and a fitting counterpart to the feared potency of females. As one of the 'women who deserve to be praised' says in *The Perfumed Garden of Sheik Nefzawi*:

> I prefer a young man for coition and him only
> He is full of courage, he is my sole ambition
> His member is ... richly proportioned in all its dimensions;
> It has a head like to a brazier.
> Enormous, and none like it in creation;
> Strong it is and hard, with the head rounded off.
> It is always ready for action and does not die down;
> It never sleeps owing to the violence of its love.
>
> (Luria and Tiger, p. 129)

Many epochs have understood that a woman of taste and appetite is best served by a delicious boy who can ejaculate many times to the older man's once. What this meant in practice in pre-revolutionary Europe was that a married woman in her twenties could take as her *cavaliere servente* a youth in his teens. Clearly in Elizabethan England, and throughout the reigns of the Stuarts, male display played an important role in heterosexual affairs. At other times men who exploited their beauty have been more likely to be homosexual and to find male protectors.

Lady Mary Wortley Montagu wrote excitedly in a letter from Vienna in 1716 when she was twenty-seven.

> I can assure you that wrinkles, or a small stoop in the shoulders, nay, grey hair itself, is no objection to the making of new conquests. I know you cannot easily figure to yourself a young fellow of five-and-twenty ogling my Lady [Suffolk] with passion, or pressing to lead the Countess of [Oxford] from an opera. But such are the sights I see every day, and I don't perceive any body surprised at them but myself. A woman, till five-and-thirty, is only looked upon as a raw girl, and can possibly make no noise in the world till about forty ... 'tis a considerable comfort to me, to know there is on earth such a paradise for old women ... (Montagu, I, pp. 269–70)

In 1755, when she was sixty-six, Lady Mary decided that 'no Man ever was in love with a Woman of 40 since the Deluge. A Boy may be so, but that blaze of straw only lasts till he is old enough to distinguish between Youth and Age, which generally happens about 17; till that Time the whole Sex appears angelic to a warm Constitution' (II, p. 98). In April 1736 she had met a handsome, cultivated, clever, 24-year-old Italian, Francesco Algarotti, and lost her 47-year-old heart. Algarotti was also admired by Lady Mary's homosexual friend Lord Hervey, and played them off against each other. In September, after Algarotti had left England, Lady Mary wrote time and again to him in France, humbling herself in repeated confessions of love; in October Algarotti replied, in time she said to save the remains of her understanding. She went on writing to him in Venice, with a most improper suggestion:

> If your affairs do not permit your return to England, mine shall be arranged in such a manner that I may come to Italy. This sounds extraordinary, and yet is not so when you consider the impression

you have made on a heart that is capable of receiving no other. My thoughts of you are such as exceed the strongest panegyric that the vainest man on earth ever wished to hear made of himself ... (II, pp. 110–11)

Algarotti, who was used to the effect his sumptuous good looks and passive charm exercised over the great and good, thought, correctly, that he could probably do better than commit himself to either of his English lovers, both of whom continued to write to him despite his slowness to reply. In March 1739 he wrote to tell Lady Mary that he could not return to her in England if she did not send him money. She did send him money and he returned to live in splendour at Lord Burlington's house, where she saw him often. In July 1739 she left England to meet him in Italy, while he set off with Lord Baltimore on a visit to Russia. On the way back he met the young Prince Frederick of Prussia, who, when he came to the throne in June of the next year, summoned him to court and gave him a Prussian peerage. When Algarotti and Lady Mary met again in Turin in the spring of 1741 she realised how misled she had been:

In you will always be found taste, delicacy and vivacity. Why is it then that I encounter only coarseness and indifference? It is that I am so dull as to excite nothing better, and I see so clearly the nature of your soul that I have as much despair of touching it as Mr Newton would have of adding to his discovery with telescopes ... (II, p. 237, author's translation from the French)

It was of no consequence that Algarotti was homosexual. Lady Mary was looking for the ideal companion with whom to share her life; she believed that Algarotti loved her taste, delicacy and vivacity, as she loved his, and that the evidence of age in her face and body was irrelevant. For many middle-aged women the most suitable choice of companion seems to be an effeminate young man who will assist her in her social life, advise her and console her, amuse and stimulate her. All kinds and degrees of affection can subsist in such a relationship. Her letters show that Lady Mary was passionately in love with Algarotti. Her other homosexual friend, Lord Hervey, on the one hand reminded Algarotti of her lack of physical attraction –

To make her lover pleased as well as kind,
She should be never mute, you always blind

(Halsband, p. 157)

– and on the other reassured Lady Mary that at fifty-two she was not too old for love and should simply choose a new love-object. Lady Mary knew better. After five years of unrequited love, the frenzy had left her for ever. She was left with what she herself called 'the passion of her life', namely her love for her daughter Mary, Lady Bute, to whom she wrote once a fortnight for more than twenty years.

Byron, himself a beautiful youth, who had no financial or social need to capitulate to the older women who wooed him, created Regency versions of the type in *Childe Harold* and *Don Juan*. The gravitation of young men towards older women principally came about because unmarried women could not risk entering the marriage market as used goods. Fornication was out and adultery was in. Our present culture of fornication and serial monogamy, though costly in terms of both money and of human suffering physical and mental, seems doomed to be with us for some time longer. It is, of course, the system that is most injurious to the interests of the older woman, who fares better even under polygamy. However much one might desire a revival of the sex culture that expected young men to be initiated by older women, in order generally to improve the quality of sexual interaction, it is unlikely to eventuate in a society where sex is not merely available but practically inescapable for the young of both sexes.

The last great work to depict the vestiges of the matching of experienced women and much younger men is Colette's masterpiece, *Chéri*. At the beginning of the novel the heroine, Léa, is fifty; for the last six years she has been having an affair with a man twenty-four years younger than she. It has been suggested that the novel was inspired by Karin Michaëlis's *The Dangerous Age* (see above, p. 93), but it was actually based on an affair of one of Colette's female friends, Suzanne Derval.

At forty-nine years of age, Léonie Vallon, known as Léa de Lonval, was coming to the end of a happy career of *courtisane bien rentrée* and *de bonne fille* whom life has spared flattering catastrophes and noble regrets. She concealed the date of her birth; but she confessed

readily, letting a glance of voluptuous condescension fall on Chéri,
that she had reached the age of allowing herself a few little *douceurs*.
She liked neatness, fine linen, mature wines and careful cooking.
(Colette, 1920, p. II, author's translation)

Among the *douceurs* Léa has permitted herself is Chéri, barely twenty
at the beginning of the liaison, now twenty-six. The affair was initiated
by the boy. Léa is not slim; she does not pretend to be younger than
she is, by contrast with Chéri's eventual mother-in-law, Marie Laure.
Her *nourrisson méchant* loves her partly because she is motherly; he
sleeps always with his head pillowed on her left breast, unaware that
she is often awake. Léa deliberately insists upon her seniority; Chéri is
not to call her *ma chère*, as if she were his chambermaid, or a girlfriend
of his own age; she is *madame* (p. 68). Her household is perfectly run;
the champagne she chooses for him as old as she is. Her love for him
is the love of a connoisseur … Colette keeps reminding us that Léa is
overripe; her eyelashes are still dark, but … her eyes still a striking blue,
but … In two years she will have the chin of Louis XVI. 'She had a
good body, guaranteed to last, a big white body flushed with rose, long
legs, a flat back, *la fesse à fossette*, and a high-slung bosom, all guaranteed
to see her out until Chéri was married' (p. 14).

As the novel turns out, Léa is wrong. Chéri is not just a love that
she has conducted with great pleasure and impeccable taste. When he
leaves her to be married, for the first time in her life Léa feels grief, grief
that grows more painful and bitter with every passing day. She goes
away, leaves no forwarding address, travels around France, ostensibly
amusing herself, in reality bored and desperate, but at no time does she
contemplate trying to make contact with Chéri. At this point she is
absent from the novel, for Colette is concerned with its hero, the young
man. If Léa's situation is difficult, Chéri's is tragic.

Chéri, unable to play the role of husband, longing for his cradle in
Léa's bosom, returns to Léa. She admits that by selfishly keeping him
by her side she has prevented him from growing up. They are both
defeated in the end by the twenty-four years that separate them; for
a moment Léa allows herself to believe that they have some time left,
but Chéri knows better. He has come back to a different Léa. The
morning after their reunion in her enormous bed of polished steel and
brass, he does not jump up as he used to, demanding his coffee and

brioches, but pretends to be still asleep. He watches her 'not powdered yet, a thin twist of hair dangling on her neck, her double chin and her devastated neck' (p. 229). She is quick to understand the alteration in him: 'You have come back to an old woman' (p. 245). She begs his pardon for having loved him 'as if they were both to die an hour after' and not thinking of his eventual destiny. In a moment of cutting psychological realism, after she has watched Chéri pause on the doorstep, and allowed herself vainly to hope that he might be about to turn back, she catches sight of herself gesticulating in the mirror. 'A panting old woman in the mirror repeated her gesture, and Léa asked herself what she could have had in common with that madwoman' (p. 251).

In *La Fin de Chéri*, Chéri, still unable to adjust to the role of returned serviceman and husband, commits the folly of calling on Léa in a new apartment, smaller, different from their love-nest in every way. He discovers a huge white-haired old woman, as jolly and unaffected as an old man, who expresses concern for his worn face and attributes his misery to his kidneys, suggesting a good restaurant where he might be able to eat the kind of food that would make him well in soul and body. Only her laugh seems to belong to his Léa; he waits in a sort of mad hope that the real Léa will jump out of this vast fleshy stranger who slaps her thigh as if it were the crupper of a horse. Ultimately Chéri cannot handle time's revenges; he shoots himself.

Colette does not give us the answers to Chéri's anguished questions. When did Léa stop dyeing her hair? When did she leave off her corset? When *Chéri* was published, Colette was forty-nine. She had been working on the idea since 1911; it was not until 1921 that she fell in love with her husband's son by his first marriage, Bertrand de Jouvenel, who was to be the model for Phil in *Le Blé en Herbe*. The relationship lasted until late 1924. *Chéri* made it possible for women of Colette's generation to take young lovers; if *La Fin de Chéri* proved that taking young lovers was a blood sport, the possibility did not deter the rash young men who entered freely into relationships with the likes of Colette and her friend, Marguerite Moreno. In 1924, while she was finishing *La Fin de Chéri*, Colette met Maurice Goudeket; she was fifty-two, he thirty-six. He had a jealous mistress, and the situation was strained at first, but Colette assumed command. She wrote to Marguerite Moreno: 'I got that crazy confidence that people get, when they fall from a belfry, and stroll for a moment in the air *dans un confortable féerique*, and feel no pain anywhere.'

Evidently Colette was thinking, as most women in her situation would do, that the love affair with Goudeket would soon come to a bruising end. While the play of *Chéri* was on tour Colette and Maurice used to meet in the property he had rented in the south of France, and she was amused by the correspondence between the fiction and her reality, but the fact was to turn out very different from the fiction. She and Maurice lived together for thirty years. In April 1935, so that they could travel together on the inaugural voyage of the *Normandie* and stay together in prudish American hotels, Colette and Maurice were married. They remained together – except for a terrible period during the war when Maurice, who was Jewish, was twice arrested, once deported and always obliged to hide – until Colette's death in 1954. In her last years she never let him see her without her powder and kohl, never exposed her devastated body to him. From 1942 she was bedridden by arthritis and her maid, Pauline, helped her to bathe and change her clothes. Maurice Goudeket has left an account of his life with Colette, which explains in some measure how she kept her charm for him; Pauline, to whom she had to show the reality behind her powdered mask, has, of course, left none.

Simone de Beauvoir devotes a significant part of *Old Age* to a discussion of the sexuality of the aged. Everybody knows, she writes, that the frequency of coitus lessens with age. The most salient factor is the marital status of the individual; the married continue to have relations, because difficulty in achieving and maintaining erection, and of satisfying a partner, are less catastrophic in a settled relationship than in a chance encounter. De Beauvoir's point of view in this discussion is, as usual in *Old Age*, entirely male-oriented. She does not appear to realise, let alone care, that she has failed to consider whether the fumblings of an aged spouse are gratifying to his wife, nor does she suggest that the frequency of coitus ought to have anything to do with a wife's desires. Worse still, though she treats masturbation as if it were equivalent as a sign of active sexuality, in this discussion there is no mention of female masturbation at all. There is never any suggestion that the changes in the female genitalia that are consequent upon menopause might make genital sexual activity not only pleasureless but painful, and that the demands for reassurance on the part of aged males who see in their penis their alter ego might be experienced by their wives as an oppression.

We have de Beauvoir's own discussion to remind us that interiorly women do not see themselves as old. Every woman being mounted by an old man with a half-erection is, in this sense, a young woman. Colette's Léa considers making love to the middle-aged men who still court her, and rejects the idea of accommodating a paunch and a wrinkled faceful of false teeth with disgust. A woman of taste would of course prefer to hold in her arms the boy of whom Lady Mary spoke, whose semen flows like tap water, the same boy as is depicted on a Greek vase in the Fitzwilliam with the legend in Greek, 'The boy, yes, the boy is beautiful.' A blaze of straw is better than no fire at all, and there is more to lovemaking than insertion of the sacred phallus. There is also closeness, sleeping together, waking together, sight, smell and touch. The sex that de Beauvoir discusses is sex without sensuality.

De Beauvoir carries her male-centred discussion even further from a female viewpoint, however. In speaking of masturbation she interpolates an observation of her own.

> When he is old he grows tired of a companion he knows too
> well, even more so since she has aged and he no longer finds her
> desirable … And no doubt many elderly men prefer their fantasies
> to their wife's age-worn body. (p. 359)

She can find no good reason for a wife's refusing to have bad sex with her husband, for she goes on, 'And then it happens either as a result of old complexes, or because consciousness of her age makes love repellent to her, the spouse refuses' (pp. 359–60). A man may be repelled by a spouse's ageing body, but a woman may not. De Beauvoir herself might have argued that this observation was not sexist but simply realistic. There do exist gerontophiles of both sexes who are poignantly attracted to and desire sexual congress with old men, but no man, says de Beauvoir, feels sexually attracted to a woman old enough to be his grandmother. She finds that there is nothing to prevent a woman remaining sexually active until the end of her days, because she does not have to fear impotence, and because she is less sensitive than a man to the appearance of her partner. She might have seen in this failure to demand an effective stimulus evidence of women's continuing oppression. We might be justified in seeing, in her failure to allow women any valid reason for rejecting sex with an aged man, a failure to recognise their right to sexual autonomy. In *Force of Circumstance* de Beauvoir had argued that the greatest success of her life was her relationship with Jean-Paul Sartre. She was to see in the years that followed that Sartre needed her less and less, and needed a succession of clever and attractive young female disciples more and more. If she suffered the jealousy that she describes in *Old Age*, her last years must have been tormented indeed. De Beauvoir needed no one but Sartre, but she could not interest him sexually and so, eventually, she lost him – if indeed she ever had him, for Sartre was never heard to say that the greatest achievement of his life was his relationship with de Beauvoir.

Simone de Beauvoir was writing on the eve of the 'sexual revolution'; the stress she placed upon coitus is part of a deliberate strategy of liberation of sexuality, a liberation which has now become promotion and even prescription. It might be argued that though there is no cultural pressure that would drive young men into the arms of older women, older women are now as free as men to look for and exploit sexual opportunities. Such an argument presupposes that women have enough money to frequent places of popular resort (can run a car for example) and present themselves in an attractive manner. Even in cases where these things are equal (and they seldom are), the older woman cannot cruise the sex scene the way that a man of the same age can. She is simply not perceived as a sexual entity, unless she makes an unsubtle display of herself, which amounts to a statement of availability, which is a turn-off to all but the least desirable partners. She then exposes herself in a buyers' market, and the results to her physical and mental health, to her very life, can be ruinous.

Susan Winter, co-author with Felicia Brings of *Older Women, Younger Men*, is full of naïve optimism.

> There are new options for love and romance. We are free to love
> the person we desire, regardless of age – theirs, or ours. Barriers
> that limit love are crumbling. The freedom to love should know
> no boundaries. As women continue to see themselves as powerful,
> deserving, and worthy, they enjoy a greater participation in all the
> world has to offer. Younger men are just one form of this expression.
> It's a choice, formerly not granted to us. It's not about sex. It's about

love. It's not about younger men seeking money or opportunity.
And, it's not about an older woman using manipulation. It's about
real love – a love that can, and does work.

Ms Winter does not say where a middle-aged woman might find
younger men who are not 'seeking money or opportunity'. As long ago
as 1954 when Noel Coward was holidaying in Capri he was fascinated by
the 'rather macabre spectacle' of 'hordes of middle-aged ladies arriving
by every boat'. The result was the comic song 'A Bar on the Piccola
Marina', where love came to Mrs Wentworth-Brewster. Romance
tourism is by no means a recent phenomenon, but few of the people
who write about it are as forbearing as Coward. Most give full vent to
sneering disgust and condescension. Jane Atkinson reported from The
Gambia in 2012 (the *Sun*, 7 December)

> The young men, some of them teenagers, target the white women.
> Marriage to a 'toubab' – a white foreigner – is their goal. They
> see them as their ticket to a new life in a country with endless
> opportunities.

The presence of the romance tourists was having a marked effect on the
decorum of social life in The Gambia.

> At the end of dinner … the women who were quietly sitting
> together rushed to the dance floor as the young Gambian men
> eagerly pounced on them. The transformation was both remarkable
> and shocking …
> The women gyrated their hips into the groins of the men –
> known as gigolos – who are often young enough to be their sons
> or even grandsons. Some even started kissing, despite The Gambia
> being a country where couples are rarely seen holding hands. This
> is a secret life for hundreds of British women who can get a package
> holiday here for as little as £400 for a week.

Atkinson gave several examples. One was a 55-year-old single mum
who used her disability allowance to visit her Gambian boyfriend up to
five times a year. Another was Helen in her late fifties, who has helped
her Gambian boyfriend to buy his own café and bar and is quoted as

saying, 'I've always wanted to set somebody up in a restaurant and now Ousman has one. He's a wonderful man, adorable. I'm so happy I've met him.' Another was a retired nurse who used her inheritance money to buy her Gambian boyfriend a house. All these women appear to have been remarkably generous to their lovers, and that generosity suggests that their lovers have been generous with them, not with money but with a kind of sensuality and tenderness that they had never known.

The photo essay of 'romance tourism' made by Sofie Amalie Klougart when she was in Kenya with ActionAid has been published and republished all over the world, which could be taken to imply that Ms Klougart is another person who has done well out of this traffic. According to *Escape Artist Travel Magazine*, 600,000 Western women travel to resorts in Africa, the Caribbean, the Pacific and the Mediterranean every year.

> Dawn met Derrick on her first trip to Negril in 2006 and has since returned twice a year to spend time with him. Derrick is now 27 and Dawn is 30 years older. 'I fell head over heels with him when we first met and he couldn't get enough of me, but I'm not daft,' she says. 'I knew he was as keen on my money as he was on me but they have nothing here and live like paupers.'
>
> Once a month Dawn sends Derrick £20 for food and when she visits the island she pays for everything, from meals, drinks and taxis to clothes and spending money. 'What do I get out of it? A lot of fun, and a beautiful body and massive cock to have my wicked way with whenever I want.' (Julie Bindel, the *New Statesman*, 29 August 2013)

Newspaper accounts of this traffic either blame the men for being prostitutes – in the Caribbean 'rastitutes', or 'bumsters' (The Gambia) or 'beach boys' (the Pacific) – or condemn the women for being randy, unattractive and overweight. It is assumed that the women are exploiting the men's poverty when in the cases quoted we can see that they were alleviating it. As the men usually have more than one woman in tow, they would seem to be doing rather better out of it than the women who imagine they're in love. The principal animus against the female romance tourist is that being old she is necessarily unattractive and therefore has no right to sexual enjoyment. It is assumed that regardless of how her bought lover behaves she is utterly unattractive, even repulsive, to him.

Men may find their sexual attractiveness actually increasing with age; very few women will find this to be the case once they have passed the less attractive phases of puberty. The commonest image of a middle-aged woman is someone who is lumpy, dumpy and frumpy, Tina Turner notwithstanding. The exceptions simply prove the rule. Many a non-lumpy middle-aged woman has had the experience of being whistled at by men in the street walking up behind her, only to have them turn to look at her face and burst out into sneering remarks because the neatness of her behind and her un-frumpy clothes misled them as to her apparent chronological age. It is not enough for a middle-aged woman to be attractive or to take care of her figure. In the competition with younger women for available men she needs to be young.

Women are far more likely than men to be attracted to individuals older than themselves. They are less susceptible to the sensual attraction of youth and much more likely to respond to the external signs of authority, power and wealth exhibited by an older man. Women are so obliging that they tend to find men not only attractive but actually sexy if they are in positions of power, regardless of what they actually look like. The women of the United States of America once voted Spiro T. Agnew the sexiest man in the country, although he was over sixty. After his disgrace, and loss of influence, his sex appeal diminished markedly and he was never mentioned in a list of sexiest men again.

Some widows and divorcees will remarry after the age of fifty, and a few of the confirmed bachelor women. Single men of the same age who are not gay, and some who are, are considered supremely eligible and much sought after as house guests and dinner-party guests. Their female counterparts are nowhere near as popular. If they have spent their adult years bringing up children and now find an empty bed as well as an empty nest, they will not find it easy to make new contacts. They are unlikely to have enough money to dress well and have the best beauty care but, even if they could make the best of themselves, they are still the same, old, selves.

Some older women do find true love, and sometimes from younger men, even much younger men. The odds are long, but other women have done it. When 49-year-old Marian Evans, aka George Eliot, first met John Cross in Rome in 1869 he was twenty-nine. She adopted the play role of his aunt and when George Lewes died in November 1878 Johnny was her chief consolation. By August 1879 they were in love. They read the *Divina Commedia* together. She wrote to him in October, on black-edged paper: 'Best Loved and loving one: the sun it shines so cold, so cold, when there are no eyes to look love on me,' and signed herself 'thy tender Beatrice'. Johnny several times asked Eliot to marry him; twice she refused. In 1877 when Thackeray's daughter Anne married Richmond Ritchie, who was nearly twenty years younger than she, Eliot wrote to Barbara Bodichon that she had known several instances of 'young men with even brilliant advantages' choosing 'as their life's companion a woman whose attractions are wholly of the spiritual order'. Lady Jebb, who was a house-guest with the newly-weds with the Bullock-Halls at Six-Mile-Bottom, wrote:

> George Eliot, old as she is, and ugly, really looked very sweet and winning in spite of both … In the evening she made me feel sad for her. There was not a person in the drawing-room, Mr Cross included, whose mother she might not have been, and I thought she herself felt depressed at the knowledge that nothing could make her young again. She adores her husband, and it seemed to me to hurt her a little to have him to talk so much to me … (Jebb, pp. 163–4)

I should rather have thought it was Johnny Cross who was more acutely aware of his wife's age; she would have found his relative youth familiar, for she had once been thirty-eight herself. Besides Johnny Cross had been treated by her as if she were his aunt, which is after all a version of a mother. They fell in love when she was mourning the death of her husband and he the death of his mother. George Eliot died before the first year of their marriage was out. Johnny Cross did not marry again. It seems fairly likely that Johnny Cross married George Eliot because of attractions 'wholly of the spiritual order', only to discover that she expected him to carry out his conjugal duty. The manner of his discovery may have been the catapult that sent him flying out of the window of the Gritti Palace.

It is seldom, or ever suggested that young men might fancy old women. I have known gay men who were sincerely gerontophile and did not fancy a man unless he was much older, but I have yet to encounter a man who sincerely lusted after women twice his age and considered himself uninterested by and impotent with younger women, though doubtless some exist. Most women would still agree with Lucy Bentham in George Moore's novel, *Lewis Seymour and Some Women*, speaking of her affair with Seymour, twelve years younger than she:

> A year and a half, nearly two years, had passed since she saw Lewis for the first time in Mr Carver's shop. She was then thirty-four, now she was thirty-six. A year of the short time allowed a woman for love had been wasted, and in ten years she would be no longer fit for love. She might keep him for ten years, but after ten years she would have to hand him over to another woman … would she suffer at this surrender of her happiness, and retire gracefully into middle age?

This is not of course a woman speaking, but a womaniser speaking in the person of a woman; nevertheless most women would accept this version of their fitness or otherwise for love. A hundred years before, Mary Wollstonecraft recalled a sprightly writer who asked 'what business women over forty have to do in the world'. Moore allows Mrs Bentham rather more time:

> She might retain him for some ten or a dozen years, till she was forty-five; at fifty a woman's life is really over, and she began to wonder how the sensual coil would break, if weariness or some accident would break it; or the arrival of another woman, a misfortune that might befall her at any moment, for she could see that all attracted him, he being a very young man. (pp. 128–9)

In the event Lucy Bentham was lucky; she got to forty-five before the blow fell.

> 'A woman dies twice,' she said, 'and in a very few years it is borne in upon us that our mouths are no longer fit for kisses. His mouth, too, will one day cease to be attractive.' (pp. 202–3)

At least Moore allows that men too eventually become unfit for love, but Mrs Bentham is unusual among female characters in novels in that she is a sensualist, and she loves Seymour for his beauty. If we accept Moore's premise that really only the young are fit for love, then we are obliged to conclude that women have mostly been forced to endure the embraces of people unfit for love. Perhaps many women are aware of being kissed rather than kissing, and feel that as long as one mouth is succulent, that is sufficient. Certainly most women could not contemplate the kind of sex in which the male is indifferent and simply allows himself to be caressed. They cannot simply wish to press greedy old mouths against firm young flesh for the sake of feeling, smelling and tasting it. It is as if women's sensuality has always been obliterated by narcissism. Even in a male brothel a woman would expect her partner to enjoy her, and would be more concerned or at least as concerned about that as about her own orgasm. We are often told that male prostitution is on the verge of becoming big business, and that female buyers exist for soft pornography displaying male bodies, and that the new kind of female executive will know where and how to find satisfaction and will have the money to pay for it, but the phenomenon never eventuates.

Old women are commonly assumed to be sexually repulsive; the mythology of temptation is full of beautiful maidens who turn into hell hags with no more gruesome attributes than the normal attributes of age. Conversely, as in *The Magic Flute*, a lecherous old hag miraculously turns into Papagena. Cronishness used to come early; it can now be indefinitely postponed. The most significant advance in the unmaking of the crone is the perfection of the art of orthodontistry. Women who are not left with toothless gums do not suffer the downward curve of the nose that meets the upward curve of the chin to create the familiar witch profile. Women do not allow bristles to sprout freely or warts and wens to proliferate. Nevertheless the fifty-year-old woman knows that her body is not what it used to be. No matter how fit she is, or how flat her belly, her skin is thinner and less elastic, her muscle tone less firm. Oestrogen replacement may slow down such changes, but it cannot stop them or undo them. It becomes more and more difficult for a middle-aged woman to undress before a stranger, especially if he does not know her age and she does not know what he expects. She may resort to subterfuge, to soft lighting and luxurious underwear, or drugs or alcohol, to blur the first impressions that she feels so crucial. And still the man, nourished on a diet of inauthentic imagery of womanhood, may take to the windowsill and chuck himself into the canal if he discovers that he has a crone to his portion.

The received opinion now is that the older woman should be having sex. The logic is that everybody has a right to sex; women have the same rights as everyone else, therefore they have a right to sex. This is probably experienced by women as a series of rather mocking demands on them, namely, that there should be someone in their lives who wants to have sex with them, and they should also be wanting sex with that person. What this means in practice is that you should be a married woman, you should have hung on to your husband and not allowed him to die or go off with someone else, and you should still fancy him. These are all tall orders, if only because they are all out of the individual woman's control. Husbands continue to die in the most inconvenient and inconsiderate fashion. Some, as they rise in affluence and influence, begin to desire more effective sexual stimuli than a familiar old wife can offer, and a female of a newer model with increased horsepower, who will be a better indicator of status than a wife who learned her cooking during the lean years; many a middle-aged woman has to accept an unwanted divorce. Others seek the divorce themselves.

Earlier discussions of the sexuality of the fifty-year-old woman have concerned themselves exclusively with the category 'married woman, husband present'. There are in Britain nearly three-quarters of a million women over the age of fifty who never married, about half as many divorcees and more than four times as many widows. Slightly more than half the female population over fifty is without a male partner. Fifty-year-old maids, widows and divorcees all have sexuality and all would be interested to know what changes they might look forward to in their sexual feelings in the course of the climacteric. The truth is that the options seem as varied as ever they were.

The sexual revolution of the late twentieth century did liberate some forms of sexual activity in theory at least from censorship and censure. Among them was lesbianism. Sexologists began to notice a new phenomenon, namely apparently heterosexual women coming out in middle age as lesbian and entering into sexual relationships with women. As a contributor to the online magazine xojane put it (2 May 2013):

> The middle-aged lesbian has become a bit of a cliché. There's even been research done to try to figure out if women are actually a little more prone to biologically shifting to homosexuality as they age …

Interest in 'late-blooming lesbianism' was at its short-lived peak in August 2010 when the American Psychological Association's annual convention in San Diego featured a session entitled 'Sexual Fluidity and Late-Blooming Lesbians'. The phenomenon is more common than many people think. Christan Moran, a researcher at Southern Connecticut State University, interviewed more than 200 women over thirty who were married to men but found themselves attracted to a woman, and concluded that heterosexual women can 'experience a first same-sex attraction well into adulthood'. Utah University professor Lisa Diamond, Associate Professor of Psychology and Gender Studies at the University of Utah, for fifteen years followed a group of seventy-nine women who reported some same-sex attraction. Every two years, 20 to 30 per cent change the way they describe themselves, gay, straight or bisexual. Seventy per cent have changed since the study began.

British newspapers were not slow to chime in, and examples were not hard to find. Mary Portas was married to a businessman for thirteen years and bore two children before falling in love with Melanie Rickey and marrying her two days after her fiftieth birthday. Susie Orbach was with Joseph Schwarz for thirty years, before falling in love with Jeanette Winterson, whom she married in 2015, being then fifty-eight years old. Elizabeth Gilbert, author of *Eat, Pray, Love*, was forty-seven and married when she realised she was in love with her best friend Rayya Ellis. Wanda Sykes, award-winning American stand-up comedian, was married to a man in 1991 and divorced him in 1998. In 2006 she met Alex Niedbalski, whom she married in September 2008; in 2009 the couple became parents of twins. Kelly McGillis was twice married to men and also had relationships with women before coming out to online magazine SheWired as lesbian in 2009, when she was fifty-two. She entered into a civil union with a woman in 2010 but the relationship broke up in 2011. Carol Leifer, fifty-three, was married to a man in the Eighties; in 1996 she met and fell in love with Lori Wolf. They have lived together since 2005, and in 2015 they were married.

Any attempt to explain these apparent shifts in sexual orientation by hypothesising about changes in hormone secretion or virilisation appear doomed to fail. As the influence of oestrogen declines it may very well be that the influence of testosterone becomes dominant but, as we have seen, our understanding of women's endocrine systems is not such as to provide a clue to these changes in sexual orientation.

As single-sex marriage has come to be seen as a human right, we are becoming used to seeing lesbian relationships as long-term, and not susceptible to loss of interest at or post-menopause. What this means is that all the discussions of menopause as the end of women's existence as sexual beings are wide of the mark. When same-sex marriage becomes possible we notice lesbian couples amongst the first seeking to give their relationships dignity and permanence, and they remain the majority of same-sex couples choosing marriage, though the margin has narrowed to 55/45. The conventional wisdom was that these relationships were more sentimental than sexual and the level of sexual activity very low. Lesbians were swift to give the lie to this easy assumption, which had probably grown out of the earlier notion that menopause equalled the end of sexual life.

Fifty-year-old Stephanie Schroeder writing for the fiftyisthenewfifty website describes how she and her 51-year-old partner remain 'as excited about sex' as they were when they first met.

> Age, it seems, has only increased our libido ... My gal and I like to 'get busy' in a sexual manner as often as possible, and when we do, sexual fervor rages ...
> There also is a large BDSM and leather sub-community within the lesbian community. And, at least here in New York City, public sex parties, thriving dungeons, casual sex, anonymous online hook-ups, polyandrous relationships, and other 'lifestyle' choices people in every category make, are alive and kicking among lesbians, too.

Lesbian relationships can be as tempestuous as any. It is in the nature of the case that we know most about celebrity couples; amongst the first lesbian relationships to founder in the glare of publicity were those of tennis great Martina Navratilova. At a lunch in 1979 23-year-old Navratilova met 37-year-old Rita Mae Brown; in 1980 the couple moved into a twenty-room mansion on the outskirts of Charlottesville; in 1981 Navratilova moved out. She was then involved with Nancy Lieberman until at a tournament in Fort Worth in 1982 she met Judy Nelson, eleven years older than Navratilova and married to a doctor for seventeen years, with two sons. They were partners for seven years. In 1991 the relationship hit a rough patch. Navratilova went off to a tournament and never came back. Nelson's credit cards and memberships were immediately cancelled. Nelson then sued Navratilova for 'galimoney' and became involved with Rita Mae Brown, who tried to make peace between the couple. Nelson eventually received an undisclosed sum in settlement.

Navratilova, already in a relationship with Olympic skier Cindy Nelson, then met Toni Layton at the Peachtree City Tennis Center. After a whirlwind courtship they went through an informal marriage; Layton had been Navratilova's 'tennis wife' for eight years when she was thrown out as suddenly as Nelson had been. The locks were changed on the house they shared and she was left homeless, penniless and with only the clothes on her back. The result was a domestic partnership lawsuit in which Layton sought and apparently won compensation. Navratilova's current partner is Julia Lemigova, Miss USSR 1990 and sixteen years younger than she. They first met at a Parisian dinner party in 2000. All Lemigova's previous relationships were with men; she did not even know same sex was possible until she left the USSR. Navratilova had always said she wasn't the marrying kind, but she and Lemigova were married in New York in 2014.

Australian actress Portia de Rossi had been married to film maker Mel Metcalfe before she met 'everyone's favourite talk show host' Ellen DeGeneres backstage at an awards ceremony in 2004. (Four years earlier DeGeneres's partner Anne Heche, who had been with her since 1997, left her for a man.) Portia and Ellen were married at their home in Beverly Hills in August 2008. Portia de Rossi has now changed her name and become an American citizen. As a celebrity couple DeGeneres and her wife have to be prepared to endure speculation about their marriage. The first threat to their union is supposed to have been caused by Portia's desire for a child. They were then said to be quarrelling about Ellen's refusal to undergo plastic surgery before the next season of her show.

Women who have entered into sexual relationships with other women after being in heterosexual relationships tend to minimise the significance of the change. Cynthia Nixon, who played Miranda in *Sex and the City*, was in a relationship with schoolteacher Danny Mozes from 1988 to 2003, and they had two children together. In 2004, Nixon began dating education activist Christine Marinoni. They became engaged in April 2009 and were married in New York City on 27 May

2012. Nixon was later quoted as saying, 'I don't really feel I've changed. I'd been with men all my life, and I'd never fallen in love with a woman. But when I did, it didn't seem so strange. I'm just a woman in love with another woman.'

All of musician Alison Goldfrapp's relationships were with men, until at the age of forty-seven she fell in love with Lisa Gunning. In a February 2010 interview with the *Sunday Times*, she rejected being called a lesbian, saying, 'I think of everything as being about a person and a relationship, and I am in a wonderful relationship with a wonderful person. It just happens to be with a lady ... It's something I've thought about for a long time and it concurs with my philosophy on life and sexuality. I don't think it can or should be pigeonholed. I've thought about this since I was a teenager. I've always found it claustrophobic to think about having to put things into categories like that. My sexuality is the same as my music and my life. Why does it need a label?'

The right of the heterosexual middle-aged woman to sexual self-expression is not one that she can exercise in the absence of an interested partner. If she has never had sex, there is not much chance that she will start getting it when she is over forty, and less chance than ever when she is over fifty, unless of course she is in one of those caring institutions where the old men and women are urged to get it on together. If she has lost her husband by death or divorce she cannot demand a replacement. It is all the more important then that she not allow herself to be convinced that without the psychic release of sex she will become a 'frustrated', bitter, cruel, dried-up, envious old stick.

The symptoms of the climacteric should not be misinterpreted as signs of mental imbalance or emotional disturbance caused by sexual deprivation. The general rule holds; doing without sex if you have been used to it is not easy, but you can do it. If you have survived so far without it, you will find life getting easier with every month that passes. Helen Gurley Brown is supposed to have said when asked what older women want in bed, 'I think many women don't want sex at all. By a certain age they heave such a sigh of relief to be done with it' (Witchel). Gloria Steinem, at age eighty, is supposed to have theorised that a dwindling libido can be a terrific advantage: 'The brain cells that used to be obsessed are now free for all kinds of great things.' British TV star Carol Vorderman, who went through six months of deep depression before finding a doctor who helped her control her symptoms by 'gels', by which she probably means HRT, now says she has had 'enough romance' in her life and is 'happily single'.

Not all cohabiting women are sexually involved with each other. One of the factors that over the centuries have driven women to cohabit has been their relative poverty. The term 'Boston marriages' was applied to this familiar phenomenon after the publication of Henry James's novel *The Bostonians*; in fact James's sister Alice for most of her life shared a house with Katharine Loring. The tendency these days is to assume that such relationships were sexual, disregarding the statements of the women involved. Other observers have assumed that though the relationships may have been 'asexual' the women were indeed lesbians. One celebrated case is that of Muriel Spark and Penelope Jardine. Spark described herself as having been 'quite menopausal' in 1968 when she met, at a Roman hairdresser's shop, 36-year-old Penelope Jardine, a student of sculpture at the Accademia di Belle Arti. When Jardine bought a house near Arezzo Spark moved in with her; they were to live and work together for more than thirty years, but Jardine insists that their relationship was not sexual.

In whatever form it might assume, one possibility remains as long as life remains: the recollected soul can always flame into love. At fifty Emily Dickinson wrote:

The Thrill came slowly like a Boon for
Centuries delayed
Its fitness growing like the Flood
In sumptuous solitude –
The desolation only missed
While Rapture changed its Dress
And stood amazed before the Change
In ravished Holiness –

(p. 629)

14

The Aged Wife

In all the editions of his *Diseases of Women: A Clinical Guide to Diagnosis and Treatment*, George Ernest Herman, MB Lond., FRCP, erstwhile president of the Obstetrical Society, repeated his opinion that

> After menstruation has finally ceased, the genital organs atrophy. The uterus becomes small, the vagina becomes smooth, and its orifice, if it has not been enlarged by child-bearing, shrinks. These changes are not important to women who have been married at the most suitable age; but to women who have been married late, to husbands younger than themselves, they may be. (pp. 582–3)

The good doctor – he seems to have been a sensible compassionate man – assumes that a woman who has married at the right age and to a person of the right age, that is, somewhat older than she, by the time she arrives at menopause has no further use for her vagina. The only woman who may be embarrassed by the unserviceability of her orifice is the one whose husband is younger than she and still makes demands on her. Or conversely, the woman whose male partner has discovered Viagra. Online gynaecologist David Eibling M.D. confesses that he cannot tell 'how many post-menopausal women end up with tears in their vaginal tissues once their partners start using Viagra' (www.mylifestages.org).

Nowadays we know better than to treat the vagina as if it were part of the furniture set aside for a husband's use; we have come to believe in female libido. Current sexual orthodoxy teaches that women have sexual desires and, not simply the right to express them, but a duty to express them in the interests of better health. Whereas Dr Herman may well have felt that there were few good reasons for continuing intercourse after menopause, nowadays there can only be bad reasons for discontinuing it. Seventy years later, Theodore Faithfull, Consultant Psychologist and Sexologist and Member of the Royal College of Veterinary Surgeons, author of *The Future of Women*, is quite certain that decline of sexual interest in the ageing female is evidence of the wrong kind of sexual interest in the first place:

> If the sex life of a married couple has been fornication, that
> is glandular relief for the male and instinctive satisfaction by
> occasional pregnancies for the female, there can be in both males
> and females in the middle years of life a lack of desire for physical
> intimacy as the glandular function decreases. (p. 104)

Faithfull has his female patients in a cleft stick. If admitting loss of interest is to admit that one's marriage has been fornication, then no woman of spirit is going to admit it. Faithfull is fairly typical in that he doesn't concern himself in the least with the ageing female who is not in a heterosexual union. For Faithfull the females who never achieved their destiny as wives and mothers are doomed to ill-health whatever they do. The females who have allowed their husbands to leave them by death or any other means are equally absent from his consideration. Though Faithfull's account of female orgasm is nonsensical and *The Future of Women* a strange and cranky book, he is by no means untypical in his treatment of female sexuality as half of that perfect whole, the couple. Most doctors nowadays would treat this case of Faithfull's in exactly the same way:

> A few years ago the wife of a man holding a responsible post in the
> teaching profession came to see me. She considered that her life was
> as good as over. The climacteric was finishing, her son would soon
> be leaving home and she felt her husband would be far happier with
> a younger woman. I told her she was talking nonsense. (p. 104)

Clearly what she is talking is not nonsense, although she may well have been wrong. But Faithfull went on:

That if she put herself right she would be a help to every young
married woman in her social circle and she and her husband would
enjoy marital intimacy for many more years. A few months later
I one day noticed a smile on her face and asked her what it meant.
'Oh!' she said. 'I suppose I must tell you. When my husband
finished last night he said my dear, you are now giving me more
happiness than in all the 25 years of married life.' (pp. 104–5)

When her husband finished what, we may ask. Whatever Faithfull
may consider he has done for this mythical female, he has not succeeded
in getting her to stop living for others. He does not explain how she 'put
herself right'. He might have felt less smug if his patient had told him
that she was standing over her husband with a whip, or walking on him
in stiletto heels, or allowing him to tie her up, beat her or defecate on
her. In this kind of discourse the husband's unexamined requirements
are assumed to be legitimate; the wife's need is to satisfy them.

In 2004 the National Social Life, Health, and Aging Project at the
University of Chicago recruited 1,550 women and 1,455 men aged
between fifty-seven and eighty-five to provide information about the
sexual activity, behaviours and problems of older adults. The results
were published in 2007 as 'A Study of Sexuality and Health among
Older Adults in the United States' in the *New England Journal of
Medicine* (Lindau et al.).

The purpose of the study was to obtain estimates of the prevalence
of sexual activity, behaviors, and problems in the older population.
We hypothesized that the profiles of activity and problems would
differ between men and women and that differences across age
groups would not be uniform for all outcomes. A second objective
was to describe the relationship between sexuality and a variety of
health conditions.

We are not surprised to learn that the likelihood of being sexually
active declined steadily with age, and was lower in women than in men,
that people in poor health were less interested in sex than well people,
that people in a relationship were more likely to have sex than people
who weren't, that old men were more likely to be in a relationship than
old women, that men were more likely to masturbate than women, and

that women were more likely to rate sex as being 'not at all important', 35 per cent of them, as compared with 13 per cent of men.

It was the more surprising then that the group led by Samuel Stroope, from Louisiana State University, Florida State University and Baylor University, reported in *The Archives of Sexual Behavior* that the lifetime decline in sexual activity between spouses slows down after fifty years and even takes an upturn: 'An individual married for 50 years will have somewhat less sex than an individual married for 65 years.' A year after marriage an average couple had a 65 per cent chance of having sex two or three times a month or more; after twenty-five years of marriage that percentage drops to 40 per cent and after fifty years to 35 per cent, but for couples surviving sixty-five years of marriage together the percentage improved to 42 per cent. It should be pointed out that 'having sex' included 'any mutually voluntary activity with another person that involves sexual contact' and that same-sex couples and people cohabiting out of wedlock were not included in the study sample of 1,600 couples aged between fifty-seven and eighty-five (Stroope et al.).

Until very recently, thinking about the sexuality of married people used to partake of a general distortion to be found in all thinking about heterosexual intercourse. Though homosexuals male and female are assumed effectively to achieve orgasm by all kinds of sex play which does not by definition involve the penetration of the vagina by the penis, heterosexuals are considered abnormal if they prefer sex in any other form than the kind guaranteed in fertile persons to result in impregnation. This is the reason the condition of the ageing woman's vaginal mucosa is crucial to her relationship with her husband. Though it has been proved time and time again that women's orgasms do not originate in the vagina and that other forms of love play are more effective in pleasuring women, and that constant exposure of the cervix uteri to the glans penis represents a health risk to women, the emphasis on intromission as the only form of heterosexual intercourse is unweakened. Not even the terrors of the AIDS epidemic have succeeded in weakening it. When we consider the question of sex between ageing spouses we assume that they will do it 'like grown-ups' in Márquez's phrase (see below). At no time in her life is a woman to be permitted to declare the vagina off-limits and take her pleasure by more certain means. If she is one of the many women who have been fucked when they wanted to be cuddled, given sex when what they really wanted was tenderness and affection, the prospect of more of the same until death do her part from it is hardly something to cheer about.

The good news is that the emphasis on intromission is weakening. Online advice to elderly lovers is likely to say this sort of thing: 'Sex can also be about emotional pleasure, sensory pleasure, and relationship pleasure. Intercourse is only one way to have fulfilling sex. Touching, kissing, and other intimate sexual contact can be just as rewarding for both you and your partner.' (Just as rewarding?) 'Holding each other, gentle touching, kissing, and sensual massage are all ways to share passionate feelings. Try oral sex or masturbation as fulfilling substitutes to intercourse.' The new orthodoxy holds that 'maintaining a sex life into your senior years is a matter of good health'. Other suggestions, that sex can burn fat, ward off common illnesses and decrease anxiety, have a whiff of overselling about them. We learn that older women require more foreplay, which is not news to those of us who think that most if not all women could have done with more foreplay. One website even tells us that there is 'evidence to suggest that vibrators may ease symptoms of menopause'.

There is a darker side still to the emphasis laid upon continuing sexual activity as the one sign of vitality in a marriage. Purveyors of pornography often justify their activities on the grounds of the services they provide for bored couples who are enabled to copulate by having their fantasy stimulated by looking at images of others doing sexy things. It is hardly necessary to scrutinise commercial pornography to register the fact that all the images are directed towards the flaccid penis rather than the dry vagina or the forgotten clitoris. Indeed it is unlikely that the unresponsive genitalia would become excited by visual stimuli in any case, for women are not yet as fetishistic as men. It cannot be too often or too clearly said that all our commercial pornography is sadomasochistic and degrades all the individuals depicted in it, the overwhelming majority of whom are women. The sex inspired by it is not just not worth having – it is fundamentally destructive.

In 1957 Maxine Davis, writer for many years on women's health for *Good Housekeeping* magazine, encapsulated the current thinking about the role of women in married sex in her bestselling book *The Sexual Responsibility of Women*. 'Ardent young couples,' she wrote, assume that 'the book of sexual life suddenly closes with the finality of the first clod of earth on a coffin' (p. 190). 'How wrong they are!' she enthuses. An old couple 'have sound reason to expect to enjoy their sex lives together after an evening spent baby-sitting for their third great-grandchild'. 'Their sexual activity naturally will not be nearly so frequent, so prolonged or intense as it used to be but it will still be possible, in a mild way, for it to be complete enough to give happiness and meaning to their lives' (pp. 190–1). This blessed couple has evidently managed to gather four generations of family around them and keep them there but, in order for happiness and meaning to enter their lives, they still need to manoeuvre the penis into the vagina. Not for Davis the suggestion that it might be rather more useful to retain the power to make each other laugh. Heaven forbid, they might laugh when they were working on the penis. A sense of the absurd in such a situation could be most inconvenient.

Life is not like Davis's paradigm. It is almost impossible to orchestrate human whims and susceptibilities so that they coincide. A perfect fit between lovers, whether sanctified or not, is so rare that no one should ever feel guilty at not having managed it. We are all like the imprisoned men in Jean Genet's film *Chant d'Amour*, straining to express tenderness through lavatory pipes and cracks in concrete walls. The ageing couple that does not celebrate its closeness by a weekly symphony on the bedsprings has nothing to apologise for. Neither does the couple that does not achieve the simultaneous orgasm of pornography.

The literature of menopause implies that loss of interest in genital congress after twenty-five years of marriage is a relatively rare and severe symptom, demanding radical intervention. Barbara Evans, writing in the Seventies, called for radical and expensive intervention, not then and not now available on the NHS.

> More serious psychological problems may call for the help of a psychotherapist and for psychotherapy. Both husband and wife may benefit from psychosexual counselling and re-education. Failure to stimulate the partner, persistent premature ejaculation on the man's part and inability to relax on the woman's part are the main factors which cause sexual activity to fail. (p. 98)

'Inability to relax' is presented as the female correlative of premature ejaculation – not itself an effective relaxant. The current orthodoxy is that psychosexual difficulties themselves may cause the formation of symptoms at menopause. If not enjoying sex with your husband is evidence of a serious psychosexual problem, the pressure is on you to submit to any kind of brainwashing to get well. Nobody wants to be permanently stigmatised as 'mentally ill'. If the menopausal woman already feels that she is losing her mind, the suggestion that her not wanting sex with her husband is a symptom of a psychosexual problem needing treatment is particularly mischievous.

'Failure to stimulate a partner' is clearly a heinous crime. Psychosexual counsellors would all claim that both partners in heterosexual intercourse should be given all necessary stimulation. They seem not to realise that the partner whose stimulation is essential to sexual intercourse is the male; once he is stimulated, especially if he is fundamentally bored, it is important to proceed to the business before his synthetic enthusiasm wanes. Stimulation moreover obeys its own law of diminishing returns, which is why some men are carried into the casualty departments of our hospitals every year with their penises flayed because they have put them into the suction nozzle of a vacuum cleaner. Just how much time, energy and money needs to be devoted to the providing of adequate stimulation is nowhere quantified. These days it is more likely to be a website than a book that instructs a wife to 'share a steamy fantasy', 'blare rock music', 'throw on a garter belt', 'massage his feet', 'arm wrestle', 'mix up a pomegranate martini', 'turn your home into a spa for the night', 'play footsie', 'wear red', 'open a box of chocolates' – oh, and – 'moan'.

Where once books instructing women how to seduce their husbands appeared on the bookstands every year, describing an array of masquerades and role-play, involving expenditure not only of money for costumes, flowers, alcohol, telegrams, etc. but of enormous amounts of time, *Fifty Shades of Grey* and its many sequels have now cornered the market. *Fifty Shades of Grey*, which sold faster than any other book in the English language, introduced a fairly innocent female readership to 'mommy porn'; the medium was as usual sadism, in this case unusually inept, if Pamela Stephenson Connolly is to be believed (the *Sun*, 11 July 2012). The equipment was an entirely reliable but invisible penis, plus leather in various forms including a riding crop, plus cable ties and baby oil, the method discipline. The woman who recoils from role play, refuses to dress up as a French maid one day, a nun the next, and a schoolgirl the next, is clearly failing 'to stimulate a partner', therefore the couple is failing to have right sex, therefore she has severe psychosexual problems, therefore she needs counselling.

If sex has never been particularly rewarding, if time and energy have been put into it and regular twice-a-week bliss-for-two has not resulted, turning fifty might be a good time to give up the struggle. If giving up sex meant giving up marriage, divorce statistics would be much higher even than they are. The re-enactment by spouses of sacramental intercourse is not necessary, although it might be pleasant. To assume that resumption of sexual activity is an infallible sign of a revivified relationship is to fall into an egregious blunder; to assert that it is a condition of revivifying marriage is tyranny. To dose women with steroids for the sole purpose of keeping them receptive to their husbands' advances is outrageous.

There are surely many middle-aged women who have husbands alive and living with them, and who desire sex with those husbands and are desired by them. If such women experience the condition of their vaginas as an obstacle to the fulfilling of their own desires, then clearly they are entitled to replacement oestrogen or anything else that works. However, if the woman wants to be able to have intercourse with her husband only so that she can have a quiet life, it is quite improper to dose her with sex steroids so that she can endure an activity that she has never much enjoyed. If a man has never been a considerate or imaginative lover, he may just conceivably become so as his own sexual potency wanes and the matter becomes less urgent. If he does not, if his expression of desire becomes more mechanical rather than less, more masturbatory rather than less, if he ejaculates earlier and falls asleep even sooner than in the first years of marriage, the middle-aged woman may quite conceivably prefer to opt out of the whole business. She might prefer to opt out too if he takes a good deal longer about it, if he wakes her up at odd times in the night, if he only feels like it after a couple of drinks or after reading some of the magazines he buys from the top shelf at the newsagent's. Or after dipping into *Fifty Shades of Grey*.

In the popular literature on menopause, a husband is assumed to have conjugal rights of access to his wife's body, when in fact he has no such rights. A husband's desire is also assumed to be more or less constant over thirty-five years. The sexologists tell us on the other hand that in men 'from adolescence onwards, there is a continuous decline in sexual interest, arousal and activity, without a sudden discontinuity in any group … sexual arousal is slower and requires more intense stimuli, ejaculations are less forceful, detumescence after orgasm is quicker and the vasocongestive increase in testicular size during sexual excitement is decreased, as is the psychosexual pleasure' (Vermeulen, p. 5). What this would seem to add up to is that the ageing male must work harder for less pleasure and his partner of many years is going to have to provide more intense stimuli, somehow, if they are to get it on at all.

Although many factors play a role in determining the frequency of sexual activity, among which impotence, boredom with the sexual partner, stress, fear of failure, or a period of forced abstinence are the most important, an age-dependent physiological decline is also undeniable. This age-dependent decrease is also observed in domestic animals, for example bulls and stallions, many of which are discarded early in life because of gradual sexual apathy (Vermeulen, p. 6). Current thinking is that about 20 per cent of men will show signs of hypogonadism in their sixties, that proportion rising to 50 per cent of men in their eighties. Opinions as to the usefulness of replacement testosterone are varied, mainly because no long-term placebo-controlled trials have ever been carried out. However clinics offering therapies for what is misleadingly called the 'andropause' are available. A first consultation at one London clinic will cost £450 (at 2017 prices), with blood tests at a starting price of £420, follow-up visits at £200 each plus blood tests; in all the initial outlay will come in somewhere between £850 and £1100. NHS Choices rejects the idea of a hormonal deficiency as causing male misery in midlife, preferring to blame stress, depression and anxiety.

Our culture encourages men to demand effective sexual stimuli; as their own sperm production declines, they need even more effective stimuli. The ruling class, which is and always has been male, has always had its pick of young flesh of both sexes. After twenty-odd years of marriage the wife of Bob Slocum, the anti-hero of Joseph Heller's second novel, *Something Happened*, published in 1974, is a more cooperative partner than she ever was, but, though her husband succeeds in responding, her willingness avails her little.

Nowadays my wife is much better. Nowadays my wife is completely different about this whole matter of sex; but so am I. She is almost

always amorous nowadays, it seems, and ready to take chances that
horrify even me. I can usually tell that she's been thinking about
it the instant I walk in, by a self-satisfied, slightly twisted smile.
I know I am right if she has left her girdle off ... (pp. 124–5)

His wife is doing everything she can to keep him interested in her;
she dresses well, looks good, is a superior 'hostess' and flirts openly
with other men. She drinks before he gets home to loosen herself up.
She has stopped asking him if he loves her. She is actually acutely
miserable; her increased libido is evidence of anything but spiritual
well-being.

My wife is unhappy. She is one of those married women who are
very, very bored and lonely, and I don't know what I can make
myself do about it (except get a divorce and make her unhappier
still). (p. 71)

Nameless Mrs Slocum displays some of the negativity of the
menopause, though, as far as we can tell, she is still a few years off it.

She thinks she has gotten older, heavier, and less attractive than she
used to be – and of course she is right. She thinks it matters to me,
and there she is wrong. I don't think I mind. (If she knew I didn't
mind she'd probably be even more unhappy.) My wife is not bad-
looking; she's tall, dresses well, and has a good figure, and I'm often
proud to have her with me. (She thinks I never want her with me.)
She thinks I do not love her any more, and she may be right about
that too. (p. 71)

Though Slocum has had many other sexual relationships and is
sexually obsessed by at least one other woman, he cannot bear the
thought that his wife might take one of his business colleagues as a
lover, but not because he is jealous.

My wife has red lines round her waist and chest when she takes her
clothes off and baggy pouches round the sides and bottom of her
behind, and I would not want anyone in the company to find that
out. (p. 509)

Slocum is not intended as a hero, nor is he some kind of archetype, nevertheless the theme of *Something Happened* is the dreadfulness of ordinariness. One is at least as likely to encounter the Slocum family in middle America as the mythical forty-year monogamous love affair that doctors imagine they are able to perpetuate through HRT. Though with a reticence rare among male novelists Heller never pretends to be able to read Mrs Slocum's mind, we may suspect that she gets half-drunk and tears at her husband's fly-buttons because she is terrified that he will abandon her. Faithfull might say that she had never enjoyed sex, because when she was younger she used to fight her husband off, and therefore she was only able to use sex as a bargaining chip.

Men who bathe and shave when they leave their wives' beds, rather than before they get into them (i.e., the majority), probably don't consider whether their wives find sex with them uncomfortable, unexciting or even revolting. It is possible that even the wives themselves have not considered the matter. When she was working on psychiatric morbidity in menopause in the Seventies, Dr Barbara Ballinger could get only 114 of her 539 respondents aged between forty and fifty-five to discuss sex with her. Of them, thirty-four said their sexual responsiveness had deteriorated and five said it had increased; twenty-four had never enjoyed sex at all; twenty-seven found sex satisfactory; five had refused to have intercourse at all for periods ranging from five to seventeen years. Only ninety of the women had husbands; of them twenty-one said the relationship was poor, twenty-five fair, and forty-four good. Only 40 per cent of the women with poor libido had good relations with their husbands, compared to 66 per cent of those with unimpaired libido (Ballinger, 1975). These figures are thought to constitute a case for hormone replacement. Get your libido fixed and your chances of a good relationship with your husband improve from 40 per cent to 66 per cent. Actually the chances are not even as good as that. Of the thirty-two women who had unimpaired libido, only twenty or so had good relations with their husbands; the impaired numbered almost twice as many. None of these discussions ever asks whether a husband is attractive, or a good lover. Loss of interest in sex is never a rational response, always a symptom. Robert A. Wilson, MD, used to put a three-pointed star on the files of the women who seemed to him to be in love with their husbands, who were only 20 per cent of his patients.

Yet the majority of women, when asked, 'Do you love your husband?' cannot give a straight answer.

'I respect him very much.'

'He is a very good man.'

'He is very kind to me.'

That's one set of responses. They don't qualify for the three-pronged star, but the prognosis is still good. Then the answers may run like this.

'He's very busy – I don't see him very much.'

'He's very tired – even falls asleep watching television.'

'He is not well – wish he would take off some weight and take better care of himself.'

Usually these remarks are uttered without any emotion. I know then something besides estrogen is needed to restore this woman to a fully feminine role. (p. 118)

The prognosis in such cases is bad, presumably. The husbands described in these terms are uninterested and uninteresting, tired, obese, distracted and worse, but it is still a sign of inadequacy in the wives that they do not find them attractive. Though as a gynaecologist Wilson cannot offer to treat these husbands, he does allow that they may need treatment:

Clearly there is something wrong here, but it is not likely to be lack of hormones in a man. More probably, it is lack of interest. The man is simply bored. The fault may be a dull mind, a dull job, or a dull wife. Whatever it is, it is unendurable and deadly. (p. 128)

The wife has already been told how to dress, how to suggest new adventurousness in sex, how oestrogen will make her breasts taut and so forth. Nobody has even suggested that her problem might be lack of interest. Hers too might be a dull mind, a dull job or a dull husband. Yet people whose minds are not stimulated are likely to have dull minds; housework is a dull job and the kinds of jobs generally done by women outside the home are dull jobs, and husbands can be very dull, especially if their best efforts have already been expended on people they consider more important, in their workplace or their playplace. The situation is as unendurable and deadly for a woman as it is for a man, and she should not be encouraged to dose herself with steroids rather than put an end to it.

An older man is by no means as likely to be unattractive to his spouse as an older woman is. Women are conditioned generally to prefer men older than themselves; they tend to look for the lineaments of a father in a husband and may very well tolerate a greater degree of physical ageing than men, who have been conditioned to desire and to demand a sexual partner younger than themselves. In September 1990 the cruise liner *Crown Princess* was launched into Brooklyn Harbour by 56-year-old Sophia Loren, resplendent in an enormous tawny wig. Her famous cleavage was well displayed in the glittering gold lamé dress she wore to the dinner on board, to be photographed hand in hand with her husband, Carlo Ponti, now eighty-one, small, sweet and frail. Though Sophia has always towered above him, and seems to come from a different breed of gorgeous humanity altogether, her name has never been linked with any other man. After he died aged ninety-four in 2007, Sophia told a interviewer that she had no intention of marrying again because for her 'it would be impossible to love anyone else'. Moreover Sophia escapes the rueful reflections of Joanne Woodward (born 1930), married to male pin-up Paul Newman, reported in *Stern* magazine in November 1990.

> While Paul is supposedly becoming more and more attractive, I'm becoming an old wreck. Anna Magnani once said that she had earned every wrinkle on her face, and when I was young I agreed with her. What a lovely old face! But when I had that old face, it stopped seeming beautiful to me … Fortunately, I inherited good skin. But I'm getting old, I'm getting wrinkles and at a certain age one stops being a pin-up. There's no female Robert Redford or Paul Newman.

There are very few male Robert Redfords and Paul Newmans if it comes to that. Most men do little if anything to render themselves presentable; if they take pains with their appearance, they are required to conceal the fact. Despite the fact that the cosmetics lobby tells us year after year that men are on the brink of wearing make-up there is still something suspect in a man's attempts at self-beautification. Though women are advised at every turn to stay attractive, men are never advised to be attractive or to behave attractively. Such was not always the case; in past epochs even British men practised the arts of flamboyant display and sexual blandishment. In the late seventeenth century and eighteenth century men painted their faces and corseted themselves in order to deny the encroachments of age, because it was understood that old men were no more attractive than old women.

The character of the *senex amans*, the old man in love, is a stock figure of European comedy from classical times. When syphilis was brought back to Europe from the Americas by the explorers at the beginning of the sixteenth century, poets sought to explain the phenomenon in a series of verse allegories in which Love and Death quarrelled, dropped their quivers and got their arrows mixed up. Some of Death's lead-tipped arrows remained in Cupid's quiver, so that young lovers were killed when he aimed at them, and Death occasionally let fly one of Cupid's gold-tipped arrows, so that an old person who should have died fell in love instead. In the popular *commedia dell'arte* the old man in love becomes the pantaloon, who exists to be mocked by the young lovers who will enjoy their right to sexual pleasure in spite of him.

In 1790, Despina, the maid in *Cosi Fan Tutte*, could get a laugh by answering Don Alfonso, when he says he has need of her, that she has no need of him. 'I want to do something for you,' he insists, and she answers again, 'For a young girl like me an old man like you can't do anything.' Yet Don Alfonso is not decrepit; he is described in the libretto as 'a man of the world'. He is witty and charming and in tune but, as he says himself, his hair is grey. That is enough to indicate to Despina that he is incapable of pleasuring her. There are two assumptions at work here and in the audience for whom Lorenzo Da Ponte wrote the libretto, one that Don Alfonso's sexual energy is not adequate to a young woman's needs, and another that he is not attractive enough to excite her.

The middle-aged theatregoers of the seventeenth and eighteenth century, who watched ridiculous figures of their own age persecuting beautiful young people with inappropriate demands and expectations, were being warned off. They were being shown how repulsive they seemed to the young people to whom they might be attracted. In so far as the ridiculous old men had financial and political power they could force their attentions upon young women, and thereby greatly increase the quantum of human misery. The comediographers were defending the rights of the young against the dead hand of paternal power and selfishness, which tried to arrogate all pleasure, including sexual pleasure, to itself. The truth is, of course, that only in the theatre could Chronos be castrated by his sons. In real life old men with money and power could take their pick of young women and did so. Poets since the time of Chaucer have dealt with the misery caused by the marriage of May and December. The outcome was usually the betrayal of the old husband by the young wife, who succumbed to a natural attraction for a younger man. This outcome could be seen as merely funny or desperately tragic, if the betrayed older man decided to avenge himself on wife and/or lover. Everything depended upon whether the audience could believe the older man capable of sexual passion. If he wasn't the story was funny; if he was the story was tragic. Sometimes, as in Leoncavallo's 1892 opera *I Pagliacci*, it was both.

By the time *I Pagliacci* was written theatregoers had stopped laughing at sex. Once sexuality had been defined as a locus of disease rather than sin, sex became deadly serious. Right sex, good sex, was credited with mystical powers, so that no one with any intellectual pretensions dared laugh at Lady Constance with forget-me-nots woven in her pubic hair worshipping the phallus of Mellors the garden god. Ordinary people, of course, continued to find sex funny, and told as many 'dirty jokes' as ever, but their common sense was banished from literature into the 'illegitimate' theatre.

For women writers the emphasis was, as might be expected, rather different. A young woman, compelled to tolerate the sexual attentions of an older man with whom she is not in love, might very well be considered to be in a more desperate situation than the young woman married to an impotent old man. Aphra Behn argues against the denial of female sexuality entailed in marrying young women to old men, rather than the oppression of submitting to the repulsive embraces of palsied eld. The most sophisticated treatment of the theme is the case of Dorothea Brook in George Eliot's novel *Middlemarch*. Dorothea does not betray her old husband; by her misplaced idealism, she betrays herself. Eliot rescues her by putting her husband to death in the nick of time, so that Dorothea can marry a man who is more likely to satisfy her sexual and emotional needs.

These commonplaces are all now outdated. What is considered obscene nowadays is the idea of age itself. We are not now allowed to call ourselves old, still less is anyone else allowed to call us old. We are now supposed to stay young, and both sexually attractive and sexually active until the utterly unmentionable end, death. We no longer refer to 'dirty old men' in the same way that we did forty or even thirty years ago. 'Dirty old men' were the ones who had a prurient and creepy interest in the sexuality of the young, although in those days we presumed that there was little that they could do about it. The 'dirty old men' were the ones who offered children sweets and talked suggestively to them, who put their hands up their granddaughters' skirts when they were sitting on their knees, who sniffed bicycle seats. They were disgusting rather than dangerous.

Now that we are not permitted to call anybody old, we must not assume that anyone is impotent either. Impotence is not a natural condition but an affliction to be treated with all the ingenuity that modern technology can assemble. There are even such things as vacuum condoms that will exert negative pressure to produce tumescence in the floppiest old penis. With it comes more cultural pressure than ever to create anxiety about loss of interest and the floppiness of the penis. Even so, there is a residue of common sense which provokes men into announcing their incapacity. Denis Thatcher, asked what he was doing in the election campaign of 1987, said, 'Helping, I suppose.' When pressed he replied rather tartly, 'Do? There's not much I can do at my age.' As a rejection of the prurience and silliness of the English gutter press his retort was quite justified, but many people must have shaken their heads over his 'negativity'. Time was when the fading of sexual desire was seen as a liberation. Consumer culture being predicated on self-pleasuring, such an attitude is untenable. Someone who is not seeking sexual pleasure is simply not playing the game.

The argument of this chapter is simply that continuing sexual interest and perfect sexual adjustment between partners who have been together for thirty years is so difficult and rare that no one should feel guilty or inadequate for not having managed it. When it has been managed it has been extraordinary and wonderful, so extraordinary that there are few accounts of it. The ones we can find are the more fascinating for that.

Forty-seven-year-old Jane Digby gave up on love in 1854, when, after three marriages, she had been rejected by her Arab lover for a younger woman and decided that she and her friend Eugenia would grow old together surrounded by their cats and dogs. She could hardly have imagined that the love of her life was about to sweep her away with him to the desert. Twenty-eight-year-old Sheik Abdul Medjuel El Mezrab, who ruled the desert around Palmyra, saw her (aged forty-eight), loved her and continued to love her for thirty years. When they were married in 1855, she said, 'If I had neither a mirror, nor a memory, I would think myself fifteen years old' (Blanch, 176). We do not know how Jane Digby El Mezrab kept the love of her dark desert king for thirty years, during which she did not live as the usual suppressed and invisible Arab wife, but rode alongside her husband like an Amazon. The sheik for his part refused to use her money and took no other wife. Isabel Burton met her in 1868 and wrote:

> She was a most beautiful woman, though at the time I write she was sixty-one, tall, commanding and queen like ... [she wore] one blue garment, beautiful hair in two plaits to the ground. (Blanch, p. 183)

Though she adopted Arab dress, Jane Digby El Mezrab kept her silver and damask and her fine bed linen; after fifteen years she succeeded in persuading her husband to use a knife and fork. She chose a Christian burial, at which her grief-stricken husband, mounted on her favourite black mare, rode up unannounced, took one last look and wheeled off into the desert.

The love of Sheik El Mezrab for the middle-aged English lady might inspire middle-aged people to think themselves into falling in love instead of talking themselves into resignation. There are some signs that a new mythology of geriatric love is springing up as the population ages; as more and more leisured elderly people reinvent the social events that were the framework of courtship, tea-dances and picnics, and sporting events of an unstrenuous nature, flirtation must ensue and old men and women must dream dreams. It would be invidious to suggest that Gabriel García Márquez had this readership in mind when he made his own highly significant contribution to the myth of geriatric love in *Love in the Time of Cholera*. The plot follows the tradition of old romances; Aucassin, in this case Florentino Ariza, must wait all his life and traverse untold hazards, mostly affairs with other women, before he can enjoy his true love, Fermina Daza. Because this is the twentieth century the fulfilment of the ancient lovers must be described in concrete terms, but Márquez, who was nearly sixty when he wrote *Love in the Time of Cholera*, has some difficulties. The first physical contact is disappointing.

> Both were lucid enough to realize, at the same fleeting instant, that the hands made of old bones were not the hands they had imagined before touching.
>   'Not now,' she said to him, 'I smell like an old woman.'
>
> (p. 329)

Admittedly these lovers are very old; Márquez is quite deliberately pitching his preposterous story as far into old age as his imagination will take him. He may be deliberately invoking images of the charnel house in insisting on the smell of the very old, who are not rotting or, as he would have it, fermenting. Old people smell less, not more, than young people, because they secrete less (see chapter 5). A clean old person is quite likely to have the same powdery smell as a baby. Nevertheless, Márquez insists that his ancient lovers smell not just bad but awful.

> Florentino Ariza shuddered: as she herself had said, she had the sour smell of old age. Still, as he walked to his cabin, he consoled himself with the thought that he must give off the same odor, except his was four years older, and she must have detected it on him, with the same emotion. It was the smell of human fermentation, which he had perceived in his oldest lovers and they had detected in him. The widow Nazaret, who kept nothing to herself, had told him in a cruder way, 'Now we stink like a henhouse.' They tolerated each other because they were an even match: my odor against yours.
> (p. 335)

So depressed are the lovers by the evidence of their own unbiological 'fermentation' that they can proceed no further in their genital affairs until Fermina drinks anisette. Then, a blow having been struck for the liquor lobby, they are off and running:

> … he dared to explore her withered neck with his fingertips, her bosom armored in metal stays, her lips with their decaying bones, her thighs with their aging veins. She accepted with pleasure, her eyes closed, but she did not tremble, and she smoked and drank at

regular intervals. At length, when his caresses slid over her belly, she
had enough anisette in her heart.

'If we're going to do it, let's do it,' she said, 'but let's do it like
grown-ups.'

She took him to the bedroom and, with the lights on, began to
undress without false modesty ...

She said: 'Don't look ... because you won't like it' ...

He looked at her and saw her naked to the waist, just as he had
imagined her. Her shoulders were wrinkled, her breasts sagged, her
ribs were covered by a flabby skin as pale and cold as a frog. (p. 338)

There is a certain perversity operating here too; if Fermina does not
want Florentino to see she ought not to undress, let alone with the
light on, which is evidently what she means by doing it 'like grown-
ups'. There is no law of taste or morality which demands that people
fuck naked or by the light of the overhead bulb. Fermina seems to be
doing her utmost to revolt Florentino, so Márquez can revolt us. How
Florentino knows that the 'flabby skin' is cold without touching it is
mysterious; Márquez's intention in invoking frogs is not. Old bodies
are not as revolting as young people think. (They are not, for example,
colder than young bodies.) Márquez's invention of heroic fucking
against tremendous odds, as if the two old people were galvanised
corpses, is actually profoundly ageist. Underlying it are two unpleasant
and invalid assumptions: that old people will only transcend their
oldness by imitating younger people, and that old people are revolting.

... she stretched out her hand in the darkness, caressed his belly,
his flanks, his almost hairless pubis. She said: 'You have skin like
a baby's.' Then she took the final step: she searched for him where
he was not, she searched again without hope, and she found him,
unarmed.

'It's dead,' he said ...

He took her hand and laid it on his chest: Fermina Daza felt the
old, untiring heart almost bursting through his skin, beating with
the strength, the rapidity, the irregularity of an adolescent's. (p. 340)

While it is probably a truism that the end of one's sexual career is as
incompetent as the beginning, it seems unduly cruel that the old lovers

have to approach each other as baldly and dispassionately as any pair of pick-ups after a town-hall dance, and that Fermina should think less of wrapping her new lover in her arms than of 'searching for him', by which I suppose Márquez means groping for his penis, and finding it 'unarmed', i.e. limp. Eventually, on the second encounter, penetration is effected.

> It was the first time she had made love in over twenty years, and she was held back by her curiosity concerning how it would feel at her age after so long a respite. But he had not given her time to find out if her body loved him too. It had been hurried and sad, and she thought: Now we've screwed up everything. But she was wrong ...
> (p. 341)

In the world of magic realism vaginas do not atrophy. Fermina Daza might well have suffered excruciating pain, and torn or bled; her lover's frail erection, for the glans penis does not often become completely turgid in eighty-year-old men, would have found penetration very difficult, if not impossible. Why the two ancient lovers have to imitate the act of generation, why they cannot pleasure each other in any of the myriad ways human beings can but must achieve 'normal' or 'grown-up' sex, seems to argue a certain lack of imagination on the part of the lovers and their creator. Márquez invents for them a normal married life in which Fermina waits as devotedly on Florentino as ever Colette's Pauline waited on her.

> ... she helped him to take his enemas, she got up before he did to brush the false teeth he kept in a glass while he slept, and he solved the problem of her misplaced spectacles, for she could use his for reading and mending ...

Locked in the boat doomed to sail for ever in the pestilential river as the corpses float by, Florentine and Fermina enact true happiness. The ending of the novel has the hollow ring of mere pious feeling. Eric Segal could hardly have written it worse.

> They made the tranquil, wholesome love of experienced grandparents ... they no longer felt like newlyweds, and even less

like belated lovers. It was as if they had leapt over the arduous calvary of conjugal life and gone straight to the heart of love. They were together in silence like an old married couple wary of life, beyond the pitfalls of passion, beyond the brutal mockery of hope and the phantoms of disillusion: beyond love. For they had lived together long enough to know that love was always love, anytime and anyplace, but it was more solid the closer it came to death. (p. 345)

After such flummery, 'love is never having to say you're sorry' sounds like hard-headedness.

Behind the prescription of unending sexual intercourse between spouses from the altar to the grave lies the domestication of passion. As we have seen, it is nowadays generally held that sex is good for you. Even though women and children are too often subject to sexual abuse, and sex is suspected as a motive in the murder of every woman and every child, the certainty that sex is at least as good for you as bran has been successfully established. The sexual revolutionaries' belief that sex was only destructive when distorted by repression has been shown to be wrong, for the incidence of all kinds of sex-related crime has risen steadily over the last twenty years. Nevertheless the belief in a domestic brand of sex, which is regular, benign, wholesome and affectionate, has completely driven out any idea of love as essentially related to death. Sex has been purged of all obsessiveness, all hostility, all jealousy, all guilt. It has been reconciled with familiarity and predictability. It is exclusive without being possessive. It is inexhaustible. To suspect, let alone believe, that this is a delusion is to be a modern heretic. To admit holding any such belief is to reveal oneself as a reactionary crone.

The version of sex as the cement of the family is a new one upon the earth and may indeed constitute a delusion, particularly as it has gained the ascendant at the same rate and at the same time that divorce has passed the level of one in two marriages in the United States, with the western European nations close behind. Older societies have acted on the principle that sex is basically unpredictable, dangerous and uncontrollable. Traditionally the sex relation between spouses has been carefully contained within a family structure, and monitored by other family members, aware of the constant potentiality for abuse and physical violence within it. Recent reporting of the frequency of spouse rape in Britain would seem to show that we cannot afford to continue pretending that sexuality has been domesticated. Most human societies have understood that young men are particularly dangerous and should be kept away from children and other men's wives, disciplined by apprenticeship or national service or the authority of an older patriarch, so that their aggressiveness did not disturb the nurturing home where women and children were meant to feel safe from outrage. The extent of our failure to ensure that mothers and children are secure can be assessed from the horrifying figures for child abuse and for wife battery and rape that every year strike us as incredible, but in which we are constrained to believe. The tiny nuclear family built about the copulating couple is unsafe for women and children. It is arguable that it is unsafe because of the primacy given to the sex relation between the couple, the maintenance of which may be thought to justify all kinds of distorted behaviour and certainly conflicts with the demands of small children.

The pressure then upon the ageing wife to continue playing the sex game with her husband, who may be still interested, or may require more effective stimuli than she can offer, or may be completely uninterested, is part of the same process that has apparently already succeeded in brutalising family life. If this is the case, which is admittedly suggested rather than demonstrated, the ageing wife would be better advised to opt out, to insist upon a different relationship with her husband in which different values were paramount. What is so clear as to be obvious is that she should have the right to opt out of the sex relationship without appearing to invite desertion.

Peasant populations generally have very clear notions about the stage in life when sexual activity should cease. For women this is usually when the first daughter reaches the age of marriage; though this may be long before menopause, it is felt inappropriate for two generations to be in the childbearing phase at the same time. And so we find very commonly in peasant populations a long period of what is called 'terminal abstinence', which is very important in limiting fertility, as it limits a potential childbearing season of thirty years to sixteen years or so (Caldwell and Caldwell, 1977; Ruzicka and Bhatia, 1982; Gajanayake, 1987).

Terminal abstinence would be considered by most developed societies an unbearable limitation on human sexual expression. In most societies that practise it, it is considered merely normal. Older people no longer feel '*la furia*'; they have other indulgences – food, alcohol, tobacco, power, money, business, politics. It is understood, moreover, that old bodies are not attractive. In some societies the powerful old men commandeer all the young women for their own use, while young men and older women alike go without. Bride-price in some societies functions as a way of supplying young women exclusively to those who can raise the payment, so that young men are obliged to watch the women of their own generation mated with the generation of their fathers. This may or may not be seen as a tyranny, largely depending upon whether there is a semi-sanctioned culture of adultery that goes along with it.

There are many different ways of organising human sexual response and human sexual relationships. Human beings are not monogamous; they are not programmed like the species that once mated can never part, none of which relies upon continual intercourse to keep them together, but only mate when they are reproducing. Human love does not depend upon the need to mate or the need for orgasm; the greatest love can survive distance and even death. When in 1750 at the age of sixty Susanna Highmore realised that she was dying, she hid notes for her husband all about their house, so that he would find them after she was gone. The notes were to tell him how deeply she loved him (*The Gentlemen's Magazine*, January 1816).

15

The Hardy Perennials

Though it is clearly not true that life begins at forty, and even more obviously absurd to claim that life begins at fifty, many women may expect to live as many years after menopause as they have already lived as adults. For some women, especially women who have felt themselves most alive when functioning as the lover and beloved of a man or men, this is by no means good news. Simone de Beauvoir inveighed bitterly against the decline not only of her sexual attractions but of her interest in sex: in *Force of Circumstance*, written in 1963 when she was fifty-five, she says:

> Never again a man. Now, not my body alone but my imagination
> too has accepted that in spite of everything, it's strange not to be a
> body any more. There are moments when the oddness of it, because
> it's so definitive, chills my blood. But what hurts more than all these
> deprivations is never feeling any new desires: they wither before
> they can be born in the rarefied climate I inhabit now. (p. 657)

There have been women who saw their influence over a man or, even more difficult, over more than one man, continue to grow long after menopause had come and gone. The essentials for such a career seem to be first of all good health, and its concomitant, good spirits, then intelligence, and then style or its equivalent. Great mistresses of the arts of civilisation continue to enchant regardless of whether they are allowing physical intimacy to one or other or all of their followers. Even courtesans, provided they were endowed with taste, wit and energy, have been able to continue living in the grand style though neither they nor the habitués of their salons were interested in sex. Such a one was the great French courtesan Ninon de l'Enclos.

In the spring of 1671, when she was fifty-one, Ninon de l'Enclos fell in love for the umpteenth time. The object of her passion was Charles de Sévigné, a smooth-faced angelic-looking young man of twenty-three. His mother, the Marquise de Sévigné, wrote to her daughter, 'Your brother wears the chains of Ninon; I wish they may do him no harm. There are minds that shudder at such ties. Ninon corrupted the morals of his father' (Letter XXV). Many years before, when the Marquis de Sévigné was a handsome rakehell who had left his virtuous wife at home to be assiduously courted by her cousin, he had caught Ninon's roving eye. As was usually the case with her, she tired of him in a few weeks and amused herself by making a conquest first of one of his wife's admirers, the Sieur de Rambouillet, and then of another, the Marquis de Vassé. Madame de Sévigné could avenge herself for this series of humiliations only in her letters. Now in middle age Ninon seduced her son, whose latest amorous exploit had been to take the actress Champmeslé away from Racine.

Mademoiselle de l'Enclos promenaded with Charles in the Cours, and let herself be seen slapping him hard for looking at other women and then kissing him to make up. Furiously jealous of the young actress, she demanded that he yield up to her Champmeslé's letters, which he did. Nothing Ninon did could awaken the spirit of gallantry in him, however. He let her exhibit him at delicious suppers in Saint-Germain but he made no attempt to hide his lack of real interest in fashionable manners and elegant conversation, at which Ninon was universally acknowledged to excel. Meanwhile his mother and her friend Madame de Lafayette were struggling to awaken in Charles some sense of the indelicacy of his position. They persuaded him to get Champmeslé's letters back, but before they could prevail upon him to give up his relationship with Ninon, she threw him out. 'He is past belief,' she said, 'with the mind of a milksop and a heart like an iced pumpkin.' The affair had lasted a month.

Ninon used to say that three months was her limit with anyone; she had had hundreds of lovers and history would go on to credit her with more. She was supposed to have taken pity on Charles Paris d'Orléans, teenaged son of the Duc de la Rochefoucauld and Madame de Longueville, who begged her to save him from his mistress, 'that fat Marquise de Castelnau'. She is thought in her sixties to have had an affair with a Swede called Jean Banier and in her nineties to have extended her favours to two licentious abbés, Gedoyn and Chateauneuf, and at the same age to have tried to seduce Bourdaloue.

Biographers have argued that Ninon gave up physical passion after Charles de Sévigné. She replied to a flattering letter from her dear friend St Evremond:

> I learn with pleasure that my soul is dearer to you than my body, and that your good sense leads you as always to the better part. To tell truth, the body is no longer worthy of attention, and the soul still does have some glow that supports it and renders it responsive to the memory of a friend, whose absence has not dimmed his image. (Colombey, pp. 119–20; author's translation)

Madame, the king's sister, the Duchesse d'Orléans, wrote to a friend:

> Now that Madame de Lenclos is old, she leads a very strict life. She maintains, so they say, that she would never have reformed if she herself had not realized how ridiculous the whole affair was. (Magne, p. 214)

Though she had given up physical passion, Mademoiselle de l'Enclos did not give up passion. She devoted herself to the cultivation and maintenance of friendship.

> Durability in friendship is at least as rare as durability in love. Time was when I cared only for the latter, now I long for the former. (Magne, pp. 214–15)

She befriended Madame de la Sablière, the unhappy wife of her old lover the Sieur de Rambouillet, and was a frequent visitor at her house in Saint-Roch, where she shared Madame de la Sablière's hospitality with the likes of Molière, La Fontaine, Mignard, Tallemant and Boileau. The same luminaries visited her exquisite house in the Rue de Tournelles, where newcomers were as astonished by the liveliness of their hostess's wit as by the freshness of her complexion. Her explanation of her youthful appearance was simply that in a lifetime of offering her guests the best wines she herself drank nothing but pure water.

She avoided late nights and all excess of eating and drinking, the sources, she was wont to say, of premature senility. (p. 229)

Saint-Simon wrote in his *Mémoires*:

Everything at Mademoiselle de L'Enclos' is done with a respect and decorum which is rarely enjoyed even by the best-loved princesses in the conduct of their affairs. She had therefore, the noblest and most attractive people at Court for friends ... it became the fashion to be received at her house, and people used to like to go there on account of the people they met. There was no gaming, ribaldry, nor brawling, and no one discussed politics or religion. Humour and elaborate wit, talk of things ancient and modern, news of everyone's love affairs, were the order of the day; but everything was discussed delicately and tolerantly, with no hint of malice, and the hostess knew how to keep conversation going by her intelligence and her great wealth of information about this and every age. (Magne, p. 231)

The Sun King himself dreaded the scalpel touch of Ninon's irony. For thirty post-menopausal years she was the arbiter of taste for *le tout-Paris*; princes, statesmen, philosophers and artists all knew that her verdict on their performances carried more weight than the screeds of bought praise that appeared in print. And some of them persisted in writing love poems to her. As for Charles de Sévigné, he became a monk.

Though Ninon was a rarity so fabulous that noble travellers in Paris insisted on being taken to meet her, she was by no means unique. The mistresses of the kings of France set a formidable precedent in durability. The Abbé Brantôme claimed to have seen the legendary Diane de Poitiers at the age of seventy 'as beautiful of face, as fresh and kindly as at thirty years'. Unfortunately for this evidence, Diane de Poitiers died at the age of sixty-six. Six months before her death, again according to Brantôme, she was lovely enough 'to move a heart of rock'; her horse had fallen with her in the streets of Orléans and her leg had been broken, but she gave no sign of pain. 'Far from it; for her beauty, her grace, her majesty, her handsome appearance were all the same as they had always been.' Above all, her skin was dazzling though she used no rouge or powder. Dreux du Radier thought her complexion the result of washing her face every morning with *eau de puits*, well water. She rose at six, rode, and then went back to bed and read till noon, and this combination of strenuous exercise and rest is thought by some to be the secret of her undiminished vitality in later life.

When Diane's lover became King Henri II of France in 1547 he was thirty-one; Diane was in her forty-eighth year. She had been a widow for fifteen years and had never changed her *petit deuil*. To the end of her life she wore only black and white. The court was quickly staffed with her associates. The king made her Duchesse de Valentinois and gave her not only an enormous sum of money with which to rebuild her own Château d'Anet, but the huge domaine of Chenonceau as well. Diane ruled him in everything; it was she who told him when to sleep with the Queen, Cathérine de Médicis; when Cathérine's children were born Diane was placed in charge of them. In 1552 the Venetian ambassador Contarini wrote:

> ... he greatly loved, he greatly loves her, and old as she is she is
> his mistress. It is true that although she has never used rouge and
> perhaps by virtue of the minute care which she takes, she is far from
> looking her age ... His Majesty ... does ... in this and in everything
> else what she wants. She is informed of everything, and every day
> as a rule the King, after his dinner, goes to her and remains an
> hour and a half to consult with her and to tell her all that happens.
> (Henderson, pp. 182–3).

In 1554, at the height of her power, 55-year-old Diane was obliged to beg the King to leave her for a time. She was unwell, and evidently did not wish him to see her at anything but her best. Her biographers do not tell us, and probably could not tell us, if her malady was connected with menopause. The king went to Saint-Germain-en-Laye. When he returned his neglected wife had arranged a ballet, to exhibit the charms of Mary Stuart's governess who, she thought, might succeed in drawing her husband away from his middle-aged lover. The King fell for his wife's stratagem and fathered a son upon the little Scotswoman, but the second part of the ruse failed. When Diane was fully recovered the King was once more by her side. When the Queen became pregnant for the eleventh time, he gave up going to her bed for good.

The love of Henri II for a woman nearly twenty years older than himself lasted until he was mortally wounded in a tournament in 1559. As he lay dying the Queen, with whom he had had no relations for the last six years, was called to his side and sworn in as regent. When Diane came to take her leave of the man she had loved for thirty years, the doors were shut against her. She was evicted from her apartments in the palace and Chenonceau was taken from her. She said that she would die with her lover; she lived on until 1566, leaving us a single realistic portrait of her in middle age to compare with the dozens of idealised depictions of her tall, graceful, long-legged, high-breasted person as the goddess Diana, in words by Marot or du Bellay, in sculpture by Jean Goujon or Benvenuto Cellini, and painted by François Clouet or Léonard Limousin.

Madame de Maintenon is an even more remarkable example of a woman's power to fascinate long after what was commonly perceived as her beauty had decayed. She was born Françoise d'Aubigny in 1635; at eighteen she married the crippled playwright Paul Scarron, who died in 1660, leaving her destitute. In 1669 Madame de Montespan appointed her governess of the children she had borne to Louis XIV of France, then living near Vaugirard; in 1674 the King decided that his children should be at court, and Madame Scarron came with them. By September 1675 she had already undermined the position of Madame de Montespan so effectively that her erstwhile patroness was sent away from the court. Meanwhile the King's architect had been sent to supervise the restoration and embellishment of the house at Maintenon that Madame Scarron had bought with the money she earned from Madame de Montespan. Her champions excuse her of all calculation in the matter.

> Her gentle nature and retiring disposition soon gained for her
> Louis's esteem; he chose her to read to him and gradually admitted
> her more and more to his confidence. In 1678 he advanced her small
> estate of Maintenon ... into a marquisate. From the first moment
> of her influence over the King she used it for the good of France
> and himself. Once she had finally succeeded in ousting Madame
> de Montespan from favour, she cleansed the Court of much of
> its looseness, made friends with the poor neglected Queen, who

trusted her and liked her, and after that lady's death was secretly
married to Louis ...

It is always romantic when a pretty young commoner marries a
powerful king. In this version of the Cinderella story the commoner
was a fifty-year-old widow who was rumoured to have been before her
marriage to the playwright no better than a prostitute. She was an old
friend of Ninon de l'Enclos, and had had a long affair with one of Ninon's
ex-lovers. Evidently Madame de Montespan did not expect her to use an
appearance of virtue to discredit her. There were many at court who saw
the Marquise de Maintenon as a designing hypocrite, among them the
King's sister-in-law, Elisabeth-Charlotte of Bavaria, Princess Palatine,
Duchess of Orléans, Madame de France, who could never bring herself
to speak of Madame de Maintenon without including the epithet 'old'.

> The old Maintenon woman amuses herself by making the King hate
> all the members of the Royal family and bend them to her will ...
> the Dauphiness is ... daily ill-treated at the old hag's instigation ...
> The old hag has already tried a dozen times to embroil me with the
> Dauphiness. (Stevenson I, p. 74)

Despite the high-bred fury of the royal families of Europe at the
unconscionable power wielded by this woman of low birth, the King
married Madame de Maintenon secretly in 1685. His sister-in-law wrote
in 1688 in answer to queries about his marriage from her aunt, the
Duchess of Hanover:

> One thing, however, is certain, the King never loved any of his
> mistresses as devotedly as he loves her. It is very amusing to see
> them together. If she is anywhere about he cannot let a quarter of
> an hour pass without whispering in her ear, or withdrawing to talk
> to her in private, and this although he has spent the whole day with
> her. (I, p. 80)

Four years later she writes again:

> On journeys like these the Great Man lives in the same house as his
> old slut, but does not sleep in the same room, and a mystery is made

of the whole affair. You will understand therefore that he has not yet acknowledged her as his wife. That, however, does not prevent him from shutting himself up with her every day when they are together and keeping the whole court waiting at the door ... (I, p. 107)

And again in 1696 she tells of the King's severity with two of his illegitimate daughters, who had been making rude songs about their stepmother:

... it appears that he did not mince his language, and he seems to have been more annoyed on Madame de Maintenon's account than because of what they said about himself. The love he bears that woman is quite extraordinary. (I, p. 45)

So unchallenged was Madame de Maintenon's power at the court of the most powerful monarch in Europe that Madame referred to her, when she was not calling her 'the old bawd', as 'the Pantocrat'. In September 1698, Madame had the satisfaction of reporting:

The Pantocrat is very powerful, but from all accounts she is not very happy and often weeps bitterly. And she often talks about Death, but I expect that is only to see how people will reply to her ... (I, p. 169)

In July 1699, Madame was displeased to discover that when she visited 'the all-powerful Dame' she was offered only a footstool to sit on, because the King visited so often and no one could be seated in a chair in his presence, except Madame de Maintenon, who was 'allowed one because of her bad health' (p. 185). In 1710 she was still 'the all-powerful Maintenon':

When the King is going neither to shoot, nor to Marly, he spends the whole afternoon with Madame de Maintenon, and he works in her room with his ministers every evening. (II, p. 55)

In 1712 Madame told her aunt:

Although the old woman is my bitterest enemy, I nevertheless wish her a long life, for the King's sake, because everything would be ten times worse if the King were to die at this juncture, and he is so devoted to the woman that he would assuredly not survive her, therefore I hope that she may live for many years to come. (II, p. 58)

When she was seventy, Madame de Maintenon 'complained to her confessor that she still very often had to lie with the old king' (De Beauvoir, 1965, p. 187n). After his death, she withdrew to the girls' school she had founded at Saint-Cyr, where she died four years later at the age of eighty-four.

In order to understand the high visibility of older women in the French court, we have to understand that the culture of pre-revolutionary France placed a high premium on refinement of taste and manners. Such depth of polish took many years to acquire; it began with discipline and after years of practice became second nature. Though everyone was aware of the bloom of young women and quick to caress them, no one visited the great *salonnières* to marvel at beauties that were more easily observed and enjoyed in milkmaids. This state of affairs still prevailed in the 1780s when, according to Madame de La Tour du Pin, the older women were 'all-powerful' (Harcourt, p. 86). After the revolution, the old ladies disappeared; 'gatherings of all the generations [became] things of the past and ... to M. Talleyrand's great regret, old ladies are no longer to be met in society' (p. 95).

Men and women alike willingly submitted to the rule of the doyennes in order to learn from them the complicated and subtle movements of the social dance. Though there were salons in England, and they were run by older women, the greater segregation in British society is manifest in that they were never central. When Molière made fun of *Les Femmes Savantes*, he was singling out women whose pedantry offended against the standards of behaviour set and observed by ladies of refinement. When women who dared to discuss matters of aesthetics and philosophy were guyed by English satirists, there was a nastier element of sheer intolerance for being expected to listen to a woman at all.

The English version of the venerable salonnière is Mary Delany, who at eighty-eight 'blushed like a girl'. When she was seventeen she was married off to a disagreeable sixty-year-old man who died five years later without making his will, leaving her without the fortune her family had hoped for. She was courted by various gentlemen, including Lord Baltimore, but she did not remarry until 1743, when she was forty-three, when Swift's friend Patrick Delany came over to England to ask her to be his second wife. He was much her inferior in rank and connections, and not a wealthy man, but she accepted him and they lived happily until his death in 1768. In her second widowhood she became a favourite of the royal family, who visited her every day. She was remarkable for her taste, her good breeding, her charm and her vivacity, which she retained until her death in 1788. George III commissioned her portrait by Opie and it hangs still in Hampton Court.

Louisa Maximiliana, daughter of Gustavus Adolphus, Prince of Stohlberg-Gedern, after eight unhappy years as the wife of the elderly, debauched and drunken Young Pretender, then living in exile as the Count of Albany, ran off with the great Italian playwright Vittorio Alfieri and lived with him as his mistress until his death in 1803, when she was fifty. Though her grief was intense, within a few months Alfieri's place at her side was filled by their mutual friend, the young French painter Fabré, who lived with her until her death in 1824 and was her sole heir.

We may speculate that these women all had attractions of other than a physical kind. In the case of Ninon and Madame de Maintenon we may judge that theirs were charms of personality. Other middle-aged women who were successful in love were so because of their rank and fortune; the most obvious example of a woman who used rank to entice into her bed men much younger than herself is Catherine the Great, who behaved as Empress in much the same way that male monarchs behaved, taking her pick of the most vigorous and attractive sex objects appearing at court.

None of the great perennials, Diane de Poitiers, Ninon de l'Enclos or Madame de Maintenon, could have had recourse to cosmetic surgery. Neither did they have hormone replacement therapy. It did not take them three or four hours to ready themselves for their public, for they were not principally valued for the effect their appearance had on strangers standing at a distance or on cameras. The dazzling old sex objects *de nos jours* are a curiously garish bunch, better to see from a distance than to come close to. They seldom state their age, though everybody knows it; they do not make a point of having triumphed over menopause. Nor are they often willing to admit being on HRT. Strange to relate, though the effects of HRT are supposed to be spectacular, or so the Masters in Menopause tell us, no one can tell from looking at her whether a woman is on HRT or not.

The making of a twenty-first-century perennial involves rather more than spring water, heredity and asceticism. Advances in surgery mean that those who can afford it can have the debris of years cleared away, leaving no trace. Wasted bosoms can be plumped, eyes widened and brightened, wrinkles erased; where once such interventions were regarded as lamentable and unconvincing, they are now *de rigueur* for any woman who does not want to be thought a failure or a slommack. Debora L. Spar, fifty-year-old President of Barnard College, explained to the readers of the *New York Times* on 24 September 2012 her own attitude to ageing and her 'beauty dilemma'.

> … for women in certain professional or social circles, the bar of normal keeps going up. There are virtually no wrinkles on Hollywood stars or on Broadway actors; ditto for female entrepreneurs or women in the news media. There are few wrinkles on the women in Congress and even fewer on Wall Street. Chief executives, bankers, hospital administrators, heads of public relations firms and publishing houses, lawyers, marketers, caterers.

The responses to what was anything but an actual confession were revealing, some horrifyingly so. Carlin Meyer, Professor Emeritus at the New York Law School, argued that 'all women face the same pressures. Not all risk losing high-paying jobs, but they face losing a spouse, or a salary, which can mean the difference between home and homelessness.' Really? Are American husbands ditching middle-aged wives because they won't accept or can't afford cosmetic surgery? Barnard alumnae wrote angrily to the *New York Times* declaring that, if the President of their alma mater were to be seen as pushing cosmetic surgery, they would no longer contribute to college funds. (It was perfectly obvious that the said President coloured her hair – a rather unforgiving donkey brown.) Part of the difficulty with the subject stemmed from the tendency of obvious acceptors of cosmetic surgery to deny the fact. In the same issue the *New York Times* ran a correction about Gloria Steinem, who had been said in an article to have undergone cosmetic surgery, which apparently she had bothered to deny. In fact Steinem herself had said in an answer to an online Q&A for *Time* magazine that when she was hosting the *Today* show in 1986 she had 'a little fat removed' from above her eyes, explaining that it was 'so I didn't look like Mao Zedong and I could wear my contacts. It looked worse afterward. It was a good warning not to do anything else.' At eighty-two Steinem still has not given up colouring her hair. Cosmetic surgery might be optional; dyeing your hair is something you owe to yourself. With dyed hair you are 'the real you'.

New York perennials did not always have to look wrinkle-free. The *arbiter elegantiarum* of New York for much of the twentieth century was the late Diana Vreeland, the 'sultana of style', who all her life dyed her hair raven black and painted her face white.

> The elaborate maquillage was eventually reduced to a fundamental scheme: matching scarlet lips and nails, shiny lids, and scarlet slashes on her cheeks, forehead, and ears. She loved to ask her companions rhetorically, 'Is it Kabuki enough?' (Collins)

Vreeland was a heavy smoker; her cigarette holders were as much a part of her style as her massive costume jewellery and her imposing nose. With chain smoking comes wrinkles and Vreeland wore hers with pride. She died in 1989 aged eighty-six.

Vreeland's successor is a good deal duller. Anna Wintour, who became editor of *Vogue* the year before Vreeland died, has been there ever since. Her power in the New York fashion world is probably greater than Vreeland's but her girlish unchanging look, as she peeps out from under a schoolgirl bob which she has worn since she was fourteen, is far less interesting.

> Rumour has it that Wintour and her hair have become so attached, that the 66-year-old style icon won't start her working day until her familiar blunt bob is chopped, blown-out and smoothed into non-movable shape by a stylist. She is, you could say, committed to her hair. (*Telegraph*, 3 May 2016)

Only the colour varies from raspberry blond to mousy. The effect of the helmet of hair is to curtain her small face from every angle except front-on. Her face is further obscured by big black sunglasses, which she always wears in public, even indoors in the dark. Her demeanour is so chilly and she is so demanding with inefficient subordinates that she is known as 'Nuclear Wintour'. If she had a menopause the fact was never mentioned, but it would have to have been around 2000, when she was dealing with a new assistant called Lauren Weisberger, who would go on to write *The Devil Wears Prada*. In the movie (2006) the Wintour role is played by then 57-year-old Meryl Streep, another hardy perennial.

Before Anna Wintour rose to power, the leading New York perennial was Helen Gurley Brown, editor of *Cosmopolitan*. For more than fifty years married to the same man, Brown was the prototype of the eternal bride. As one of her friends told James Kaplan for an article in *Vanity Fair* (June 1990), 'It must be *exhausting* to be a girl at sixty-eight.' The eternal bride has no children if she can help it, so that she can fix what Kaplan calls her 'heat-lock eyes' on her husband and give his least action her full, dazzled attention. Whenever they are likely to be observed she must gaze at him with parted lips as if they are on the brink of some kind of sex marathon, as Nancy Reagan (another perennial bride) used to do whenever she appeared in public with President Reagan. As she must appear girlish, the eternal bride does not get her bosom pumped up, though Brown did opt for breast augmentation at the age of seventy-three. Otherwise she had no body to speak of; her face on the other hand was large, stretched shiny-tight by surgery and split by a gash of lipstick and porcelain.

> But don't even mention the word menopause to Mrs. Brown
> because she says that with the high doses of estrogen she takes, and
> recommends, she never experienced its side effects. She's much
> more focused on what women can do to feel younger (sex, cosmetic
> surgery and more sex), picking up where her last best-selling advice
> book, 'Having It All' (Simon & Schuster, 1982), left off. (Witchel)

Brown worked hard to project her glamour despite her lack of hair. Her hair had always been thin and with age and years of dyeing it got thinner. She underwent at least one facelift, an eyelift, had her nose bobbed, her eyebrows tattooed, and silicone injections in her face. For women wanting to look good for a party she recommended mixing moisturiser with Preparation H. She died in 2012 at the age of ninety.

Less famous but in some ways more remarkable than either Helen Gurley Brown or Anna Wintour is Wintour's friend Barbara Amiel. Amiel had various partners including three husbands before she landed Conrad Black in 1992 at the age of fifty-two. Sarah Sands, her editor when she worked on the *Telegraph*, wrote in an article for the *Independent* (18 November 2007) that 'Amiel was more than 50 years old when she married Black, yet he was besotted by her sexiness'. That 'yet' reveals more about Sands than it does about Amiel. (Black was four years younger than Amiel.) In 2002, a year after he had been created Baron Black of Crossharbour, his Baroness granted an interview to *Vogue* in which she boasted that her 'extravagance knows no bounds' as she showed off 'a fur closet, a sweater closet, a closet for shirts and T-shirts and a closet so crammed with evening gowns that the overflow has to be kept in yet more closets downstairs', as well as a dozen Hermès Birkin bags, thirty to forty handbags made by Renaud Pellegrino and more than 100 pairs of Manolo Blahnik shoes. Amiel's 'extravagance' was not confined to clothes; she also had a large collection of jewellery, mostly diamonds and pearls. The timing of the interview was unfortunate; goaded beyond endurance, Hollinger International, the holding company for Black's media interests, began legal action in Illinois against the couple and other executives, seeking $1.25 billion in damages. In 2007 Hollinger filed for bankruptcy and Black was sentenced to six and a half years in prison; on his release he was immediately deported from the US to his native Canada and Baroness Black went with him.

Mary Beard is a perennial of a different kind. She has reached the age of sixty-three without ever dyeing her hair, never had botox or fillers or a brow lift. She has been married to the same man since 1985. Her appearances on the BBC2 series *The Romans*, in which she flew around ancient Rome on a bicycle, drew a nasty response from revered journalist A. A. Gill, who demanded that she be kept away from the 'cameras altogether' because she was 'too ugly for television'. A subsequent appearance on *Question Time* resulted in abuse that is too vile to repeat. Beard's reaction was to reply to the trolls and even to find one of them a job. She felt that the abuse was so deeply misogynist it was not actually personal, and she responded for the sake of women. Which is not to say that it was not shocking and hurtful.

Amongst the hardiest of the hardy perennials are the Dames. The order of Dames Commander of the Order of the British Empire (as it is still bizarrely known) was instituted in 1917 to reward those faithful servants of the Crown who were not eligible for knighthoods on account of being female. Most of them were members of various royal households, but gradually performers begin to appear in honours lists. Amongst the first were Nellie Melba in 1918 and Clara Butt in 1920; subsequent DBEs included Sybil Thorndike in 1931, Edith Evans in 1946, Peggy Ashcroft and Margot Fonteyn in 1956, Judith Anderson and Flora Robson in 1960, Margaret Rutherford in 1967, Anna Neagle in 1969, Cicely Courtneidge in 1972, Joan Hammond in 1974, Wendy Hiller in 1975, Janet Baker in 1976, Gracie Fields and Joan Sutherland in 1979, Celia Johnson in 1981 and so forth. Dames are apt to be perennials because the honour is usually conferred in advanced age. The most conspicuous and possibly the hardiest crop of perennials are the five best-known theatrical dames of today, Dame Helen Mirren, seventy-two, Dame Joan Collins, eighty-four, Dame Judi Dench and Dame Maggie Smith, both eighty-three, and Dame Barbara Windsor, eighty. All five have worked through menopause and far beyond, and none has attempted to deny or belie her advancing years.

Helen Mirren was damed in 2003 when she was only fifty-eight, which is young for a great dame. (At forty-six Maggie Smith was even younger.) She is best known to non-theatregoers these days as the face of the L'Oréal Age Perfect range in which she is made to say lines like these, 'It's the science I trust to help me look like me. Nourish and indulge your skin, and show those age spots who's boss. Grow another year bolder. Look and feel more radiant. Our perfect age is now. So are we worth it? More than ever' – as if she meant them. Her fine skin is more genetic than cosmetic; once you have an age spot L'Oréal is not going to get rid of it for you.

Dame Joan was sixty-seven in 2000 when she met Percy Gibson in New York, not long before she was due to tour in a play. Percy was to be the producer. Collins's own account of their courtship given to the *Guardian* in 2013 describes Gibson as 'kind, loving and funny':

Eventually we began a passionate affair. I was in my 60s and he was in his 30s, but the age difference never posed a problem. We talked it through and he didn't want children. He adores my children and grandchildren. We've been married for 11 years, but when I look at him across a room, my heart still skips. I don't think about the future and we never discuss what might happen in 20 years. If he dies, he dies!

In fact Dame Joan and Percy are still together sixteen years after they were married in 2002. Dame Joan told the *Daily Express* in 2014 how she managed this.

In my opinion, HRT is the miracle drug. Although many doctors still pooh-pooh or condemn it completely, it can prevent brittle bones, increase energy levels, improve memory and concentration levels, and make dull skin glow again. As I have experienced myself, HRT can keep your bones as strong as they ever were.

HRT isn't a magic pill that will turn you into a young girl again, but it can most certainly improve the quality of your life in many ways. So run, don't walk to your nearest physician. If he turns out to be one of the nonbelievers, find a doctor who is a believer.

Dame Judi Dench was told at her first-ever audition that everything was wrong with her face. She was fifty-three in 1987 when Peter Hall asked her to play Cleopatra for the Royal Shakespeare Theatre production; she refused, pointing out that 'a menopausal dwarf' like herself would be absurdly miscast in the role. Hall insisted, and the result was a triumph. She was made a Dame the very next year. While Dame Joan's public image is two-thirds wig, Dame Judi has worn the same undyed 'cropped chop' hairstyle since long before menopause, and has never had any form of cosmetic surgery. Her audiences in cinemas and theatres or in front of the TV like her just the way she is. Her macular degeneration is so far advanced that she can no longer read a script, but even so she is never out of work. Widowed in 2001, she now steps out with farmer and conservationist 72-year-old David Mills. She has also got a new tattoo.

According to her autobiography published in 2001 *EastEnders* star Barbara Windsor, born August 1937, divorced her first husband in 1985, married her second in 1986, divorced him in 1995 and married Scott Mitchell in 2000 when she was sixty-two and he was just thirty-seven. The pair who go everywhere together can be seen to be still happy together. Dame Barbara turned eighty this year. She is clear about looking good for her age: 'It's my genes. My dad looked incredibly young, so did my mother. And a younger husband helps. Scott is only forty-five. If he hadn't come along, I don't know what I'd have done.' She still wears heels to add to her 4'7" and extravagant wigs. Now she campaigns to raise awareness of the availability of cataract surgery, having had treatment in both eyes herself.

Dames are a heartening list because they have all made significant contributions in their various fields, and they all look like continuing to do so, with a modicum of luck. The importance of a sense of vocation has been adumbrated in some of the most sensible accounts of women's ageing, and these women can all give testimony to it. People who waste time tend to get wasted by it. This life-course trajectory is not available to American women; American hardy perennials have rather different tales to tell, as is illustrated by the career of Jane Fonda, whose fight against advancing eld has been verily heroic.

It has been said that if you are to fight age you have to decide between the face and the body. A cruder version says, 'It's either your ass or your face.' In 1982 when Jane Fonda was forty-five she released the first of her twenty-three hugely successful exercise videos. In 1991 54-year-old Miss Fonda became engaged to be married to the President of CNN; to mark the occasion she shared with her public the fact that to go with her opal and diamond ring she had had augmentation mammoplasty. Fonda soon realised that Turner was a womaniser, but the marriage held on until 2001. For six years she did not date, then in 2009 she moved in with 67-year-old record producer Richard Perry, who told her then that he had been diagnosed with Parkinson's disease. She told a journalist in 2009 that she was 'happier than ever and the sex is better'. In 2016 she announced that she was about to go under the knife again so that she can look as young as she feels. In January 2017, Fonda and Perry split up.

Fifty-five-year-old Conservative MP Teresa Gorman probably had ambitions to become a perennial when she set up the Amarant Trust in 1986. The purpose of the charity was to develop a chain of HRT clinics; three years later she published *The Amarant Book of HRT*. As the inaugural chairman of the Amarant Trust her heavily made-up face appeared in an airbrushed photograph on the front page of its first newsletter, which urges women to demand HRT as a right. Mrs Gorman was vociferous about her own hormone replacement and evidently sure that her own appearance was encouraging. *She* magazine cooperated in what seems now an extraordinarily risky promotional campaign, featuring Mrs Gorman in a full-page colour photograph with all the lustre that make-up, hair-lacquer, pale pink jacket, diffused lighting and airbrush could bestow. The result was less encouraging than Mrs Gorman clearly hoped. Though she may have thought she looked terrific, others might easily have disagreed, especially when they saw her in the televised sessions of the House of Commons when she had not had the attentions of make-up artists, hairdressers and lighting cameramen. On the one hand, Mrs Gorman's contribution in the Commons was neither so judicious nor so venturesome as to inspire emulation and, on the other, if Mrs Gorman had developed a malignancy or a thrombosis or gallstones and been as public about it as she was about her HRT, the consequences for Ciba-Geigy, Organon, Schering and all could have been disastrous.

Attitudes to Teresa Gorman were often condescending and at times downright bitchy. In *A Woman's Place* published in 1997 Edwina Currie sneered that 'Teresa Gorman had at last succumbed to advancing years, stopped taking the tablets and shrunk to a benign little granny.' In fact no such thing had happened. At eighty-one Gorman claimed that HRT was keeping her 'very sexually active'. Her husband James Gorman died in 2007; in 2010 she married again, after placing an ad in *Private Eye*, 'Old trout seeks old goats. No golfers. Must have own balls' and got 128 replies. In 2010 she married widower Peter Clarke, who was sixteen years younger than she.

Generally, women in high places are ashamed to admit that they are taking replacement hormones and far less willing to function as advertisements for it than Mrs Gorman. Mrs Thatcher told us about the practitioner who gave her electric tingles in her bath but not about her patchet – if she had one. Mrs Gorman successfully sued for libel when she was incorrectly quoted as saying that Mrs Thatcher was a user of replacement hormones. Mrs Thatcher did not sue any of the sources that said that she was, but she herself refused to divulge whether she was or not. It would have been worth rather more than a king's ransom to the pharmaceutical multinationals if Mrs Thatcher could have been persuaded to announce that she was on HRT. Once she had retired from politics there was nothing to stop her doing a deal, but by then she would have proved to be more of a liability than an asset. Funnily enough, the Amarant Trust newsletter features an editorial by Teresa Gorman, MP BSc which asks:

> Can we grow old with grace and dignity like the Queen Mother or must we face the indignity of declining health with the prospect of ending life in a home incapable of living an independent life?

Did she mean to say that the Queen Mother was on HRT or that HRT confers all the benefits that accrue from the Queen Mother's income? Certainly, Mrs Gorman would have been ill-advised to associate HRT even so indirectly with the image of the Queen, who stopped smiling at menopause, while the Queen Mother's smile, in the manner of the Cheshire Cat's, outlasted the century. The implication that hormone replacement can guarantee good health in extreme old age is absurd. In Mrs Gorman's confused editorial there is little evidence of the mental tonic effect claimed for HRT by the Masters in Menopause. The main reasons only 2 per cent or so of British women took up HRT were not after all their own timorousness and the reluctance of doctors to take their problems seriously, but their own inbuilt scepticism and common sense.

The heroine of the most enduring twentieth-century romance has to be the woman who was born Camilla Shand and is now the Duchess of Cornwall and the wife of the Prince of Wales. She may be thought to have yet to prove herself as a hardy perennial, as she has turned seventy only last year, but she has had to contend with a lifetime's worth of vicissitudes. The truth seems to be that she and the Prince of Wales have been in love for forty-five years. At first they were deliberately separated. In 1973 she was married by the rites of the Catholic Church to Andrew Parker Bowles, to whom she bore two children. Prince Charles is godfather to her son. When the prince's favourite uncle was killed by the IRA in 1979 he turned to Camilla for support, and there are those who think the forbidden relationship was revived at that time. The 'firm', as the court is known, had decided on a child bride for Charles; Diana Spencer was fourteen years younger than Camilla and fifteen years younger than Charles, who made a go of the marriage as far as siring the heir and the spare, but there was no escaping his love for Camilla and his growing dislike for his wife.

In 1992, when Diana told the world about her overcrowded marriage, Camilla found herself battered by a storm of public loathing, which was made more humbling by the release a few months later of the tapes of intimate phone conversations between her and Charles recorded in 1989. This was the same time as she was observing the decline of her mother, crippled by acute osteoporosis. In 1994 her mother's long suffering ended. So did Camilla's marriage to Parker Bowles. What is not clear is whether the original Catholic marriage has been annulled, and on what grounds. The Catholic Church does not countenance divorce. Camilla may still be the wife of Andrew Parker Bowles in the eyes of the Catholic Church. It is notable that she was married to Prince Charles only in a civil ceremony and that some of the privileges of being the wife of the heir apparent are still being withheld.

In the Nineties Camilla's friends in the leafy shires were said to be worried for her. She was said to be desperately unhappy and to cry every day, as the nation's hatred was flung in her face. She bought her own house and took refuge there with her children and her horses, as Charles's marriage too came to an end. The next year brought the shock of the death of the people's princess, and the orgy of public lamentation that ensued. Camilla was by then deep in the peri-menopause. Because her mother and grandmother had both suffered from crippling osteoporosis she had little choice but to use HRT. Meanwhile the gossip columnists and the talk show hosts impudently wondered aloud whether the heir to the throne would or should marry his 'poxed up old slag'.

It was nearly two years before Charles and Camilla appeared in public together. Insults did not stop coming; the reporting of Camilla's wedding to her prince was full of snide innuendo, which continues to this day. The Duchess of Cambridge is said to despise her stepmother-in-law and to have banned her from having anything to do with Prince George and Princess Charlotte. In January 2016 Camilla was rumoured to have decided to dump Charles as a loser and demand a divorce settlement of anything from £175 to £400 million, apparently in the belief that the Queen will abdicate and name Prince William as her successor. The sources for all this scuttlebutt are not close to the royal family or indeed Britain. Gossip-mongering is what we must expect from the tabloids, but more gratuitous is the sneer that emanated from the saintly *Guardian* (5 March 2007) when it was announced in 2007 that the Duchess of Cornwall was to undergo a hysterectomy, which scribbling medico Ann Robinson decided was necessitated by a 'massive prolapse'. This is her verdict.

Clearly, Camilla is unlikely still to be having periods. So, she is most likely to be having her hysterectomy because her womb is full of large, painful fibroids which are non-cancerous lumps in the muscle of the womb, or because the womb has prolapsed and is trailing southwards. According to gynaecologist Nick Morris,

> 'Camilla's probably got a stage IV prolapse and an enterocele and hysterectomy's the only option.' In other words, a womb that's descended so far, it's protruding out of the vagina and loops of bowel that bulge into the vagina.

Nick Morris is a gynaecologist in full-time private practice, who shortens and tidies up labia at the Cadogan Clinic for a mere £4,000 a pop. Ann Robinson on the other hand is a GP who should know better than to think that fibroids are typically 'painful'. Her considered opinion about the causes of prolapse does not inspire confidence either.

> Coughing, constipation, heavy lifting and obesity add extra strain and make prolapse more likely. Hunting isn't mentioned, but I can't imagine that jigging up and down on a horse helps.

'Jigging up and down on a horse'? – a technical term, obviously. It is to be hoped that Robinson makes a better GP than she does a writer, but her willingness to speculate suggests otherwise.

Dancing keeps the body strong; Margot Fonteyn danced with Nureyev from 1962 when she was forty-two until her retirement in 1979. Martha Graham gave her last performance in 1970, when she was seventy-six. The most remarkable hardy perennial among ballerinas has to be the Cuban Alicia Alonso. Alicia was practically blind from the age of nineteen; diagnosed with a detached retina, she underwent a series of operations that made the condition worse. Each time she was made to stay in bed and avoid movement until her eyes had completely healed, in case her recovery was affected. Nevertheless, in 1943, within months of being allowed to dance again, and virtually blind, she was asked to stand in for the injured prima ballerina of the New York City Ballet Theatre and dance the lead in *Giselle*. The critics were unanimous; a star had been born. She danced all over the world to great acclaim until, in 1959, at the invitation of Fidel Castro, she returned to her native Cuba, where she founded the Ballet Nacional de Cuba. I saw her dance in Havana in 1985 aged sixty-four, relying on nothing to guide her but her male partner's encircling arms. Until recently she continued to direct the ballet and to teach Cuban dancers.

Singing too is strenuous exercise. Montserrat Caballé was fifty-four when she recorded 'Barcelona' with Freddy Mercury in 1987. Birgit

Nilsson was in her fifties when she sang in the opening concert of the Sydney Opera House in 1973. Mirella Freni gave her last performance at the Washington National Opera in 2005, at the age of seventy, singing the role of the teenager Ioanna. Christa Ludwig was sixty-six in 1994 when she gave her final performance at the Metropolitan Opera singing Fricka in *Die Walküre*; she and her old sparring partner Elisabeth Schwarzkopf are still teaching masterclasses.

The hardy perennials would all admit that they have been lucky, but their careers illustrate the concomitant truth that without hard work and dedication, that luck could well have come to nothing. At Christmas 2016 a quango called Public Health England informed the nation that eight out of ten forty- to sixty-year-olds were living an unhealthy life, eating too much, drinking too much and not getting enough exercise. A campaign was launched called One You, aimed at the 87 per of men and 79 per cent of women in that age bracket who are overweight or obese, exceed the chief medical officer's guidelines and are physically inactive. The PHE was quoted as saying that middle-aged people eat 'a lot of fast food and sweets' and engage in binge-drinking alcohol. No hard evidence was produced for the assertion, but it does suggest that forty to sixty is a testing time, when far too many people give up on the future. The greatest of the hardy perennials are all enjoying deeper satisfactions and greater successes in their sixties, seventies and eighties than were theirs in those difficult middle years.

16

The Old Witch

Witches are to be found in every human society, throughout history, all over the world. Though young women and men have been accused of sorcery and paid the price, the archetypal witch is both old and female. Women who outlive their husbands, or worse, their children, are anomalies in societies where high maternal mortality has been the norm. Their very survival has something in it of the not-natural; it is inevitable that illiterate villagers will assume that childless, widowed women who live long have thrived at the expense of others, that the younger people who sickened inexplicably and died have been eaten up by them. The old women may even believe it themselves. For peoples who have no other explanation of infertility, sickness and death, belief in witches is a necessity. The ideal candidate must be somebody who will function as a scapegoat. She must therefore be without allies and expendable. In 1563 Johann Wier, in *De Praestigiis Daemonum*, argued that witches were 'poor, mindless old women', 'childish old hags', 'old women of melancholic nature and small brains' to be pitied rather than feared. According to Reginald Scot in *The Discoverie of Witchcraft* published in 1584:

> One sort of such as are said to be witches are women which be commonly old, lame, blear-eyed, pale, foul, and full of wrinkles, poor, sullen, superstitious and papists or such as know no religion, in whose drowsy minds the devil hath gotten a fine seat, so as, what mischief, mischance, calamity or slaughter is brought to pass, they are easily persuaded the same is done by themselves ...

French demonologist Jean Bodin agreed: 'For every male witch there are fifty female witches ...' (fol. 245–245ᵛ). The Mosaic law is quite clear on the correct treatment for witches: 'Thou shalt not suffer a witch to live' (Exodus 22:18; Leviticus 20:27).

The view which seems to have been dominant in the minds of the superstitious was that, in the words of the *Malleus Maleficarum*, the first witch-hunt manual, published in Cologne in 1487, 'To disbelieve in witches is the greatest of heresies.' Although this went against the official Catholic position, and there is a persistent belief that the book was actually banned by the Vatican, it was printed many times and read all over Europe. Even so, by the beginning of the eighteenth century enlightened men like Joseph Addison were arguing that there had never been such things as witches, only superstition, timorousness and prejudice, to which mischievous old women added by their own irrational and meddlesome practices. Yet, at the time that Addison was writing to deplore the cruelty and superstition that led to their persecution, witches were still being sentenced to death by fire.

There should be no more shame in being a witch than in being old, for witches have a long and distinguished history that reaches far back beyond the invention of writing, to the time when women protected the birthplace and the dangerous transitions between life and death. Much of the story is the story of the criminalisation of female power and the discrediting of female knowledge, in order to corrode and eliminate the rights and privileges of mothers. In a society where there is still a degree of matrifocality we are not surprised to find positive images of the powerful old woman. A remarkable example is the folk-tale of Mwipenza the Killer as it used to be told by the Hehe people of Southern Tanzania. Mwipenza is overcome by a very old woman, who was old twenty years before when Makao, the female protagonist of the tale, had gone with her mother to get a medicine for her sister who was dying. The old woman's dark powder had saved the girl's life. Now Makao needs a medicine for her mother but she is attacked by Mwipenza, who lies in wait for her outside the old woman's hut. Her husband finds Makao dying, but before he can pull out the stick that is pinning her to the ground, the old woman comes out of her hut and calls to him for help.

As soon as Makao's husband started towards her the old woman stopped crying and in a very excited voice called out to him, 'I was

just trying your tender heart … You were coming to help me first
and now I will help your wife for you.' (Mvungi, p. 69)

Only then does he see that Mwipenza is lying dead on the ground
transfixed by a pole, killed evidently by the old woman's magic. The old
woman smears a green fluid on Makao's wounds and she is miraculously
made whole. The young couple turns to the ancient woman to ask how
she overcame the killer; she only 'laughed and said, "You two go along
with your child"' (p. 69).

The story is clearly not meant to be taken literally; the ancient
witchdoctress is rather a figure of the matriarchy or the sororal principle
which places the group above the individual and even the couple. She
has something in common with the legendary anchoresses of the early
Christian Church, who emerged from their caves and huts only to
perform prodigies. In *The Manufacture of Madness* Thomas Szasz gives a
useful précis of the witch's role in pre-industrial society.

> Because of the nature of the human bond between suffering peasant
> and trusted sorceress, the good witch becomes endowed with
> great powers of healing: she is the forerunner, the mother, of the
> mesmeric healer, the hypnotist, and the (private) psychiatrist. In
> addition, because she is actually a combination of magician and
> empiricist, the sorceress acquires, by experimenting with drugs
> extracted from plants, a genuine knowledge of some powerful
> pharmacological agents. So advanced is her knowledge that, in 1527,
> Paracelsus, considered one of the greatest physicians of his time,
> burnt his official pharmacopoeia declaring that 'he had learned
> from the Sorceresses all that he knew'. (pp. 84–5)

Witch, healer, shaman, the older woman has another, immensely
important function in pre-literate societies.

> In those tribal communities where birth is aided, the assistant is
> most commonly the woman's own mother. In fact, mother and
> daughter may travel quite a distance to be together at this time.
> The second most common assistants at a tribal birth are women
> from the mother's family, her grandmother, her sisters and/or other
> female relatives from her clan … In tribes that have made the

transition from matrilineal clan to patriarchal family, the mother-in-law may assist … (Goldsmith, pp. 23–4)

Though mothers still need mothering, their mothers are no longer permitted to carry out this important function. Any man who claims to have sired the child, and some who do not even go so far, can assist a woman in childbirth. Any mother who demanded the right of entry to her daughter's labour room would be regarded as overprotective, interfering, even mischief-making. Mother–daughter relationships have decayed so far in our society that there is no reason to expect that a mother's presence would ease rather than exacerbate a daughter's anxiety. There is nothing that a mother knows about childbirth that could be of benefit to her labouring daughter. She certainly would not be allowed to perform her traditional duties of providing physical support at the mother's back, or massaging her abdomen, or keeping her clean and cool. The important change that would be felt, when the woman cradling her daughter between her thighs, supporting her back in her labour, urging her through her contractions, giving birth as it were by proxy to her own grandchild, sees her first grandchild emerge into the light, cannot happen so dramatically. Nowadays the mother's mother will probably not even be the first person to be telephoned or to learn of her changed status. It is hardly necessary to point out that the father's mother would be as welcome in the birthplace as the wicked fairy at the christening of Snow White. We are not surprised to read that a high proportion of the women arraigned in the witch-hunts of the sixteenth and seventeenth centuries were midwives.

As patriarchal society evolved, the real power of women decayed. More and more they were obliged to make do with fantasy power, either to manipulate those with power over them, or to invent fantasy antidotes for real oppression, by casting spells or preparing potions. The realm in which these magical preparations worked was the imagination; a powerless person could be rendered powerful by an amulet or a philtre. He had only to wait for some misfortune to befall his oppressor to feel thoroughly avenged and give (dis)credit to the witch. The old woman who muttered the magic words or collected the moon-drenched herbs was not a cynical manipulator of the credulity of others; all too often she believed in her occult power herself and, as women have always done, shouldered the burden of communal guilt. The women who voluntarily accused themselves at witch-trials, however, represent only the tiniest proportion of women who strove for power over the imagination, most of whom were loved and revered as the tellers of tales.

In tutoring the imagination of the very young, the old wives romanticised and spiritualised a life that was in reality utterly monotonous and dreary. They filled the woods with yearning, sighing souls instead of wind currents and gossamer trails; they put out saucers of milk for the spirits of dead children that clung to the houses where they died young (so very, very many), and lo! in the morning the good sweet milk was gone and the hearth was swept clean and polished by their grateful hands. Grandmothers' fables made the world as thrilling a place as Steven Spielberg's fantasies do now, and did so in a fashion that stimulated the child's creative fantasy, rather than deadening it by repetitive overstimulation. Those who take Addison's view of their activities, and object that old wives' tales fill children with trepidation and make them timid, have misunderstood both how important it is that a child experience suspicion and how children love to be scared out of their wits.

> It has often been pointed out that myths, rhymes, fairy tales
> and children's games shelter vestiges of the old religions. Out of
> northern myths and rites come Mother Goose and her nursery
> rhymes. A turn-of-the century book-cover betrays the bird original
> of Mother Goose. From the letter 'M' of 'Mother' in the title hangs
> a pair of goose feet. Mother Goose herself is shown riding with her
> bird. The broomstick she rides is a whittled-down version of the
> sacred tree, the revered connection between sky and earth. She may
> not be as graceful as Aphrodite, but why should she be? She has
> fallen into a world turned away from nature, a world that in the
> sixteenth and seventeenth centuries ... used fire and water to purge
> away all memory of her former position and of her very existence.
> (Johnson, p. 85)

What wiped out the domestic witch was the spread of literacy. Children have not needed any more to listen at grandmother's knee to fables of the rewards of good children and the deliciously hideous punishments of naughty ones, since education was compulsory and their imaginations given into the control of the printed page. In all societies the illiterate elders begin to lose authority once their children learn to read. When the pace of social change is as dizzy as it has been since the end of the Second World War, having been around longer is a positive disqualification for knowing anything. A grey head is known to be stuffed with obsolescent notions. The fact that university researchers are now tramping the world looking for oral historians can be taken as a sign that oral histories have become a matter for academics and not for the communities who should be listening to them and learning from them. We have lost all the art forms of old women: the lullaby vanished, leaving not one authentic strain behind; the folk song was collected when it was well cracked in the ring; the fairy tale was stolen, distorted, printed and discredited.

In *Persuasions of the Witches' Craft*, Tanya Luhrmann describes a modern, bookish version of the witch:

> [Nature] was the Great Goddess whose rites Frazer and Neumann –
> and Apuleius – recorded in rich detail. Witches are people who read
> their books and try to create, for themselves, the tone and feeling
> of an early humanity, worshipping a nature they understand as
> vital, powerful and mysterious. They visit the stone circles and pre-
> Christian sites and become amateur scholars of the pagan traditions
> behind the Easter egg and the Yule log. (pp. 45–6)

What is being described here is organised witchcraft, which is not the witchcraft of every woman who hangs up a fatty bone for the finches, who tries to be sure to greet the full moon face to face as a mark of respect, who collects firewood on a waning moon and sows seed on a waxing one, who says good morning to the magpie and warns the bees of a birth or a death in the family. Those of us who are gardeners do not need to train ourselves to be aware of the seasons, intuitively or any other way, for the seasons have us by the throat. One kind of witch gathers in pubs and cellars to talk of Isis and Osiris; another kind of red-cheeked, wild-haired witch is to be found tramping along the hedgerows in the wind and rain, followed by her old dog or, even, her cat.

Real witches never had to learn their lore from Frazer, Neumann and Apuleius; real witches were not people who read books to find out what to do and when. Witchcraft is not a matter of generalisations, if only because it has to be closely allied to the spirit of place. Serious mistakes are made in herbal medicine because people do not understand that a herb that grows in a particular way in one place exercises a different function from the same herb growing in different conditions, only a few miles away. The proportions to be used and the methods of preparation must reflect these differences. Certain combinations and decoctions can be helpful in one environment and noxious in others. The meaning of the winds, of dew, of moonshine is different on different sides of the same hill. The books of witchlore that have tried to systematise this vast body of knowledge and extract general principles from it have produced meaningless prescriptions. The kind of mistake they make can be illustrated from a modern example. Researchers in Bangladesh were trying to extract the active principle from an abortifacient used with great efficacy in a particular area. None of their extracts seemed to have any emmenagogic qualities at all. Eventually an old practitioner explained that the women brewed the abortifacient potion in fermented rice water in a copper vessel; the synergistic compound that resulted from that procedure was too dangerous to be included in any modern pharmacopoeia, but it certainly worked.

No witch these days would be allowed to hang out a shingle or practise as a healer, except perhaps upon herself and her animals. Yet in the Seventies, in sophisticated Tuscany, people with intractable ailments still went to the wise woman who was called by the modern version, *strega*, of her classic name *Strix*. She would charm warts away, charm straying love back again, prescribe a gentle wash for skin ailments or a posy of herbs to be fed to cows in the spring to clear their blood, and try a little conservative prediction now and then. She might instruct a young woman with cystitis to arise from her bed at first light and to go out, without urinating or breaking her fast, to find the young basal rosette of *Verbascum thapsiformis*, and, squatting low, to urinate upon it. In the only case I know of the cystitis was cured and never came back. I thought the walk with a full bladder was the most important part of the treatment; the patient was sure that an exhalation arose from the plant and entered her bladder. In the case of an older woman's cystitis the white witch prescribed a mild decoction of lime flowers and camomile to be drunk in quantity, the copious urine that resulted to be cast out where the evil humour would afflict slugs and snails instead of the patient. As an indirect assurance that the old lady would reverse the habit of a lifetime and drink enough water to dilute the acid urine that was irritating her bladder, this portentous to-do could hardly have been bettered.

Mostly, though, the white witch is limited to activities like those of Australian poet Rosemary Dobson's grandmother, 'Amy Caroline', who like the classic Strix is half bird:

> My grandmother, living to be ninety, met
> Whatever chanced with kindness, held her head
> On one side like a sparrow's, had a bird's
> Bright eyes. At dinner used to set
> An extra place for strangers. This was done
> She said in Bendigo and Eaglehawk, it was
> A custom she observed. In her thin house
> That spoke aloud of every kind of weather
> She put out food for lizards, scattered crumbs
> For wrens beside the pepper-tree and saved
> The household water for geraniums.

The outdoor witches of England far outnumber the 30,000 or so who gather in subterranean gloom to burn incense and cast spells, and even the thousands more who dabble in the occult. When Maureen and Bridget Boland published their *Old Wives' Lore for Gardeners* in 1976, old wives rushed to buy it, and their children to buy it for them. Though, as the Boland sisters confessed, they were not old wives but old spinsters, their book contained 'the sort of lore their grandmothers passed down to them' which they wished to pass 'on to those who are not afraid of finding a certain amount of superstition mingled with good sense'.

In 1934 the great psychologist Helene Deutsch, then fifty years old, left Vienna and went to live in America. When it became clear that she and her family could never return to Vienna, they looked for a farm. After one false start they found a dilapidated property in New Hampshire. They renamed it for the Polish witch Babayaga. Considering this forty years later in *Confrontations with Myself*, Deutsch writes:

> What is the relationship of Babayaga to me, the would-be farm-wife immersed in her scientific and professional work? Babayaga is

me, and the legend of this Polish witch leads directly back to my childhood. In Polish folklore, Babayaga is a good witch, who is especially kind to children; she is also a rustic witch, usually seen carrying on her back a load of wood, and sometimes children. Thus both my love for my grandchildren and my fantasies about being a countrywoman have fitted in very well with this figure; she is the prototype of the kind grandmother, even though her mode of transportation is a broom and her passageway the chimney. I told the children many stories about my role as a witch, and I think that Babayaga is to them, even today, associated with their real granny and beloved 'Gruhu'. (p. 193)

On the next page Deutsch, who never mentions her own menopause, describes a period of conflict between her 'emotional preoccupations' and her 'intellectual self'.

I felt like the personification of a children's song my grandsons loved: A peculiar creature turns up in a chicken yard. She feels out of place and unwanted, and moves on to the goose yard. But there too she is greeted by protesting cackles. In despair she asks herself, 'Who am I? I am not a chicken. I am not a goose. I am a chirkendoose.' My grandsons enjoyed this song without knowing how much their grandmother identified with this strange animal. (p. 194)

'Unconscious motives play an especially large role' in the apparently haphazard juxtaposition of themes in writing. The paragraph that follows this deals with Deutsch's pet hen, Jenny, and would have been followed by accounts of other woman–animal identifications if Deutsch had not been 'ashamed' of what the man who ran the farm for her (her superego) would 'think'. The solution is the identification with her land and her animals, the role that she finds in the *genius loci*, the white witch Babayaga.

In December 1949 British psychiatrist Morris Carstairs went to live for a year in a village near Udaipur in Rajasthan. His next-door neighbours were Dhapu, a widow, her son, his wife and their baby. It was months before Carstairs discovered that Dhapu, a forceful woman with a foul temper and an inexhaustible vein of obscene abuse, was believed to be a *dakan* who had been blinding people and causing deaths and disease in the village for at least twenty years. The villagers believed that she had the power to know whenever her name was mentioned and would punish anyone who identified her. Carstairs tried to sympathise with the poor old woman, whom he saw as victimised by a suspicious community, but he was repelled by her vicious hostility towards her co-villagers, by her mendacity and because 'She seemed unable to accept my assurance that I did not believe that she was a witch and that I thought it unfair that she should be so regarded' (p. 21). Carstairs could not quite imagine that a woman would accept the role forced upon her, or that she would glory in her power over the imaginative life of the whole village.

Many of the confessional interrogatories, or penitentials, of the early Middle Ages include questions to be put by the priest regarding the practice of sorcery. This ranged from harmless foolishness like the placing of a fish between the labia to marinade, as it were, for a day or two before cooking it and serving it to a man whose affections one wanted to engage, to flying about at night and attending witches' sabbaths. Burchard's penitential, written at the beginning of the eleventh century, asked:

> Have you believed what many women, turning back to Satan,
> believe and affirm to be true; as that you believe that on the silence
> of the quiet night … you are able, while still in your body, to go
> out through the closed doors, and travel through the spaces of the
> world, together with others who are similarly deceived; and that
> without weapons you kill people … and together cook and devour
> their flesh … if you have believed this, you shall do penance on
> bread and water for fifty days and likewise in each of the seven years
> following.

Clearly Burchard did not share the witches' delusion; the sin that was being confessed was not making a pact with Satan but believing that you had made a pact with Satan. Though Burchard's punishment was harsh, it was enlightened compared to the summary vengeance wreaked on Dhapu. Six months after Carstairs left the village he learned that, as a result of the raving of a feverish woman who was thought to have been possessed by her, Dhapu, who had been beaten several times before, had been hit repeatedly about the face with an axe. The bones of her left forearm, flung up to protect herself, were smashed. As she sank unconscious to the ground, the ravings of her supposed victim ceased. Three days later Dhapu the *dakan* died. Interestingly, Carstairs was anxious that her murderers should not receive too harsh a sentence. In fact two of the killers got six months, of which they served a month, and the third eighteen months, of which he served a year. The woman involved got off scot-free. Meanwhile in the village 'the tension and mistrust seemed to have gone'. Dhapu's death, called 'tragic' by Carstairs, was entirely unregretted and unavenged, even by her son.

The priestly authorities of the Middle Ages, anxious to erect their own law in the place of mob law, rather than punish the witches themselves, punished those who killed witches, by stoning, immersion, or flaying or burning them alive. Perhaps they understood that the witch functioned by the consent and with the complicity of her community. As long as the people respected her occult power, they were failing to respect the visible power of church and state. Societies that make use of witches to exert control over the uncontrollable are the same societies that need to use extremes of brutality in eradicating them.

There would be no point in disembowelling a witch, and parading her intestines through her village, if she had not been a powerful individual. Witchhood brings real power. The old woman whose very shadow can blight anything it falls upon need no longer play the meek, obliterated wife–mother. Her face is uncovered; her death-dealing eye looks out of her head, powerfully penetrating her environment, rather than being penetrated and mastered by it. The representatives of the ruling class have always been sceptical about such power and refused to capitulate to the popular superstition that needed to see witches magically routed by dismemberment or burning. The same lordly view, that old women's power over others was merely a senile delusion on their part and crass credulity on the part of their clients, was widely held until 1921, when Margaret Murray published *The Witch-Cult in Western Europe*, which argued that witches were adherents of an ancient pagan fertility cult. The argument held until 1969, when the anthropologist Lucy Mair pointed out that what witches have in common all over the world is that they are not defined by their adherence to religion but by their rejection of the prevailing moral and social order. In 1975 Norman

Cohn demolished Murray's sources and exposed the ancient fertility religion as a fraud.

The element that remains underemphasised in modern discussions of witchcraft is the extent to which the assumption of a witch role represents a coherent protest against the marginalisation of older women and a strategic alternative to it. Studies of spirit possession have been much more perceptive. In *Case Studies in Spirit Possession*, edited by ethnopsychiatrist Vincent Crapanzano and Vivian Garrison, 'twelve of the fifteen cases presented involve women, and the theme of female powerlessness, as well as the manner in which possession phenomena permit both temporary and long-term increases in women's power and control, is conspicuous in most of the histories' (pp. xi–xii).

'Possession,' argues Crapanzano, 'is found most frequently among people of inferior, marginal, ambiguous or problematic status, especially women' (p. 29). The anthropologists can see quite clearly that spirit possession forms part of a strategy on the part of powerless marginalised people seeking a central role in the life of their community. They agree generally that the strategy is unconsciously adopted, but conscious–unconscious is a continuum rather than a contrast. People in general, and uneducated people in particular, may and do know and not know at the same time. A woman of strong personality reacting against her increasing irrelevance to the world of men and younger women may make a conscious decision to enter the realm of witchcraft, but thereafter certain consequences entail themselves and she may well be carried along upon a momentum that she herself has not generated. Every time an angry woman thinks of her persecutors and says to them in her heart, 'Just you wait. You'll be sorry,' she involves the age-long tradition of witching. When ill befalls them, as sooner or later it must, if her heart rejoices at their being brought low, she is affiliated for ever to the black art.

It makes sense that women, once released from their bondage to their fathers, husbands and sons after a lifetime of being told that they are unstable, unreliable, irrational creatures, should avenge themselves by making a principle out of instability and unreason, working through the superstition and credulity of beings weaker than themselves to positions of real power, well able to subvert duly constituted authority both religious and secular. It makes sense too that they should take as their allies in this strategy other defamed creatures for which society has no use, the owl and the bumble-bee of Daniel Defoe's famous parallel in Appleby's Journal (quoted by Nina Auerbach in *Woman and the Demon*).

> Horrible! Frightful! Unsufferable! An OLD MAID! I had rather
> be metamorphosed into an Humble Bee, or a Screech Owl; the
> first, all the boys run after it to Buffet it with their Hats, then pull
> it a Pieces for a poor dram of Honey in its Tail; and the last, the
> Terror and Aversion of all Mankind, the fore-runner of Ill-luck, the
> foreboder of Diseases and Death. (pp. 110–11)

The witch's familiars are, like her, actually harmless, serviceable creatures, subjected to unreasonable abuse because they are considered unappealing and their real usefulness is unrecognised. Once in league with owls and toads, the old woman can both reject the world's devaluation of her and, by frightening her enemies, revenge herself against them. However, the male authority that the witch subverts by hobnobbing with creatures as unattractive and unnerving as herself may revenge itself with exemplary savagery.

With the exaltation of the natural that follows the triumph of empiricism all evidence of the supernatural or preternatural has to be seen as fraudulent at best, and most likely diabolical. To the convinced empiricist like Addison all invocation of magical power is subversion. The belief that women who have a special understanding of animals must be evil only grows up as distrust of animal nature deepens; that distrust is the product of male supremacist culture and there is no good reason why women should share it. Traditionally women have tended animals, especially small animals and birds. They have bred, fed, prepared and cooked them for their mutual masters' tables while those masters were acquiring the 'enlightened' rationalist education that would deliver the created world into their control.

In 1609, 79-year-old Maria de Zozaya was turned over to the Spanish Inquisition as a witch …

> … when the young priest of the town came home without a single
> hare after having been out hunting all day even he blamed Maria de
> Zozaya. In this case, however, she got no more than she deserved,
> for when the priest passed her house she would say: 'See that you
> catch plenty of hares, Father, so the neighbors can have jugged

hare.' ... Maria de Zozaya confessed to the inquisitors that as
soon as the priest had passed by she turned herself into a hare and
ran ahead of him and his hounds the whole day long so that they
returned home exhausted. This, she added, had occurred eight times
during 1609. (Henningsen, p. 159)

Maria was to die in prison nine months later. It is but a short step
from the old woman's imagining herself to be a hare outrunning the
hounds until they died of exhaustion, to the huntsmen imagining
that a particular hare is not a real hare but a witch transmogrified,
as Wodrow records in his *Analecta* of one Elspey in 1698 (Black,
p. 81). Fourteen years later Addison deplored the fact that 'If a hare
makes an unexpected escape from hounds the huntsman curses Moll
White ... I have known the master of a pack of hounds upon such an
occasion send one of his servants to see if Moll White had been out
that morning.' Though we can only guess at the justification or lack
of it for suspecting Moll White of disrupting the hunt, we can see in
the work of literate women of rank a similar attempt at subversion.
The extraordinary Duchess of Newcastle wrote an extraordinary poem
on 'The Hunting of the Hare' and published it herself in 1653. After a
moving account of the hare's desperate attempts to outrun the hounds,
she turns on man the hunter.

Yet Man doth think himselfe so gentle, mild,
When he of creatures is most cruell wild,
And is so Proud, thinks only he shal live,
That God a God-like Nature did him give.
And that all Creatures for his sake alone,
Was made for him, to Tyrannize upon. (Greer et al., p. 70)

Anne Finch, Countess of Winchilsea, loved to roam on a summer
night, with none but owls and glow-worms for company.

When nibbling sheep at large pursue their food,
And unmolested kine rechew the cud;
When curlews cry beneath the village walls,
And to her straggling brood the partridge calls;
Their short-lived jubilee the creatures keep,

Which but endures whilst tyrant man does sleep ...
(Lonsdale, p. 23)

The Countess would have been astonished, and displeased perhaps, if anyone had pointed out the similarity between her nocturnal carnival of the animals and a witches' sabbath. The Countess's ideals are nothing if not lofty; nevertheless, as she announces her intention to gad about the fields all night, she gives the slightest hint of a witch-like urge to eschew human intimacy and associate with members of the lower orders of creation. In seeing herself and the other animals in 'A Nocturnal Reverie' as inhabitants of a twilit world unknown to the controller man, Anne Finch was lightly sketching in an important change in attitudes, which is an integral part of the gradual demystification of female power. Imaginative or spiritual affinity with the lower orders was not always considered evil. The Celtic princess Melangell, who is revered as a saint, fled into the wilds of Powys to live as an ascetic. A hare pursued by the Prince of Powys and his huntsmen dashed into the glade where she was praying and took refuge in her skirt. When the royal party rode up and the hare peered forth from Melangell's skirt, the hounds fell back whining. When the master of the hunt lifted his horn and blew, no sound came out. The prince was so impressed by this extraordinary circumstance, which he, less enlightened than the Spanish Inquisition or Joseph Addison, took to be evidence of great sanctity, that he granted the forest to Melangell. Ever thereafter hares congregated there and the people called them 'Melangell's lambs'.

This is only one of many stories of the early saints exercising power over and on behalf of animals. According to *Butler's Lives of the Saints* both St Pharaildis and St Werburga are supposed to have restored a plucked and roasted goose to life and full plumage. St Milburga could command the birds of the air; St Bee was fed by seabirds; St Thecla's feet were licked by the lions that should have killed her in the amphitheatre; St Ulphia commanded the local frogs to be silent, and so they are to this day; Blessed Viridiana had two snakes that fed from her plate; all kinds of animals ate out of the hand of St Colette; St Catherine of Vadstena was saved from a rapist by a stag.

Some of the legends that associate saints with animals may represent survivals of older nature religion and goddess worship; the St Gertrude who is never pictured without mice running up and down her staff or playing on her distaff is thought to be a survival of Freya. St Walburga, the great healer, has her feast day on the witches' great festival, the first of May or Walpurgisnacht. As the animal world lost its sacredness and wonder faded into the daylight of rationalism, the women who had power over animals lost their prestige. As man asserted his superiority over the other animals and his right to use and abuse them as he pleased, he persecuted their protectors. Addison would have thought any woman praying in a glade a demented enthusiast. Less advanced thinkers would have suspected her of praying to the tree, or having sexual congress with the green man, now dethroned as a nature-god and a figure of Satan himself.

If we consider the stories of the female saints that are to be found in collections like the *Golden Legend* of Jacopus de Voragine, we cannot fail to be struck by the similarity of their supernatural powers to the proscribed activities of witches. There is hardly a female saint who doesn't have the gifts of prophecy and of reading hearts. Female saints come to people in dreams and appear to crowds in visions with less effort than it took a necromancer to conjure up a single imp. Magical virgins do not scruple to foretell dire punishments that will light upon their enemies, and the hagiographers gleefully recount the disasters that befell all who gainsaid them, whether they were blinded, or fell from a great height, or burst into flames or agonising plague sores; the difference between a saint's prediction of divine retribution and a witch's curse is to the victim merely academic. Virgin martyrs can be dropped into boiling lead or stuck with poniards to the hilt and feel as little as any witch with a bodkin driven into her witchmark. Some saints, like St Christina the Astonishing, could fly; others, like St Mary of Egypt, could walk on water; still others could and did sail across the sea on a leaf. St Martha overpowered a dragon and led him about like a dog with her girdle as a leash. Most of these superwomen were young and virgin. The older woman in search of a role model will find little to emulate in their spectacular careers, in which far too much time was spent fighting off the lewd advances of earthly tyrants who revenged themselves by inflicting the most elaborate and ghastly mutilations and torments. The magical virgin's martyrdom is the precursor of the immolation of the witch; in the case of Joan of Arc, the two coalesced.

The mother of both the female saint and the witch is the sibyl. Representations of sibyls give us virtually the only examples of positive images of older women, whether they be Michelangelo's muscular examples in the lunettes of the Sistine Chapel or the musical versions by Orlandus Lassus. The name 'sibyl' is so ancient that no one knows its derivation. It is thought that sibyls are descendants of the traditional female seers of the Orient, who entered Greek religion through Judaic influence. Only fragments of the original Greek sibylline verses that were revered by the Romans as oracles can now be identified.

> The Romans thought enough of these obscure Greek hexameters
> to scour the Mediterranean world for replacements after a fire had
> destroyed the originals in 83 BC ... Under the Empire, consultation
> of the Sibylline verses stored in the temple of Apollo on the Palatine
> was sporadic. Tiberius vetoed one attempt, but Nero consulted
> them after the great fire of AD 64. The last known consultation
> was made by Julian the Apostate in AD 363, and the books were
> destroyed by Stilicho in about 408. (McGinn, pp. 9–10)

The eight books of Greek hexameters that were believed by the patristic authors, and by medieval and Renaissance writers, to be Oracula Sibyllina were in fact written between the mid-second century BC and about AD 300 and collected and edited by scholars in the late fifth and sixth centuries. The ten sibyls of Varro, namely the Persian, Libyan, Delphic, Cimmerian, Erythraean, Samian, Cumaean, Hellespontic, Phrygian and Tiburtine, became twelve to match the apostles, and were credited with foretelling the birth of Christ. They were supposed to have prophesied the outcome of the Trojan War to Agamemnon and to have led Aeneas through the underworld. Augustine numbered them among the few pre-Christians who would see Heaven. Thus transmogrified into precursors of Christianity, the ancient sibyls were much quoted and painted.

> Having made this adaptation from pagan prophetess to Christian
> seer, the Sibyl was not able to effect a similar transition to the
> modern world where the acids of historical criticism exposed the
> pious forgeries of the past. On the mythic level at least, the image

of the Sibyl, the wise and beautiful old woman inspired by God, deserves our respect and consideration. (McGinn, p. 35)

If we are to be well, we must not cast the old woman out, but become her more abundantly. If we embrace the idea of witchhood, and turn it into a positive, assertive, self-defining self-concept, we can exploit the proliferation of aversion imagery to our own advantage. It is after all no shame or embarrassment to us to know that lager louts find our presence inhibiting. Perhaps we do spoil things for all the boys together propping up the bar in the local pub or littering our highways and byways with their cans or bashing and knifing each other at football matches. So much the better. Why not wear an invisible T-shirt that says 'A glance from my eye can make your beer turn rancid'? Some of the work being done with elderly female patients exhibiting the distorted behaviour associated with senile dementia has found that the old ladies screaming obscene abuse and deliberately soiling themselves have cause for bitter rebellion. Workers are at last considering the possibility that their bizarre behaviour is not evidence of brain decay but of frustrated protest which, if it can be verbalised and externalised, may be to some extent mollified.

Janice Boddy, Professor of Anthropology at the University of Toronto, writing about the Zar cult of Northern Sudan in 1989, came to the conclusion, although tentatively, that 'spirit possession is a feminist discourse, though a veiled and allegorical one, on women's objectification and subordination. Additionally, the spirit world acts as a foil for village life in the context of rapid historical change and as such provides a focus for cultural resistance that is particularly, though not exclusively, relevant to women.' The expression of malevolence through the fantasy outlet of maleficium could be a kind of psychoprophylaxis for the corrosive resentment felt by disenfranchised old women who are denied the right to express any of the hostility and contempt that the younger generation assumes as its birthright. The stereotype of the snowy-haired granny beaming affectionately at her apple pie needs to be balanced by her dark side, with 'tangled black hair, long fingernails, pendulous breasts, flowing tongue between terrible fangs'. That, according to P. F. McKean, is what the Indonesian witch Rangda, 'the mother who is also widow, the one who represents the beginning and end of fertility, or of life' (p. 280), looks like. Rangda does not creep; she dances.

Mary Ellman tells us in *Thinking about Women* that 'the preternatural female is extinct, and none of her former manifestations carries conviction now'. Among the superfemales who have vanished from the earth she lists the 'domestic witch'.

> Traditionally, magic was divided between men and women, exactly as the professions and trades continue to be divided. Male magic was intellectual, female magic was manual. The men pored over portentous charts and symbols and were visited by high-ranking devils. The women cackled and mixed vile broth in pots. (p. 141)

Thinking about Women is a book written with the lightest of scalpel strokes. Ellman's half-serious distinction between male and female magic is based upon a real historical distinction between the black arts of necromancy and conjuration, with their elaboration in satanism, all of which relied upon the cabbalistic texts, and the traditional witching activities of illiterate women, who dealt in divination, charms and healing. However, Ellman's view of witchcraft itself, being based upon literary caricature, is libellous.

As long as illiteracy survives, witchcraft will survive. Until traditional healers and birth-attendants have all been criminalised and punished for competing with institutionalised medicine, the domestic witch will survive. The Western world had to burn its witches out before the Addisons of the eighteenth century could declare confidently that they had never existed. The rest of the world still fears and respects the occult power of wise women. As any health worker knows who has to deal with migrant workers and their families, migrant women refuse to accept the explanations of illness that doctors give them, refuse to carry out modern treatments and struggle to take their sick children home so that the evil influences responsible for their illness can be counteracted by the necessary magic.

Ellman might have been surprised to find how many witches are still in business even in Europe. Italian *streghe* still cast the beans or the *cordella* and still collect porcupine spines for love philtres. English fortune-tellers reading the tea-leaves, interviewees crossing their fingers, women blowing on knotted string to cause impotence in a straying lover, are all helpless people struggling to gain by magic some control over their destiny. Girls sleeping with wedding-cake under their pillows are remembering old sympathetic magic from the same box of tricks as the mixing of a drop of menstrual blood in the beloved's food, or the murmuring of magic rhymes and looking in the mirror on midsummer night to see the shape of their husband-to-be. The experts in these non-religious rituals are of course the old women.

A first step on the road to witchhood is to say, 'You are wrong, my dear fellow. I am old. I am as old as the hills.'

> Witchcraft has not a pedigree
> 'Tis early as our breath
> And mourners meet it going out
> The moment of our death –

(Dickinson, p. 694)

Some ancient crones after all look good, very good. They are the white-bodied witches who tempt the ascetics in the patristic writings, the witches who turn into wrinkled hags during the act of love, as if age was a mark of satanism. Those people who deny to the fifty-year-old woman that she is old are the very people who find age shameful and obscene. They beg us to lie about it for their own comfort.

When Karen Blixen was preparing a speech on African women for the Danish Women's Association in 1937 she wrote:

> All old women had the consolation of witchcraft; their relations with witchcraft were comparable to their relations with the art of seduction. One cannot understand how we, who will have nothing to do with witchcraft, can bear to grow old. (Thurman, p. 317)

Even those of us who look good know that the secret marks of age, the witch-marks, are there. The proliferation of moles and wens, the sags and wrinkles at knees and elbows, the pads on our knuckles, the spurs on our heels, the thinning of our hair, the bristles that sprout on our chins, all are easily hidden, but we know that they are there. If we were to be hauled off and stripped naked at our own witch-trial, they would be seen. So let us assume the witches' right and cackle in our turn. Let us as freely express our malice toward ageists as they towards us. Let us make caricatures of them as relentlessly belittling as their caricatures of us.

In 1985 we began to hear that 'Webs of Crones' had been established by American women who have not been afraid to grow old. Barbara Walker's book *The Crone: Woman of Age, Wisdom and Power* of 1985 is still in print. It and myriad other links and resources can be found on a website called elderwoman.org. There is also Crones Counsel, Inc., which is 'dedicated to claiming the archetype of Crone through the creation of gatherings that honor and advance the aging woman's value to society'. The first meeting of Crones Counsel, with 130 attendees, was held in 1993 at the Snow King Resort, Jackson Hole, Wyoming; the next, twenty-sixth meeting will be held in Bellingham, WA in September 2018.

The Pagan Council of the UK lists eighteen covens none of which appears to be led by older women. Many of them offer training and initiation which would appear to place them close to the mainstream of male-oriented secret societies; one is a Brotherhood for UK Pagan Gay Men. Another is led by a 'high priest'. Whereas the American Crones Counsel (no apostrophe) is a creative, spontaneous, informal get-together in which women bear witness to female experience, the pagan covens appear highly ritualised and even sectarian, being Druid, Wiccan, Hekatean, Alexandrian, Eclectic, Dianian, Gardnerian, Norse or 'Traditional Brythonic'. According to a website on 'how to become a witch' 'modern witches are very social creatures. There are always events and gatherings going on in most major metropolitan areas.' Another site tells would-be witches, including solitary witches, to read all the books they can get their hands on. And that some 'paths have oath-bound information which is held in secret'. None of which is going to appeal to a post-menopausal hedge witch, who will find nothing new or intriguing in hocus-pocus and mumbo-jumbo.

The second number of *Women in Politics* (1986) was devoted to 'Women as Elders: Images, Visions and Issues'. Gert Beadle of the Kelowna Web of Crones contributed an article on 'The Nature of Crones':

> It is in the nature of a Crone to lean to overview, for she is in a
> reflective period of her life and the big picture has her attention.
> She has walked in many moccasins not her own and has observed
> all that pinch and restrict the desire for freedom. (Beadle, p. xiii)

Freedom is not what organised witchcraft is about. Freedom is what you are left with when your subservience to employer, home and family is no longer needed. Freedom is what the Duchess of Newcastle's hare was seeking as he fled the hounds. Freedom was what the Countess of Winchilsea felt as she roamed the darkened fields while her husband slept. Freedom is what the old people who walk out of care homes every week are seeking.

Why not walk in the aura of magic that gives to the small things of life their uniqueness and importance? Why not befriend a toad today?

Witchcraft was hung, in History,
But History and I
Find all the Witchcraft that we need
Around us, every Day –

(Dickinson, p. 656)

17

Serenity and Power

When Karen Blixen was forty-six she came out of Africa back to Denmark. Her coffee plantation in Kenya had gone broke. When it was auctioned off to pay the accumulated debts, the stockholders lost more than £150,000. Her unfaithful husband, whom she had forgiven for giving her syphilis, had insisted on a divorce which she had agreed to with reluctance. All her hopes of pregnancy had been dashed, and she had quarrelled with her lover, who had been killed in a plane crash days later. She had attempted suicide at least once during this turbulent time. She was so thin and frail that her friends had suggested that she go to a clinic in Montreux; there she found out that her syphilis, which had been supposed cured, had become syphilis of the spine, tabes dorsalis. The course of the disease was well known: locomotor ataxia meant she would never again walk properly; anorexia meant that food would nauseate her; she would develop perforating stomach ulcers, and her face would soon take on a deadly pallor and be covered with a grid of tight wrinkles. Her greatest bereavement was the loss of Africa, which left her with a physical longing for the light, the sky and the bush that never faded. Crates of treasured possessions followed her to Denmark, but she did not open them for thirteen years.

Baroness Blixen's way of dealing with her intense physical and mental pain at this crisis time, a climacteric in every sense of the word, was to be reborn as Isak Dinesen. Isaac was the post-menopausal child of Abraham and Sarah, who said when he was born, 'God hath made me to laugh, so that all who hear will laugh with me.' Dinesen was

Blixen's maiden name. She herself called this time her fourth age, saying she began to write 'in great uncertainty about the whole undertaking, but, nevertheless, in the hands of both a powerful and happy spirit' (Thurman, p. 476).

In 1933 this new 48-year-old writer produced *Seven Gothic Tales*. In the first of the tales, 'The Deluge at Norderney', a group of travellers, menaced by a flood tide, take refuge in a barn, where Malin Nat-da-Nog, like a *précieuse* of old, organises them into a salon. For most of her life Malin has been a virginal spinster, until she begins to invent a rakish past for herself and voluntarily to confess to every kind of perversion and every lecherous excess. The night, which ends with the old noblewoman demanding a kiss of a young man, before placing the dripping hem of her skirt in his hand, for the water is rapidly rising round the barn, is a figure of woman's life. The old woman's heroic exercise of imagination on the brink of being overwhelmed is as clear a statement as Blixen ever made of the motivation of her own struggle. She is describing Malin Nat-da-Nog in this passage, but she might as well have been describing herself:

> What changed her was what changes all women at fifty: the transfer
> from the active service of life – with a pension or the honors of
> war, as the case may be – to the mere passive state of a looker on.
> A weight fell away from her; she flew up to a higher perch and
> cackled a little. (Dinesen, 1934, p. 20)

The imagery of the caged bird is important in this collection; it recurs again and again at climactic moments in the stories. Women are seen as caged by their conditioning, by religion and convention; when they are older their grief and rage at their confinement are converted into passionate indignation when they see other creatures caged. In 'The Supper at Elsinore', one of the De Coninck sisters, 'spiritual courtesans' in their early fifties who conduct their own version of a salon, learns that she is soon to meet the ghost of her dead brother:

> Her misery drove her up and down the avenues like a dry leaf
> before the wind – a distinguished lady in furred boots, in her own
> heart a great mad wing-clipped bird, fluttering in the winter sunset.
> (p. 250)

In the story called 'The Monkey', the old Prioress actually changes bodies with her pet monkey. She is determined to procure a marriage between two of her younger kinsmen. The intended groom has a sudden glimpse of the kind of energy that older women can deploy:

> Boris kissed her hand … and then all at once he got such a terrible
> impression of strength and cunning that it was as if he had touched
> an electric eel. Women, he thought, when they are old enough to have
> done with the business of being women, and can let loose their strength
> must be the most powerful creatures in the whole world. (p. 61)

The Prioress, of course, is caged by her religious vocation. As when she escapes she is merely a monkey, her power must remain latent. Karen Blixen had every reason to believe that she had, as she said in a letter to Lady Daphne Finch Hatton, 'one foot in the grave', but once the first book of her fourth age was translated into Danish from the English in which she wrote it she was ready to write her masterpiece. *Out of Africa* is about the Africa she lost, and with it the love, hope, health and light that she would never know again; it is imbued with the elegiac feeling that is the reward for having been able to mourn and to let go. Hannah Arendt explains the importance of story-telling in Blixen's struggle to defy her dreadful illness:

> Without repeating life in imagination you can never be fully alive,
> 'Lack of imagination' prevents people from 'existing'. 'Be loyal to
> the story', as one of her storytellers admonishes the young, means
> no less than Be loyal to life, don't create fiction but accept what
> life is giving you, show yourself worthy of whatever it may be by
> recollecting and pondering over it, thus repeating it in imagination;
> this is the way to remain alive. And to live in the sense of being
> fully alive had early been and remained to the end her only aim
> and desire. 'My life, I will not let you go except you bless me, but
> then I will let you go.' The reward of story-telling is to be able to let
> go: 'When the story-teller is loyal … to the story there, in the end,
> silence will speak.' (Arendt, p. 99)

Karen Blixen exerted her old woman's power many times, enchanting several younger and stronger men into acting out her fantasies for years at a time. In these relationships, although she did not permit herself physical intimacy, she was as exacting as any lover. Using her emaciated appearance and her stark-white, fantastically wrinkled pixie face, with its huge, glittering, kohl-encircled eyes, she fascinated her prey and kept them subject to her whims by binding them fast with the yarns she spun. Racked by her cruel disease, Karen Blixen remains a virtuosa of the art of ageing.

There are not many women who took the art of ageing to such heights of refinement. Possibly the greatest was Madame de Maintenon, who became 'Epouse du Roi' when she was forty-eight (see above, p. 372). Her explanation of the strange joy of old age, so unlike the mixture of unexamined conflicting emotions that afflict us when we are still battling with women's sexual and reproductive destiny, would have been perfectly understood by Karen Blixen, who conscientiously imitated what she imagined was the manner of the *grandes salonnières*: at the end of her life Madame de Maintenon described her feelings in these words:

> I have no regret for the loss of my youth. I do not see anything that makes us happier than detachment and, because to achieve detachment it is necessary to have played one's part in the world, one burns one's youth in accumulating a small store of ecstasy and pain. Believe me, one is well content to find one's soul rich enough to be able to dispense with exaggerated feelings and vain agitations. What satisfaction to know that the drama is played out, and to enter into indifference.

People who are still being made miserable by the play of 'exaggerated feelings and vain agitations' persist in the irrational belief that their torment is what makes life worth living. In 1836 Anna Jameson wrote to her dear friend Ottilie von Goethe, whose on-again off-again love affair with a handsome young English guards officer had resulted in the clandestine birth of an illegitimate third child, sixteen years after her second (legitimate) child:

> Your life has been one of passion and suffering and intervals of *tranquillity* have been to you intervals of *ennui*. When the storm of sensation and emotion is over, you feel as if your heart were dead, but it is not so and I will prove it to you one day. (Erskine, p. 149)

The older woman, who can offer nothing but abiding affection and loyalty to her friend, has to endure many rejections. The very fact that she can be relied upon means that she will be forgotten in the storm of sexual relationships and must wait quietly and unreproachfully until she is required to comfort and console. Anna Jameson persevered in her friendship with Ottilie. The attachment grew stronger and endured until Jameson's death in 1860.

Karen Blixen used to say, 'One must in this lower world love many things to know finally what one loves the best ...' It is simply not true that the ageing heart forgets how to love or becomes incapable of love; indeed it seems as if, at least in the case of these women of great psychic energy, that only after they had ceased to be beset by the egotisms and hostilities of sexual passion did they discover of what bottomless and tireless love their hearts were capable.

In 1862, Christina Rossetti, herself thirty-two, wrote a sonnet about the transformation of one woman, probably her mother, who would then have been in her late fifties. The woman's present condition is seen from the perspective of a younger woman, and is hardly encouraging, but the poet's conviction that a kind of spiritual grandeur resides in the winning of the struggle against negative emotions is genuine.

Ten years ago it seemed impossible
    That she should ever grow as calm as this,
    With self-remembrance in her warmest kiss
And dim, dried eyes like an exhausted well.
Slow-speaking when she has some fact to tell,
    Silent, with long unbroken silences,
    Centred in self yet not unpleased to please,
Gravely monotonous like a passing bell.
Mindful of drudging daily common things,
    Patient at pastime, patient at her work,
Wearied perhaps but strenuous certainly.
Sometimes I fancy we may one day see
    Her head shoot forth seven stars from where they lurk
And her eyes lightnings and her shoulders wings.

                          (Rossetti, vol. 3, p. 286)

Rossetti does not see in this monumental figure the calm of the Blessed Virgin, or any other passive saintly female figure; the figure she describes is that of a sexless Archangel.

Simone de Beauvoir rejected the characterisation of old age as a time of calm, and even more the idea that ageing people should strive for a measure of detachment and tranquillity. She regarded the serene older woman as a perpetuation of the stereotype, a mere continuation of the submissiveness of the feminine woman, and no more authentic. De Beauvoir herself never abandoned the role of consort, although she had in reality increasingly rare opportunities of playing it. She never looked to solitude and found it freedom, because she insisted to such a large extent on living through Jean-Paul Sartre. In cultures where women spend less of their time with men than with children and other women, the role of consort does not bulk so large. The ideal of a peaceful, contemplative third of one's life is more devoutly wished for by agricultural labouring women the world over than it could ever be in our cartoon-comic-strip world where all aunts babble, all old maids gnash their shaky teeth and grandmothers are black beetles equipped with death-dealing handbags and umbrellas. In African village life the large, strong woman plays a very important role. In matrilocal societies, family life revolves about the senior female. Where outwork has taken fathers far away, their mothers must keep their wives and children safe. Older women play an important part in the struggle for the liberation of black Africa. The effects of slavery on the black family are such as to intensify its reliance upon the older woman. The Afro-American woman bears a strong family resemblance to her queenly African counterpart, even when she is forced to live in a menial condition. In *An Unfinished Woman*, Lillian Hellman describes her old nurse, Helen:

> Other people always came in time, to like and admire her, although her first impression of them was not always pleasant. That enormous figure, the stern face, the few crisp words did not always seem welcoming, as she opened a door or offered a drink, but the greatest clod among them came to understand the instinctive good taste, the high-bred manners that once they flowered gave off so much true courtesy. And in the period of nobody grows older or fatter, your mummie looks like your girl, there may be a need in us

for the large, strong woman, who takes us back to what most of us
wanted and few of us ever had. (p. 179)

Though aged writers do not often write about the greatest adventure
of all, growing old, the subject seems to enthral and appal writers on the
threshold of the ageing process, especially in the pre-menopause. This
strengthens the impression of ageing as an external phenomenon, only
identifiable from outside, that is, by the young. There is a certain truth
in this, for one's age is always the centre from which one looks forward
and back, and one has no realisation of the objective fact of one's age.
Perhaps it is the young who need to define age, to push it off and away.
I wonder if I am older or younger than the blue-tit I can see feasting
off horse-chestnut flowers full of dew. He shall certainly die long before
I do, so I guess I am younger after all. I look at women in Tesco and
I cannot tell if I am older or younger than many of them. Younger than
the ones who smoke, older than the ones who don't drink, younger than
the ones who are obese and older? No, younger than the ones who have
less to do. Australians when they are annoyed by someone's behaviour
often snap, 'Oh, be your age!' Though one cannot be anything else, one
cannot consciously be one's age.

Vita Sackville-West was approaching forty when she wrote *All Passion
Spent* for her sons, in order to give them some perspective on growing
old. The account she gives of the last year in the life of the widow of a
'great man' is quietly and subtly subversive. Lady Slane, who had never
lived independently in her life but had always quietly acceded to the
wishes of others, did not like her children or grandchildren very much,
was repelled by their graspingness and ambition, their noisiness and lack
of sensitivity. Rather than accept their rather grudging care, she went
to live in a house in Hampstead with her best friend, her French maid.
There she made new friends of her own generation who understood her
much better than her children, much better indeed than her husband.
One of these is Mr Bucktrout, who owns the house she takes, principal
apologist for their naughty lifestyle:

'The world, Lady Slane, is pitiably horrible, it is horrible because it
is based upon competitive struggle – when I first went into business
… I was fierce … When did I give up these principles? Well, I set
a term on them; I determined that at sixty-five business, properly

speaking should know me no more. On my sixty-sixth [birthday]
I woke a free man.' (pp. 120–3)

Though she makes a valiant attempt at entering the experience of an
old woman, Vita Sackville-West was perhaps too young to get it quite
right. Lady Slane's relationship with her old body seems topsy-turvy.

Her body had, in fact, become her companion, a constant resource
and preoccupation; all the small squalors of the body, known
only to oneself, insignificant in youth, easily dismissed, in old age
became dominant and entered into the tyranny they had always
threatened. Yet it was, rather than otherwise, an agreeable and
interesting tyranny. (p. 194)

Aches and pains are by no means 'insignificant in youth' but
intolerable, unbearable. The young experience pain as an affront,
and often as a source of anxiety, so that pain is complicated by a
psychological dimension that makes it much worse. Part of the battle
for pain relief is simply to remove attention from the pain, rather
than to prevent the pain signal being sent. The young, outraged by
their pain, refuse to ignore it, probe and pick at it; older people
register it and forget it. Young people find certain squalors, flatulence
for example, frightfully embarrassing. An old lady can accept the
fact that she may occasionally belch or fart. Most of the aches
and pains of eld cause no anxiety, being merely the creaking of an
ageing frame. We acknowledge them, salute them like old friends,
and learn gradually to accommodate them. They do not ask to be
irritably rooted out, nor do they insist upon the taking of medicines
to obliterate them. They can be ignored. It becomes a kind of contest
with oneself to see how thoroughly one can forget the sore hip and
the tender knucklebone. To begin to complain of a pain that must
simply be endured is to give it the upper hand, and simply to annoy
the people, if there are any such, who care about one and grieve that
they cannot help. One finds oneself marvelling at the seriousness with
which younger people take minor ailments, the way they dramatise
colds and exaggerate tummy upsets, and demand treatments of no
known efficacy. They do not suspect that 'never mind' is actually a
useful piece of advice.

Mr Bucktrout not only does not regret his own youth, he finds youth itself rather tiresome.

'I find that as one grows older one relies more and more on the society of one's contemporaries and shrinks from the society of the young. They are so tiring. So unsettling. I can scarcely, nowadays, endure the company of anybody under seventy. Young people compel one to look forward to a life full of effort. Old people permit one to look backward on a life whose effort is over and done with. That is reposeful. Repose, Lady Slane, is one of the most important things in life, yet how few people achieve it? The old have it imposed upon them. Either they are infirm or weary. But half of them still sigh for the energy which once was theirs. Such a mistake.' (p. 98)

To the middle-aged woman, repose may seem a long way off. Repose is not torpor or oblivion, but the cessation of fever and fret, of snatch and grab. It has been said that the mark of a gentleman is that he never hurries; it is the paradox of ageing that to hurry is to waste time. If you wish to grasp the present, you must slow down and give the task in hand your full, wide-eyed attention. It is difficult to learn not to hurry, especially when time seems to pass more and more rapidly as one grows older. The way to slow it down is of course to slow oneself down.

Mr Bucktrout reminded Lady Slane how choppy life is at twenty:

'... It is terrible to be twenty, Lady Slane. It is as bad as being faced with riding over the Grand National Course. One knows one will almost certainly fall into the Brook of Competition, and break one's leg over the Hedge of Disappointment, and stumble over the Wire of Intrigue, and quite certainly come to grief over the Obstacle of Love. When one is old, one can throw oneself down as a rider on the evening after the race, and think, Well, I shall never have to ride that course again.'

Lady Slane demurred.

'But you forget, Mr Bucktrout ... when one was young, one enjoyed living dangerously – one desired it – one wasn't appalled.'

Vita Sackville-West had not learned her own lesson herself; still embroiled in slightly pointless *Sturm und Drang*, she imagined that the contemplative life of older people was a grisaille version of the multicolour of youth.

> They were too old, all three of them, to feel keenly; to compete and circumvent and … Those days were gone when feeling burst its bounds and poured hot from the foundry, when the heart seemed likely to split from complex and contradictory desires; now there was nothing left but a landscape in monochrome, the features identical but all the colours gone from them and nothing but a gesture left in place of speech. (p. 117)

The time when the landscape is monochrome is the time of obsession when unmanageable feeling colours all perception. The author has reversed her own image; when the molten matter issues from the foundry it casts on everything its lurid glow. Everything is ruddy and presents only a single glinting lit face to the observer. The lens, moreover, is distorted, for the self interposes between the observer and the thing seen. 'What about me?' it screams. 'Where do I fit in?' It is not possible to answer, 'But this is not about you.' When you are young, everything is about you. As you grow older, and are pushed to the margin, you begin to realise that everything is not about you, and that is the beginning of freedom. Elizabeth Jennings (born 1926) wrote for a collection published in 1972 as *Relationships* a poem called 'Let Things Alone':

> You have to learn it all over again,
> The words, the sound, almost the whole language
> Because this is a time when words must be strict and new
> Not concerning you,
> Or only indirectly,
> Concerning a pain
> Learnt as most people some time or other learn it
> With shock, then dark.
>
> The flowers will refer to themselves always
> But should not be loaded too much

With meaning from happier days.
They must remain themselves,
Dear to the touch.
The stars also
Must go on shining without what I now know.
And the sunset must simply glow. (p. 104)

While one is still the heroine of one's own tale one cannot understand, let alone accept, the rigour of this argument. In fact only by triumphing over self-consciousness can the feminine victim become the female hero.

As the ideal woman, the feminine type is the stepdaughter of masculine civilization, living the consequences of the cultural practices of sexualization and devaluation. Her estrangement from her real self is accommodation to a culture from which she is alienated. Her suffering is both a criticism of that culture and the price she has paid for a flight into dependent safety that 'protects' her from opposing conditions that oppress her. (Westkott, p. 199)

Marcia Westkott is here summarising Karen Horney's theory of the function of psychotherapy, which is to deconstruct the feminine woman's distortion of herself to fit the conflicting demands and expectations of male supremacist culture. Whether we accept Horney's theory of conditioning or not, we cannot but be aware that the middle-aged woman no longer has the option of fulfilling the demands of patriarchal society. She can no longer play the obedient daughter, the pneumatic sex object or the madonna. Unless she consents to enter into the expensive, time-consuming and utterly futile business of denying that she has passed her sell-by date, she has sooner or later to register the fact that she has been junked by consumer culture. She is on her own; as menopause usually cures uterine dysfunction, it also cures the anguish of the feminine supermenial. Horney expected the younger woman to make the heroic pronouncements that are forced on the ageing woman:

First, I (and nobody else) am responsible for my life, for my growth as a human being, for the development of whatever talents I have. It is of no use to imagine that others keep me down. If they actually do, it is up to me to fight them.

Secondly, I (and nobody else) am responsible for what I think, feel, say, do, decide. It is weak to blame others and it makes me weaker. It is useless to blame others, because I (and nobody else) have to bear the consequences of my being and my doing. (p. 200)

The woman ejected from feminine subjection by the consequences of her own ageing can no longer live through others, or justify her life by the sexual and domestic services that she renders. She must, being in free fall, take a long look at the whole landscape that surrounds her and decide how she is going to manage to live in it, no matter how chill the wind that buffets her ill-equipped person. At first she may cling to her old life, trying to claw back something of what she poured into it so unstintingly, but eventually, her grieving done, her outrage stilled, she must let go. Only if she lets go can she recover her lost potency. The younger woman needs her love objects too desperately to love them without hostility in an undestructive way. When the older woman releases or is forced to release her desperate stranglehold and feels herself dropping away, real love will bear her up.

Elizabeth Jennings explores her theme of letting things alone in a series of elegant and tough poems that speak directly to the woman who is turning back into herself, for example, the sonnet called 'Growing' from a 1975 collection called *Growing-Points*:

Not to be passive simply, never that.
Watchful, yes, but wondering ... (p. 106)

The woman new-born after the climacteric can say to herself as Jennings does in 'Accepted' from the same collection:

You are no longer young,
Nor are you very old.
There are homes where those belong.
You know you do not fit
When you observe the cold
Stares of those who sit

In bath-chairs or the park
(A stick, then, at their side)

Or find yourself in the dark
And see the lovers who,
In love and in their stride,
Don't even notice you.

This is a time to begin
Your life. It could be new.
The sheer not fitting in
With the old who envy you
And the young who want to win,
Not knowing false from true,

Means you have liberty
Denied to their extremes
At last now you can be
What the old cannot recall
And the young long for in dreams,
Yet still include them all. (p. 141)

In its beautifully spare diction, with no surface shimmer of effect and
no display of technical virtuosity, this poem is the authentic utterance of
the female survivor, not passive, never that, looking on and loving what
she sees in a way more passionate because uneloquent. This voice is the
idiom of 'disinterest', a word whose real meaning we have forgotten;
her 'disinterest' means that the female hero values the life around her
not because of any use she may make of it, but for itself. As Jennings
said in 'Growing',

The poem leaves you and it sings. (p. 106)

Jennings learned this early, earlier than most of us who only open the
eyes of the soul when we are forced to. From very early in her career her
poems were not about her, nor was she displaying herself in them. In
1986 she wrote in the preface to her own selection from her previously
published collections:

When I re-read my past work I can see a development; to such an
effect indeed, that some of them seem to be no longer any part

of me. But of course once a poem is published it ceases to have much to do with oneself. Art is not self-expression while, for me, 'confessional poetry' is almost a contradiction in terms. (p. 13)

Not all Jennings's later poems manifest the same serenity and power; indeed, any poem is the record of a struggle to achieve its own resolution between disparate and warring elements. Some of Jennings's poems adumbrate a worse bereavement than the one that prompted *Relationships*, as if the poet's detachment had been corroded by the deliberate assault of one who dispossessed her even more brutally than by dying, this time by lying.

The self-possessed woman walking in the golden light of her high detachment excites a certain kind of predator who longs to tumble her back into the darkness of need and hostility masquerading as real life. If she is taken unawares by this last encroachment on her integrity, the older woman can suffer even more bitterly than ever the younger woman writhed in the bonds of sexual passion. It may take her longer to realise the extent of her spiritual disease than it did when she was young, for the soul ages much as the body does, but the devastation is difficult to reverse. The recovery of serenity and power after such infection is painfully slow.

When she was in her early sixties Elizabeth Bishop wrote a deceptively simple poem called 'One Art' that makes a similar point to Jennings's 'Let Things Alone':

> The art of losing isn't hard to master;
> so many things seem filled with the intent
> to be lost that their loss is no disaster.

> Lose something every day. Accept the fluster
> Of lost door keys, the hour badly spent.
> The art of losing isn't hard to master.

> Then practise losing farther, losing faster;
> places and names, and where it was you meant
> to travel. None of these will bring disaster.

The point of the poem is, of course, that the art of losing is hard to master. As for it not bringing disaster, we must conclude with R. D.

Laing that the 'disaster has already happened'. Every menopausal woman panics at her hopeless short-term memory, imagining that Alzheimer's is upon her, when in fact she has never known where she put her keys. The problem is not the losing but the fear of losing; most of what we are afraid of losing is already gone and we have survived. Our illusions of omnipotence and perfectibility were never anything but illusions. That is the dreadful thing that has already happened. Now we can relax and let things slip through our fingers.

Once we lose our sense of grievance everything, including physical pain, becomes easier to bear. As the inflammatory response in the body slows down, so does the inflammation of the mind. As we hoist in the fact that happiness is not something we are entitled to, or even something we are programmed for, we begin to understand that there is no virtue in being miserable. We can then begin to strive for the heroism of real joy. As Dorothy L. Sayers reminded her readers in an essay called 'Strong Meat':

> 'Except ye become as little children', except you can wake on your fiftieth birthday with the same forward-looking excitement and interest in life that you enjoyed when you were five, 'ye cannot enter the kingdom of God'. One must not only die daily, but every day we must be born again. (p. 15)

The lifting up of the heart is a strenuous business and we must work our way into it gradually. This is not a joy that comes from lack of awareness or refusal to contemplate the pain of the world. It comes rather from the recognition of the bitterness of the struggle, not just for ourselves, but for everyone, and the importance of survival. When silly death-wishes and juvenile self-destructiveness are at length driven out, the spiritual athlete can pile on the weights and smile genuinely in her own triumph over a nobler kind of pain than the pangs of self-pity that once beset her. George Eliot wrote in a letter in 1876, when she was fifty-seven:

> Anyone who knows from experience what bodily infirmity is – how it spoils life even for those who have no other trouble – gets a little impatient of healthy complainants, strong enough for extra work and ignorant of indigestion. I at least should be inclined to

scold the discontented young people, who tell me in one breath
that they never have anything the matter with them, and that
life is not worth having – if I did not remember my own young
discontent. It is remarkable to me that I have entirely lost my
personal melancholy. I often, of course, have melancholy thoughts
about the destinies of my fellow-creatures, but I am never in
that mood of sadness which used to be my frequent visitant even
in the midst of external happiness. And this notwithstanding a
very vivid sense that life is declining and death close at hand.
(Haight, 1954, Vol. 6, p. 310)

The discontent of youth passes when you realise that the music you
are hearing is not about you, but about itself. The important thing is
not you listening to the music, but the self-realising form of the music
itself. Then you can begin to understand that beauty is not to be found
in objects of desire but in those things that exist beyond desire, that
cannot be subordinated to any use that human beings can make of
them. Emily Dickinson may have been only thirty-four when she wrote
the following poem, which was discovered and printed only after her
death, but it describes with great fidelity the ageing woman's discovery
of beauty.

As imperceptibly as Grief
The Summer lapsed away –
Too imperceptible at last
To seem like Perfidy –
A Quietness distilled
As Twilight long begun,
Or Nature spending with herself
Sequestered Afternoon –
The Dusk grew earlier in –
The Morning foreign shone –
A courteous, yet harrowing Grace –
As Guest, that would be gone –
And thus, without a Wing
Or service of a Keel
Our Summer made her light escape
Into the Beautiful. (pp. 642–3)

Only when a woman ceases the fretful struggle to be beautiful can she turn her gaze outward, find the beautiful and feed upon it. She can at last transcend the body that was what other people principally valued her for, and be set free both from their expectations and her own capitulation to them. It is quite impossible to explain to younger women that this new invisibility, like calm and indifference, is a desirable condition. At first even the changing woman herself protests against it; she may even take steps to reverse it, by wearing more revealing or garish clothes, but sooner or later she will be forced to accept it. Some of the evidence seems to show that women who have been short-changed by our education system, so that their minds are undeveloped and their imaginations unstimulated, never manage this transition but remain blind and embittered. When they are at the mercy of a mass culture that celebrates older women who 'still remain youthful', that is, spend enormous sums of money in the attempt to fashion themselves into ghastly simulacra of youthful bodies, they have less chance than ever of surmounting the shock of invisibility. They are mocked by the endless succession of stories about middle-aged film-stars becoming engaged to be married, equipped like Jane Fonda and Cher with new silicone breasts to keep the new husbands entertained. Most middle-aged women are shrewd enough to notice that each new marriage of such celebrities breaks up rather sooner than the last. What is not so obvious is that often the husbands have to be paid off; marriage with an ageing box office property is a nice little earner. The shine in the wide eyes of the 55-year-old Hollywood fiancée can also be seen as the white stare of desperation.

Most of us do not have the money that such self-delusion costs. We have to make use of other resources, spiritual resources. Even the woman whose mind and soul have been ignored by everyone, including herself, has within her the spiritual resources to make something of her new life, though she may have some difficulty in getting at them. If no one has ever cared what a woman thought, she may have begun to doubt whether she did actually think. Under the pressure of brutalising work in the home or out of it, she may have indeed stopped thinking; nothing deadens the soul more effectively than a dreary routine of thankless tasks. It may be necessary to break that routine quite violently to free the soul from the weight of petty cares. It may be necessary to disappear for a while, to go bush, in order to begin to reflect. Many of the tales of menopausal women's bad behaviour are simply descriptions of this process. There may be danger in taking time to be alone to reflect, and perhaps to grieve for times that can never return and, worse, bitterer, time that was wasted, but there is more danger in not taking it.

Religion is one of the easier ways that the ageing woman can unlock the door to her interior life. If she has been an unreflective Christian or Hindu or Muslim or Jew or Buddhist she may find it easiest to find her interior life by entering more deeply into the implications of her religion. Examples of the piety of older women are to be seen on all sides; what is not so easy to discern is the joy that entering into the intellectual edifices of the great religions can give, to those who have faith. Women who do not adhere to a particular creed will nevertheless find that in the last third of their lives they come to partake of the 'oceanic experience' as the grandeur and the pity of human life begin to become apparent to them. As one by one the Lilliputian strings that tie the soul down to self-interest and the short view begin to snap, the soul rises higher and higher, until the last one snaps, and it floats free at last. That last string is probably the string of life itself, but you must not ask me to be more precise. My own gyves have not yet quite fallen away – I cannot see so far.

There is nothing original in this view, that:

> An aged man is but a paltry thing,
> A tattered coat upon a stick, unless
> Soul clap its hands and sing, and louder sing
> For every tatter in its mortal dress …
>
> (W. B. Yeats, 'Sailing to Byzantium')

Yeats was one who, in Seamus Heaney's phrase, did not whine at death but withstood it. He knew that he had to gather all his spirituality to confront the inevitability of decay; when 'Sailing to Byzantium' was written his greatest poems were still to write.

Some may prefer a more prosaic formulation of the same idea, which does not invoke religious notions of the 'immortal soul' as a storehouse of grace. More acceptable terms for modern ears are 'self' for soul, and 'energy' for grace, as they are deployed in 'A Philosophy of Energy' by Stanley Jacobs, consultant to the London Borough of Southwark,

Lewisham and the ILEA. Jacobs sees 'self' as the 'source of all energy', of 'infinite worth and value':

> And yet we still believe the most extraordinary things about ourselves – that we are unworthy and unlovable and unable to give love; that we are incomplete and inadequate, bad or mad; that we have been irreparably damaged by certain experiences of life – but self (soul) has always been and will forever be ... (p. 2)

Jacobs cites Camus, of all people, saying that 'in the midst of winter I finally learned that there was in me an invincible summer'.

When I first came to East Anglia, in 1964, I was twenty-five years old. I did not notice the huge skies. I had no time to stand and stare. I would have been surprised to learn that on a typical Mid-Anglia day, you can see on one side a great boil-up of cloud, black and lowering, trailing skirts of precipitation or flirting edges of blinding silver foam, while, turned the other way, the gaze may lose itself in a deep blue vault with chalky chunks of cloud floating in it, while at the zenith crinkled skeins of cirrus are shaken out by a high frigid air stream. Though I saw the obvious things – the green snouts of the crocuses poking through the snow, the red mist in the hedgerows as spring drew on, the flambeaux cast by the chestnuts – I was unaware of the titanic weather war being fought over my head. I could not feel immensity. I could not give in to wonder, because there in my mind's eye was I. Like all young people I was preoccupied with inventing myself. In order to survive I had to fashion a self and project it. A woman, any woman, has to fashion a self that will attract; in every situation, every encounter, she has to be self-conscious. She may be aware of the process that holds her captive, but she cannot escape it. Though I protested about it as a thirty-year-old feminist, I was still its victim and its beneficiary.

I walk the same paths now that I walked fifty years ago, but now I am not aware of the figure I am cutting. I neither expect nor hope to be noticed. I am hoping only to take in what is happening around me even on the bleakest winter day, the blood-warm glow of the upturned clods in the ploughland, the robin's greedy whistle, the glitter of the stubble against a dark sky. I want to be open to this, to be agog, spellbound.

And to do that I have to shake myself free of footlingness. Lady Slane would have known what I mean:

> Certain Italian paintings depicted trees – poplar, willow, alder –
> each leaf separate, and sharp, and veined, against a green translucent
> sky. Of such a quality were the tiny things, the shapely leaves, of
> her present life, redeemed from insignificance by their juxtaposition
> with a luminous eternity.
>   She felt exalted, she escaped from an obvious pettiness, from a
> finicking life, whenever she remembered that no adventure could
> now befall her except the supreme adventure for which all other
> adventures were but a preparation. (pp. 195–6)

You may say that the thrill of discovering such things is only important to Lady Slane and me because we feel nothing else. I would answer that I never knew such strong and durable joy before. Before I felt less on greater provocation; I lay in the arms of young men who loved me and felt less bliss than I do now. What I felt then was hope, fear, jealousy, desire, passion, a mixture of real pain, and real and fake pleasure, a mash of conflicting feelings, anything but this deep still joy. I needed my lovers too much to experience much joy in our travailed relationships. I was too much at their mercy to feel much in the way of tenderness; I can feel as much in a tiny compass now when I see a butterfly still damp from the chrysalis taking a first flutter among the brambles. In her widowhood Willa Muir answered her own anguished cry, 'How shall I live without love?' in this wise.

> Where is my Love, my Dear
> In my heart, in my head,
> Not here,
> Not in my bed.

> Where is my Love, my Dear?
> In my memory, in my mind,
> Not here,
> Not among humankind.

Where is my Love, my Dear?
In poems, in the air,
Here, here,
Nowhere and everywhere.

The feeling may well be elegiac. Though at fifty I did not make every third thought a thought about my death, I was aware of mortality as I never was before. I did not squander my time then and I don't squander it now; I would never dream of bartering an hour of a spring morning to lie in bed. If I am sleepless I go out into the darkness to join the short-lived jubilee of the other creatures. As Mr Bucktrout said:

'Life is so transitory, Lady Slane, that one must grab it by the tail
as it flies past. No good in thinking of yesterday or tomorrow.
Yesterday is gone, and tomorrow problematical.' (p. 126)

'What,' asked the men who were just now making me a new driveway, 'what do you reckon is the best time of life?' They were boys from the black stuff, with a good deal of gypsy in their make-up, so I was less surprised by the question and less suspicious of it than I would have been in different circumstances.

'I reckon it were eighteen', said the older of the two. 'I'm no good for anything now.'

'You might have been good for it then,' said the other, 'but London to a brick you couldn't get any.'

I found myself saying, 'The best time in life is always now, because it is the only time there is. You can't live regretting what's past, and you can't live anticipating the future. If you spend any amount of time doing either of those things you'll never live at all.' Such a commonplace cannot entirely explain my passion for being alive and my hunger to gather up each moment. The theme chimes over and over in Shakespeare's sonnets.

In me thou see'st the glowing of such fire,
That on the ashes of his youth doth lie,
As the death bed, whereon it must expire,
Consumed with that which it was nourished by.

This thou perceivest, which makes thy love more strong,
To love that well, which thou must leave ere long.

(Sonnet 73)

If we continue to see our own age through the eyes of observers much younger, we will find it impossible to understand the peculiar satisfactions of being older. If we can conquer our own lack of interest in ourselves and our kind, and turn to older women's writing about being older women, we will find stated again and again the theme of joy. In 1741 when Mary Chandler, who had suffered all her life from a crooked spine, was fifty-four, she got her first proposal of marriage. This is how she answered it:

At fifty-four, when hoary age has shed
Its winter's snow, and whiten'd o'er my head,
Love is a language foreign to my tongue.
I could have learned it once, when I was young,
But now quite other things my wish employs.
Peace, liberty and sun, to gild my days ...
I want no heaps of gold; I hate all dress,
And equipage. The cow provides my mess ...
I'd rather walk alone my own slow pace,
Than drive with six, unless I choose the place ...
And, when I will, I ramble, or retire
To my own room, own bed, my garden, fire;
Take up my book, or trifle with my pen;
And, when I'm weary, lay them down again:
No questions asked; no master in the spleen –
I would not change my state to be a queen.

(Lonsdale, p. 154)

Chandler, who supported herself by working as a milliner, experienced her solitude as liberty. Women who have lived all their lives in houses filled with noisy other people, responding automatically to the demands of others, might find the sudden silence deafening and frightening, especially if it falls just when menopause is disrupting sleep patterns and mood control. Chandler did not have to shift her focus radically to slide into old maidism, for she had always been alone. Nevertheless, her recipe – peace, liberty and sun – is not a bad one.

Besides liberty, the other important source of delight for the select band of older women who survived fifty years and wrote about it is friendship. For some, like the circle of wise and happy old ladies that surrounded Joanna Baillie and Hannah More, friendship signified society. For others a single relationship was important, as in 'Boston marriages', in which two women pledged a lifelong commitment to each other. The two women agreed to live together, two being able to live as cheaply as one, and to represent for each other emotional security and support in their intellectual or creative endeavours. Many such relationships, like that of Willa Cather and Edith Lewis, Sarah Orne Jewett and Sally Fields, the Ladies of Llangollen and the women who called themselves 'Michael Field', began when the women were young. Some of them were clearly sexual liaisons, scarred with all the betrayals and infidelities that sexual relationships usually suffer. For some middle-aged women friendship flowered into deep sisterly attachment, less interesting to a modern mind but more durable and hardly less deep than the passionate attachments of younger women.

Charlotte Mary Yonge had a bad time in her mid-forties when severe headaches virtually crippled her. She was probably enduring a difficult pre-menopause at the same time that she had to bear the stress of her mother's long decline before she died of softening of the brain in 1868. Yonge was fifty when Gertrude Walker came to live with her and help her with her correspondence. The relationship was probably the happiest time of Charlotte's life; Gertrude, who was crippled, liked to call herself 'Char's wife'. They were to remain together until Gertrude's death in 1897, nearly a quarter of a century later (Coleridge, pp. 270–81).

Once we are past menopause we are all oddballs. We need feel no embarrassment about looking for relationships that do not follow the accepted paradigm. We may find the companionship that may have seemed to be lacking even when we were in the midst of family matters very close by, in a sister or brother we have not seen much of since we both lived in the same house, in a niece, a stepchild, or a home help. Stevie Smith lived with her maiden aunt, Margaret Annie Spear, in a house in Palmer's Green from the time she was three until her death, aged sixty-eight, in 1971. She instructed her biographers not to say 'because I never married I know nothing of the emotions. When I am dead you must put them right. I loved my aunt' (Braybrooke, 1971).

That love, which was not easily come by, is celebrated in her poems:

> My spirit in confusion
> Long years I strove
> But now I know that never
> Nearer shall I move,
> Than a friend's friend to friendship,
> To love than a friend's love.

(Smith, 1985, p. 186)

In the culture of coupledom where no love is worth the name that is not sanctified by genital congress, Stevie Smith's love for her lion-aunt is seen only as a kind of boarding-school substitute for real life. Stevie Smith was well aware of the intolerance that 'normal' or 'ordinary' people would unthinkingly feel about a life as oddly uneventful or 'unfulfilled' as hers, but she had no such feelings herself.

'I love my Aunt. I love her,' she said, 'I love the life in the family, my familiar life' (Smith, 1979, p. 27). For Stevie Smith happiness was 'to have a darling Aunt to come home to, that one admires, that is strong, happy, simple, shrewd, staunch, loving, upright and bossy ...' (p. 28) with 'lionish kind eyes' (p. 30) or 'an eagle managing eye'. Her aunt was 'the Begum Female Spider who has devoured her Suitors and who lives on and makes these crocodile-like pronouncements, and who is like a lion with a spanking tail who will have no nonsense' (p. 38).

Stevie Smith's is not the paradigm of adult life that we have been taught to revere. There is nothing here of Marquez's making love 'like grown-ups'. The 'immaturity' of Stevie Smith's style is the expression of her rejection of the notion of female life that is considered normal, right and proper. She is forced to use the literary instrument shaped by centuries of male elitist culture, but she does so in a deliberately childish way, so that at the same time as she uses it, she subverts it. Her distorted prosody, and the strange bluntness and simplicity of her vocabulary, enact and re-enact her wry refusal to fit her emotions and her sexuality to the contours of a man.

Now I am old I tend my mother's sister
The noble aunt who so long tended us,
Faithful and True her name is. Tranquil.
Also Sardonic. And I tend the house.

It is a house of female habitation
A house expecting strength as it is strong
A house of aristocratic mould that looks apart
When tears fall; counts despair
Derisory. Yet it has kept us well. For all its faults,
If they are faults, of sternness and reserve,
It is a Being of warmth, I think; at heart
A house of mercy.

(p. 410)

When you see that lumpy figure walking on the skyline with her dog, just think, you can never know how happy she is. And as for her, she doesn't feel the need to tell you. People who are really happy do not concern themselves with convincing others of the fact.

While the anophobes draw frightful caricatures of the untreated menopausal woman, and the hormone replacers rend their garments and bemoan the tragedy of the cessation of ovulation, women themselves remain silent. Let younger people anxiously inquire, let researchers tie themselves in knots with definitions that refuse to stick, the middle-aged woman is about her own business, which is none of theirs. Let the Masters in Menopause congregate in luxury hotels all over the world to deliver and to hearken to papers on the latest astonishing discoveries about the decline of grip strength in menopause or the number of stromal cells in the fifty-year-old ovary, the woman herself is too busy to listen. She is climbing her own mountain, in search of her own horizon, after years of being absorbed in the struggles of others. The way is hard, and she stumbles many times, but for once no one is scrambling after her, begging her to turn back. The air grows thin, and she may often feel dizzy. Sometimes the weariness spreads from her aching bones to her heart and brain, but she knows that when she has scrambled up this last sheer obstacle, she will see how to handle the rest of her long life. Some will climb swiftly, others will tack back and forth on the lower slopes, but few will give up. The truth is that fewer women come to grief at this obstacle than at any other in their tempestuous lives, though it is one of the stiffest challenges they ever face. Their behaviour may baffle those who have unthinkingly exploited them all their lives before, but it is important not to explain, not to apologise. The climacteric marks the end of apologising. The chrysalis of conditioning has once for all to break and the female woman finally to emerge.

Works Cited

Abbott, D. (1981) *New Life for Old: Therapeutic Immunology* (London, Frederick Muller)

Aksel, S., Scomberg, D., Tyrey, L., and Hammond, C. (1976) 'Vasomotor symptoms, serum estrogens and gonadotrophin levels in surgical menopause', *American Journal of Obstetrics and Gynecology*, 126:2

Allbutt, T. C., ed. (1896–9) *A System of Medicine by Many Writers* (London, Macmillan)

American Cyclopaedia of Obstetrics and Gynaecology (1887)

Anderson, M. (1983) *The Menopause* (London, Faber & Faber)

Anon. (1851) 'Woman in her psychological relation', *Journal of Psychological Medicine and Mental Pathology*, p. 35

Arendt, H. (1973) *Men in Dark Times* (Harmondsworth, Penguin)

Ashwell, S. (1844) *A Practical Treatise of the Diseases peculiar to Women* (London, Samuel Highley)

Asso, Doreen (1983) *The Real Menstrual Cycle* (Chichester, Wiley)

Auerbach, N. (1982) *Woman and the Demon: The Life of a Victorian Myth* (Cambridge, MA, Harvard University Press)

Austen, J. (1978) *Emma*, ed. R. W. Chapman (Oxford, Oxford University Press)

Avis, Nancy, Coeytaux, R. R., Levine, B., Isom, S., and Morgan, T., (2016) 'Trajectories of response in acupuncture for menopausal vasomotor symptoms: the Acupuncture in Menopause Study', *Menopause*, 23:6

Aylward, M. (1973) 'Plasma tryptophan levels and mental depression in post-menopausal subjects: Effects of oral piperazine-oestrone sulphate', International Research Communications System, Vol. 1, p. 30

Ballinger, C. B. (1975) 'Psychiatric morbidity and the menopause: Screening of general population sample', *British Medical Journal*, 3(5797): pp. 344–6

—— (1976) 'Psychiatric morbidity and the menopause: Clinical features', *British Medical Journal*, i, pp. 1183–5

—— (1977), 'Psychiatric morbidity and the menopause: Survey of a gynaecological outpatient clinic', *British Journal of Psychiatry* 131: 83–9

Banner, L. M. (1990) *The Meaning of Menopause: Aging and its historical context in the twentieth century* (Milwaukee, University of Wisconsin Center for Twentieth Century Studies)

Barentsen, R., Van De Weijer, P. H. M., Van Gend, S., Foekema, H. (2001) 'Climacteric symptoms in a representative Dutch population sample as measured with the Greene Climacteric Scale', *Maturitas*, 38:2

Barnett, R. C., and Baruch, G. K. (1978) 'Women in the middle years: A critique of research and theory', *Psychology of Women Quarterly*, 3:2

Barrett-Connor, E., Wingard, D., and Criqui, M., (1989) 'Postmenopausal estrogen use and heart disease factors in the 1980's', *Journal of the American Medical Association*, 261:2095–2100.

Bart, P. B. (1971) 'Depression in middle-aged women', *Woman in Sexist Society: Studies in Power and Powerlessness*, ed. V. Gornick and B. K. Moran (New York, Basic Books)

——, and Grossman, M. (1978) 'Menopause', *The Woman Patient: Medical and Psychologcal Interfaces*, ed. M. Notman and C. Nadelson (New York, Plenum Press)

Beadle, Gert (1986) 'The nature of crones', *Women and Politics*, 6:2

Bean J. A., Leeper, J. D., Wallace, R. B., Sherman, B. M., and Treloar, A. E. (1979) 'Variations in the Reporting of Menstrual Histories', *American Journal of Epidemiology*, 109:2

Beyene, Y. (1986) 'Cultural significance and physiological manifestations of the menopause: a biocultural analysis', *Culture, Medicine and Psychiatry*, 10:1

Billington, Rachel (1979) *A Woman's Age* (London, Hamish Hamilton)

Bishop, E. (1984) *The Complete Poems 1927–1979* (London, The Hogarth Press)

Black, G. F. (1938) *A Calendar of Witchcraft in Scotland 1510–1727* (New York, New York Public Library)

Blanch, L. (1954) *The Wilder Shores of Love* (London, John Murray)

Boddy, Janice (1989) *Wombs and Alien Spirits: Women, Men, and the Zar Cult in Northern Sudan* (University of Wisconsin Press)

Bodin, J. (1587) *De la demonomanie des sorciers* (Paris, Jacques du Puys)

Bodnar, S., and Catterill, T. B. (1972) 'Amitriptyline in emotional states associated with the climacteric', *Psychosomatics*, 13:2

Boivin M. A. V., and Duges, A. (1834) *A Practical Treatise on Diseases of the Uterus and its Appendages* with notes by G. Heming (London, Sherwood, Gilbert & Piper)

Boland, M. and B. (1976) *Old Wives' Lore for Gardeners* (London, The Bodley Head)

Boland, N. C., and LaVelle, L. (2006) *Menopause: Just the Facts Ma'am* (AuthorHouse)

Boorde, A. (1547) *The Breuiary of Helthe* (London, Wyllyam Myddleton)

Braybrooke, N. (1971) 'Poet Unafraid', *Daily Telegraph*, 14 March, p. 11

Bright, T. (1586) *A Treatise of Melancholie* (London, John Windet)

Brizendine, Louann (2010) *The Female Brain* (New York NY, Broadway Books)

Brown, P. S. (1977) 'Female pills and the reputation of iron as an abortifacient', *Medical History*, 21:3

Browning, E. B. (1911) *The Poetical Works of Elizabeth Barrett Browning* (London, Oxford University Press)

Bucknill, J. C., and Tuke, D. H. (1858) *A Manual of Psychological Medicine: containing history, nosology, description, statistics, diagnosis, pathology, and treatment of insanity, with an appendix of cases*, int. F. J. Braceland (London, Churchill)

Burch J. C., Byrd B. F., Jr, and Vaughan, W. K (1974) 'The effects of long-term estrogen on hysterectomized women', *American Journal of Obstetrics and Gynaecology*, 118:6

Burn, Gordon (1990) *Somebody's Husband, Somebody's Son: The Story of the Yorkshire Ripper* (London, Pan Books)

Burton, R. (1989) *The Anatomy of Melancholy*, ed. T. C. Faulkner, N. K. Kiessling and R. L. Blair (Oxford, Clarendon Press)

Bush, T. L., Barrett-Connor, E., Cowan, L. D. et al. (1987) 'Cardiovascular mortality and noncontraceptive use of estrogen in women: results from the Lipid Research Clinics Program Follow-up Study', *Circulation*. 75: 1102–1109

Butler's Lives of the Saints (1956) ed. H. J. Thurston & D. Attwater (London, Burns & Oates)

Caldwell, J. C., and Caldwell, P. (1977) 'The role of marital abstinence in determining fertility: a study of the Yoruba in Nigeria', *Population Studies*, 31:2

Campagnoli, C., Morra, G., Belforte, P. and L., and Tousijn, L. P. (1981) 'Climacteric symptoms according to body weight in women of different socioeconomic groups', *Maturitas*, 3:3–4

Campbell, S., ed. (1976) *The Management of the Menopause and Postmenopausal Years* (Lancaster, MTP Press)

Campbell, S., McQueen, J., Minardi, J., and Whitehead, M. I. (1978) 'The modifying effect of progestogen on the response of the postmenopausal endometrium to exogenous oestrogens', *Postgraduate Medical Journal*, 54:2

Caplan, P. (1984) *Class and Gender in India: Women and their Organisations in a South Indian City* (London, Tavistock Publications)

Carpenter, J. S., Gass, M. L., Maki, P. M., Newton, K. M., Pinkerton, J. V., Taylor, M., and Utian, W. U. (2015) 'Nonhormonal management of menopause-associated vasomotor symptoms: 2015 position statement of The North American Menopause Society', *Menopause*, 22:11

Carstairs, G. M. (1983) *Death of a Witch: A Village in North India 1950–1981* (London, Hutchinson)

Chakravarti, S., Collins, W., Newton, J., Oram, D., and Studd, J. (1977) 'Endocrine changes and symptomology after oophorectomy in premenopausal women', *British Journal of Obstetrics and Gynaecology*, 84:10

Chandernagor, F. (1984) *The King's Way: recollections of Françoise d'Aubigné, Marquise de Maintenon, wife to the Sun King*, translated by Barbara Bray (London, Collins)

Chari, S., Hopkinson, C. R. N., Daume, E., and Sturm, G. (1979) 'Purification of inhibin from human ovarian follicular fluid', *Acta Endocrinologica*, 90:2

Chattha, R., Kulkarni, R., and Nagarathna, R. (2008) 'Factor analysis of Greene's Climacteric Scale for Indian women', *Maturitas*, 59:1

Chen, R. Q., Davis, S. R., Wong, C. M., and Lam, T. H. (2010) 'Validity and cultural equivalence of the standard Greene Climacteric Scale in Hong Kong', *Menopause*, 17:3

Cohn, N. (1975) *Europe's Inner Demons: an Enquiry inspired by the Great Witch-hunt* (London, Chatto, Heinemann for Sussex University Press)

Coleridge, C. (1903) *Charlotte Mary Yonge: Her Life and Letters* (London, Macmillan)

Colette (1920) *Chéri* (Paris, Arthème Fayard)

—— (1926) *La Fin de Chéri* (Paris, Flammarion)

Collins, Amy Fine (2011) 'The Cult of Diana', *Vanity Fair*, 11 July

Colombey, G. (1968) *Correspondance authentique de Ninon de l'Enclos* (Geneva)

Comfort, A. (1956) *The Biology of Senescence* (London, Routledge & Kegan Paul)

Cooper, Sue Ellen (2004) *The Red Hat Society: Friendship and Fun after Fifty* (Warner Books)

—— (2005) *The Red Hat Society's Laugh Lines: Stories of Inspiration and Hattitude* (Warner Books)

Cooper, W. (1987) *No Change: A Biological Revolution for Women* (London, Arrow Books)

Crane, Maggie Rose (2008) *Amazing Grays: A Woman's Guide to Making the Next 50 the Best 50 *Regardless of your hair color* (FTA Press, San Diego, CA)

Crapanzano, V., and Garrison, V., eds (1977) *Case Studies in Spirit Possession* (New York, London, Wiley)

Crichton Miller, H. (1924) 'The Emotional Basis of Physical Disorder', the *Lancet*, 23 February

Culpeper, N. (1826) *Culpeper's Complete Herbal and English Physician* (Manchester, Cleave & Son)

Cummings, S. R., Black, D. M., and Rubin, S. M. (1989) 'Lifetime risks of hip, Colles', or vertebral fracture and coronary heart disease among white postmenopausal women', *Archives of Internal Medicine*, 149:11

The Cyclopaedia of Practical Medicine: Comprising Treatises on the Nature and Treatment of Diseases, Materia Medica and Therapeutics, Medical Jurisprudence ..., ed. J. Forbes, A. Tweedy and J. Conolly (1833–5) (London, Sherwood, Gilbert & Piper)

D., H. (1956) *Tribute to Freud* (New York, Pantheon)

David, K. (1980) 'Hidden powers: cultural and socio-economic accounts of Jaffna women', *The Powers of Tamil Women*, ed. S. S. Wadley (Syracuse NY, Maxwell School of Citizenship and Public Affairs)

Davis, Donna Lee (1986) 'The meaning of menopause in a Newfoundland fishing village', *Culture, Medicine and Psychiatry*, 10:1

Davis, M. (1957) *The Sexual Responsibility of Women* (London, Heinemann)

Davis, P. (1988) *Aromatherapy: An A–Z* (Saffron Walden, the C. W. Daniel Company)

De Beauvoir, Simone (1962), *The Prime of Life*, trans. P. Green (London, André Deutsch and Weidenfeld & Nicolson)

—— (1965) *Force of Circumstance*, trans, R. Howard (London, André Deutsch and Weidenfeld & Nicolson)

—— (1977) *Old Age*, trans. Patrick O'Brien (Harmondsworth, Penguin)

—— (1984) *The Second Sex*, trans. and ed. H. M. Parshley (Harmondsworth, Penguin)

Dege, K., and Gretzinger, J. (1982) 'Attitudes of families towards menopause', *Changing Perspectives on Menopause*, ed. A. Voda, M. Dinnerstein and S. O'Donnell (Austin, University of Texas Press)

Dement, W., Richardson, G., Prinz, P., Carskadon, M., Kripke, D., and Czeisler, C. (1986), 'Changes of sleep and wakefulness with age'. In *Handbook of the Biology of Aging*, 2nd edn, ed. C. E. Finch and E. L. Schneider (New York, Van Nostrand Reinhold), pp. 721–43

Dennerstein, L. (1987) 'Depression in the menopause', *Obstetric and Gynaecologic Clinics of North America*, 14:1

Deutsch, H. (1945) *The Psychology of Women* (New York, Grune & Stratton)

—— (1973) *Confrontations with Myself: An Epilogue* (New York, Norton)

—— (1984) 'The Menopause', *International Journal of Psycho-Analysis*, 65, Pt 1

Dewees, W. P. (1833) *A Treatise on the Diseases of Females* (Philadelphia, Lea & Blanchard)

Diamond, Lisa M. (2010) *Sexual Fluidity: Understanding Women's Love and Desire* (Cambridge MA, Harvard University Press)

Dickinson, E. (1970) *The Complete Poems*, ed. T. H. Johnson (London, Faber & Faber)

Dinesen, I. (1934) *Seven Gothic Tales*, int. D. Canfield (New York, Harrison Smith & Robert Haas)

—— (1942) *Winter's Tales* (London, Putnam)

Dobson, R. (1965) *Cock Crow* (Sydney, Angus & Robertson)

Donegan, J. (1986) *Hydropathic Highway to Health. Women and Water-cure in Ante-bellum America* (New York, Greenwood Press)

Donovan, J. C. (1951) 'The menopausal syndrome. A study of case histories', *American Journal of Obstetrics and Gynaecology*, 62:6

Drake, E. F. (1902) *What Every Woman of Forty-five Ought to Know* (Philadelphia, Sylvanus Stall)

Dreifus, C. (1977) *Seizing Our Bodies* (New York, Vintage Books)

Dworkin, A. (1987) *Intercourse* (London, Secker & Warburg)

Eisner, H., and Kelly, L. (1980) 'Attitude of women toward the menopause', Paper presented at Gerontological Society Meeting, San Diego, California

Eliot, G. (1895) *Adam Bede* (Edinburgh and London, Blackwood)

Elkins, G., Fisher, W., Johnson, A., Carpenter, J., and Keith, T. (2013) 'Clinical hypnosis in the treatment of postmenopausal hot flashes: A randomized controlled trial', *Menopause*, 20:3

Ellman, M. (1968) *Thinking about Women* (London, Macmillan)

English, O. S., and Pearson, G. H. J. (1958) *Emotional Problems of Living: Avoiding the Neurotic Pattern* (London, George Allen & Unwin)

Erikson, E. (1951) *Child and Society* (New York, Imago)

Erskine, B. E. S. (1915) *Anna Jameson: Letters and Friendships* (London, T. Fisher Unwin)

Evans, B. (1988) *Life Change: A Guide to the Menopause, its Effects and Treatment*, 4th edn (London, Pan Books)

Exton-Smith, A. N. (1986) 'Mineral metabolism', *Handbook of the Biology of Aging*, 2nd edn, ed. C. E. Finch and E. L. Schneider (New York, Van Nostrand Reinhold)

Fairfax family, *Arcana Fairfaxiana Manuscripta* facs, int. G. Weddell (Newcastle-on-Tyne, Mawson, Swan & Morgan)

Fairfield, L. (1923) 'An Address on the Health of Professional Women', the *Lancet*, 3 July

Fairhurst, E., and Lightup, R. (1980) *Being menopausal: women and medical treatment*. Paper presented to the medical sociology group of the British Sociological Association at the University of Warwick, 1980

Faithfull, T. (1968) *The Future of Women and other Essays* (London, New Age Publishers)

Floyer, John (1702) *The ancient psychrolousia revived: or, an essay to prove cold bathing both safe and useful. In four letters* ... (London, Sam. Smith and Benj. Walford)

Fothergill, J. M. (1885) *The Diseases of Sedentary and Advanced Life: A Work for Medical and Lay Readers* (London, Baillière & Co.)

Frankenhaeuser, M., Lundberg, U., and Chesney, M. (1991) *Women, Work and Health: stress and opportunities* (New York, Springer Science)

Freud, S. (1987) *On Psychopathology, Inhibitions, Symptoms and Anxiety*, Pelican Freud Library, Vol. 10 (Harmondsworth, Penguin)

Furuhjelm, M. (1966) 'Urinary excretion of hormones during the climacteric', *Acta Obstetrica Gynecologica Scandinavica*, 45:3

Gajanayake, I. (1987) 'Cessation of childbearing in the absence of contraception in Sri Lanka', *Journal of Biosocial Science*, 19:1

Gardanne, C. P. L. (1816) *Avis aux Femmes qui entrent dans l'âge critique* (Paris, Gabon)

Gaskell, E. C. (1954) *Cranford* (London, J. M. Dent)

Gath, D., Cooper, P., and Day, A. (1982) 'Hysterectomy and psychiatric disorder: Levels of psychiatric morbidity before and after hysterectomy', *British Journal of Psychiatry*, 140:4

Geokas, M. C., and Haverback, B. J. (1969) 'The aging gastro-intestinal tract', *American Journal of Surgery*, 117:6

Gerard, J. (1985) *Gerard's herball: The Essence thereof Distill'd by Marcus Woodward from the edition of Th. Johnson, 1636* (London, Bracken Books)

Ginsburg, J., Swinhoe, J., and O'Reilly, B. (1981) 'Cardiovascular responses during the menopausal hot flush', *British Journal of Obstetrics and Gynaecology*, 88:9

Gleason, R. B. (1870) *Talks to my Patients* (New York NY, Wood and Holbrook)

Goldsmith, J. (1984) *Childbirth Wisdom from the World's Oldest Societies* (New York, Condon & Weed)

Goodale, Jane C. (1980) *Tiwi Wives. A Study of the Women of Melville Island, North Australia* (Seattle and London, University of Washington Press)

Gordon, T., Kannel, W. B., Hjortland, M. C., and McNamara, P. M. (1978) 'Menopause and coronary heart disease: the Framingham Study', *Annals of Internal Medicine*, 89:2

Grant, E. C. (2013) 'Memories of Thatcher', *British Medical Journal*, p. 246

Grasshoff, Malika (2005) 'The central position of women in the life of the Berbers of Northern-Africa exemplified by the Kabyles: the four seasons life cycle of a Kabyle woman', paper delivered to the second world congress on matriarchal studies, San Marcos and Austin TX

Greenblatt, R. (1974) *The Menopausal Syndrome* (New York, Medcom Press)

Greene, J. G. (1984) *The Social and Psychological Origins of the Climacteric Syndrome* (Aldershot, Gower)

—— and Cooke, D. J. (1980) 'Life stress and symptoms at the climacteric', *British Journal of Psychiatry*, 136:5

Greer, G., Hastings, S., Medoff, J., and Sansone, M. (1989) *Kissing the Hod: An Anthology of Seventeenth Century Women's Verse* (London, Virago Press)

Guinan, M. E. (1987) 'Osteoporosis and estrogen replacement therapy – the jury is still out', *Journal of the American Medical Women's Association*, 42:3

Gullette, Margaret (1997) 'Menopause as Magic Marker: Discursive Consolidation in the United States and Strategies for Cultural Combat', *Reinterpreting Menopause: Cultural and Philosophical Issues*, ed. Paul A. Komesaroff, Philipa Rothfield and Jeanne Daly (New York & London, Routledge)

Haight, G. S. (1954–6) *The Eliot Letters* (London, Oxford University Press)

—— (1969) *George Eliot: A Biography* (Oxford, Oxford University Press)

Hallström, T. (1979) 'Sexuality of women in middle age: the Göteborg study', *Fertility in Middle Age: Proceedings of the Eighth IPPF Biomedical Workshop*, ed. A. S. Parkes, M. A. Herbertson and J. Cole. *Journal of Biosocial Science*, 11: Suppl. 6 (London, Galton Foundation)

Halsband, R. (1960) *The Life of Lady Mary Wortley Montagu* (New York, Oxford University Press)

Hammond, C. B., Jelovsek, F. R., Lwee, K. L., Creasman, W. T., and Parker, R. T. (1979) 'Effects of long term estrogen replacement therapy', *American Journal of Obstetrics and Gynaecology*, 133:5

Hancock, E. (1989) *The Girl Within* (New York, Fawcett Columbine)

Hanifi, M. J. (1978) 'The family in Afghanistan', *The Family in Asia*, ed. M. S. Das and P. D. Bardis (New Delhi, Vikas)

Hannon, L. F. (1972) *The Second Chance: The Life and Work of Dr Paul Niehans* (London, W. H. Allen)

Harcourt, Felice, trans. (1969) *Memoirs of Madame de la Tour du Pin* (London, Harvill)

Harmon, Amy (2016) 'Dog test drug aimed at humans' biggest killer, age', *New York Times*, 16 May

Hausman B. B., and Weksler, M. E. (1986) 'Changes in the immune response with age', *Handbook of the Biology of Aging*, 2nd edn, ed. C. E. Finch and E. L. Schneider (New York, Van Nostrand Reinhold)

Hayley, W. (1785) *A Philosophical Historical and Moral Essay on Old Maids* (London, T. Cadell)

Heller, J. (1974) *Something Happened* (London, Jonathan Cape)

Hellmann, L. (1972) *An Unfinished Woman* (Harmondsworth, Penguin)

Henderson, H. W. (1928) *Dianne de Poytiers* (London, Methuen)

Henningsen, G. (1980) *The Witches' Advocate: Basque Witchcraft and the Spanish Inquisition* (Reno, University of Nevada Press)

Herman, G. E. (1898) *Diseases of Women: A Clinical Guide to their Diagnosis and Treatment* (London, Cassell)

—— (1903) *Diseases of Women: A Clinical Guide to their Diagnosis and Treatment*, rev. edn (London, Cassell & Co.)

—— (1907) *Diseases of Women: A Clinical Guide to their Diagnosis and Treatment*, new and rev. edn (London, Cassell & Co.)

—— and Maxwell, R. D. (1913) *Diseases of Women: A Clinical Guide to their Diagnosis and Treatment* (London, Cassell & Co.)

Horney, K. (1967) *Feminine Psychology*, ed., int. H. Kelman (London, Routledge & Kegan Paul)

Hunter, D., Akande, O., Carr, P., and Stallworthy, J. (1973) 'The clinical and endocrinological effect of oestradiol implants at the time of hysterectomy and bilateral salpingo-oophorectomy', *British Journal of Obstetrics and Gynaecology*, 80:9

Hutton, J., Murray, M., Jacobs, H., and James, V. (1978) 'Relation between plasma oestrone and oestradiol and climacteric symptoms', the *Lancet*, i, pp. 678–81

IHF (International Health Foundation) (1969) *A Study of the Attitudes of Women in Belgium, France, Great Britain, Italy and West Germany* (Brussels, IHF)

—— (1975) *The Mature Woman: A First Analysis of a Psychosocial Study of Chronological and Menstrual Aging* (Geneva, IHF)

Jackson, S. H. (1798) *Cautions to Women respecting the State of Pregnancy* (London, G. G. & J. Robson)

Jacobs, Stanley (1989) 'A Philosophy of Energy', *Holistic Medicine*, 4:2

Jaszman, L., Van Lith, N., and Zaat, J. (1969) 'The peri-menopausal symptoms: the statistical analysis of a survey', *Medical Gynaecology and Sociology*, 4:3

Jebb, C. L. [1960] *Dearest Love to All: The Life and Letters of Lady Jebb*, ed. M. R. Bobbitt (London, Faber & Faber)

Jennings, Elizabeth (1986) *Collected Poems* (London, Carcanet)

Jensen, A. K., Kristensen, S. G., Macklon K. T., et al. (2015) 'Outcomes of transplantations of cryopreserved ovarian tissue to 41 women in Denmark', *Human Reproduction*, 30:12

Johnson, B. (1988) *Lady of the Beasts: Ancient Images of the Goddess and her Sacred Animals* (San Francisco, Harper & Row)

Jorden, E. (1603) *A Briefe Discourse of a Disease called the Suffocation of the Mother* (London)

Kapur, P., Sinha, B., and Pereira, B. M. J. (2009) 'Measuring climacteric symptoms and age at natural menopause in an Indian population using the Greene Climacteric Scale', *Menopause* 16:2

Karacan, I., Rosenbloom, A. L., Londono, J. H., Salis, P. J., Thornby, J. I., and Williams, R. L. (1973) 'The effect of acute fasting on sleep and sleep-growth hormone response', *Psychosomatics*, 14:1

Kaufert, P. A., and Gilbert, P. (1986) 'Women, menopause and medicalisation', *Culture, Medicine and Psychiatry*, 10:1

King, J. [1844] *Observations on Hydropathy* (London)

Kisch, E. H. (1926) *The Sexual Life of Woman in its Pathological and Hygienic Aspects* (London)

Kligman, A. M., Grove, G. L., and Balin, A. K. (1986) 'Aging of human skin', *Handbook of the Biology of Aging*, 2nd edition, ed. C. E. Finch and E. L. Schneider (New York, Van Nostrand Reinhold)

Knopp, R. H. (1988) 'Cardiovascular effects of endogenous and exogenous sex hormones over a woman's lifetime', *American Journal of Obstetrics and Gynaecology*, 158:6 (Part 2)

Koster, A. (1990) 'Hormone replacement therapy: use patterns in 51-year-old Danish women', *Maturitas*, 12:4

Kraepelin, E. (1896) *Psychiatrie; ein Lehrbuch für Studierenden und Aertzen* (Leipzig, Barth) 1907

—— (1904) *Lectures on Clinical Psychiatry* (London, Baillière & Co.)

Kreamer, Ann (2007) *Going Gray: How to Embrace Your Authentic Self with Grace and Style* (New York, Little, Brown)

The Ladies Physical Directory or a Treatise of all the Weaknesses, Indispositions and Diseases Peculiar to the Female sex from Eleven Years of Age to fifty or Upwards (1727, at author's appointment at the Gentlewoman's at the Two Blue Posts)

Lahdenperä, M., Lummaa, V., and Russell, A. F. (2005) 'Menopause: why does fertility end before life?', *Climacteric* 7:4

Laszczynska, M, Brodowska, A., Starczewski, A., Masiuk, M., and Brodowski, J. (2008) 'Human postmenopausal ovary–hormonally inactive fibrous connective tissue or more?', *Histology and Histopathology*, 23:2

Lauritzen, C. (1973) 'The management of the pre-menopausal and the post-menopausal patient', *Frontiers in Hormone Research*, 2:1

—— (1990) 'Clinical use of oestrogens and progestogens', *Maturitas*, 12:3

Lee, John R., and Hopkins, V. (online) 'Soy Milk Estrogen and Menopause: The Light and Dark Sides of Soy'

Lessing, Doris (1973) *The Summer Before the Dark* (London, Jonathan Cape)

Lethaby, A. E., Brown, J., Marjoribanks, J., Kronenberg, F., Roberts, H., and Eden, J. (2007) 'Phytoestrogens for vasomotor menopausal symptoms' (The Cochrane Database of Systematic Reviews (4): CD001395)

Levine, M. E., Lu, A. T., Chen, B. H., Hernandez, D. G., Singleton, A. B., Salfati, E., Manson, J. E., Quach, A, Kusters, C. D. J., Kuh, D., Wong, A., Teschendorff, A. E., Widschwendter, M., Ritz, B. E., Absher, D., Assimnes, T. L., and Horvath, S. (2016) 'Menopause accelerates biological aging', *Proceedings of the National Academy of Sciences*

Levinson, D. J., Darrow, C. H., Klein, E. B., Levinson, M. H., and McKee, B. (1978) *Seasons of a Man's Life* (New York, Knopf)

Lindau, S. T., Schumm, L. P., Laumann, E. O., Levinson, W., O'Muircheartaigh, C. A., and Waite, L. J., (2007) 'A Study of Sexuality and Health among Older Adults in the United States', *New England Journal of Medicine*, 357:8

Linnaeus, C. (1753) *Species Plantarum* (Stockholm, Laurentius Salvius)

Lock, M. (1985) 'Models and practice in medicine; menopause as syndrome or life transition', *Physicians of Western Medicine*, ed. R. A. Hahn and A. D. Gaines (Boston, D. Reidel)

—— (1986) 'Ambiguities of aging: Japanese experience and perceptions of menopause', *Culture, Medicine and Psychiatry*, 10:1

Lonsdale, R., ed. (1989) *Eighteenth-Century Women Poets: An Oxford Anthology* (Oxford, Oxford University Press)

Luhrmann, T. M. (1989) *Persuasions of the Witch's Craft; Ritual Magic and Witchcraft in Present-Day England* (Oxford, Basil Blackwell)

Luria, G., and Tiger, V. (1976) *Everywoman* (New York, Random House)

McCay, C. M., Crowell, Mary F., Crowell (1934) 'Prolonging the Life Span', *The Scientific Monthly*, 39:5

MacFadyen, U. M., Oswald, I., and Lewis, S. A. (1973) 'Starvation and human slow-wave sleep', *Journal of Applied Physiology*, 35:3

McGinn, B. (1985) 'Teste David cum Sibylla: The significance of the Sibylline tradition in the Middle Ages', *Women of the Medieval World: Essays in Honor of John H. Mundy*, ed. J. Kirshner and S. F. Wemple (Oxford, Basil Blackwell)

McGrady, P. (1969) *The Youth Doctors* (London, Barker)

McKean, P. F. (1982) 'Rangda the witch', *Mother Worship: Themes and Variations*, ed. J. J. Preston (Chapel Hill, University of North Carolina Press)

Mackenzie, R. (1985) *Menopause: A Practical Self-help Guide for Women* (London, Sheldon Press, SPCK)

Magne, E. (1926) *Ninon de L'Enclos*, trans. and ed. G. S. Stevenson (London, Arrowsmith)

Mair, Lucy (1969) *Witchcraft* (London, Weidenfeld & Nicholson)

Makara-Studzinska, M. T., Krys-Noszczyk, K. M., and Jakiel, G. (2014) 'Epidemiology of the symptoms of menopause: an intercontinental review', *Menopause Review* 13:3

Mankowitz, Ann (1984) *Change of Life: A Psychological Study of Dreams and the Menopause* (Toronto, Inner City Books)

Maresh, M., Metcalfe, M. A., McPherson, K., et al. (2002) 'The UK VALUE hysterectomy study: description of the patients and their surgery', *British Journal of Obstetrics and Gynaecology*, 109:3

Márquez, Gabriel García (1988) *Love in the Time of Cholera*, trans. E. Grossman (London, Jonathan Cape)

Mattson, M. P. (2005) 'Energy intake, meal frequency, and health: a neurobiological perspective', *Annual Review of Nutrition*, 25:237–60

Menville de Ponsan, C. F. (1840) *De l'Age Critique chez les Femmes, des maladies qui peuvent survenir à cette epoque de la vie, et les moyens de les combattre et les prévenir* (Paris, Baillière)

Metz, S. A., Deftos, L. J., Baylink, D., and Robertson, R. P. (1978) 'Neuroendocrine modulation of calcitonin and parathyroid hormone in man', *Journal of Clinical Endocrinology and Metabolism*, 47:1

Michaëlis, K. (1912) *The Dangerous Age*, with an introduction by Marcel Prévost (London, New York, John Lane)

Miles L. E., and Dement, W. C. (1980) 'Sleep and aging', *Sleep*, 3:2

Montagu, M. W. (1967) *The Complete Letters of Lady Mary Wortley Montagu*, ed. R. Halsband (Oxford, Clarendon Press)

Moore, G. (1917) *Lewis Seymour and Some Women* (London, William, Heinemann)

Moran, Christan (2008) 'Mid-life sexuality transitions in women – A queer qualitative study' (thesis 1456263) Southern Connecticut State University

Moreau de la Sarthe, J. L. (1803) *Histoire naturelle de la femme* (Paris, Dupart)

Morton, R. A., Stone, J. R., and Singh, R. S. (2013) 'Mate choice and the origin of menopause', *PLOS Computational Biology*, 9:e1003092

Muir, W. (1969) *Laconics, Jingles and other Verses* (London, Enitharmon Press)

Murdoch, Iris (1987) *Bruno's Dream* (Harmondsworth, Penguin)

Mulley, G., and Mitchell, J. (1976) 'Menopausal flushing: Does oestrogen therapy make sense?', the *Lancet*, i, pp. 1397–9

Murray, M. (1921) *The Witch-cult in Western Europe: A Study in Anthropology* (Oxford, Clarendon Press)

Mvungi, M. A. (1985) 'Mwipenza the killer', *Unwinding Threads: Writing by Women in Africa*, ed. C. H. Bruner (London, Heinemann)

Nachtigall, L. E. and L. B. (1990) 'Protecting older women from their growing risk of cardiac disease', *Geriatrics*, 45:5

Nash, Denis, Magder, Laurence S., Sherwin, Roger, Rubin Robert J., and Silbergeld, Ellen K. (2004) 'Bone density-related Predictors of Blood Lead Level among Peri- and Post-menopausal women in the US', *American Journal of Epidemiology*, 160:9

Nathanson, C. (1980) 'Social roles and health status among women: the significance of employment', *Social Science and Medicine*, 14a:5

Neugarten, B. L., Wood, Viviane, Kraines, Ruth J., and Loomis, Barbara (1968) 'Women's attitudes towards the menopause', *Middle Age and Aging* (Chicago, University of Chicago Press)

—— and Kraines, R. (1965) 'Menopausal symptoms in women of various ages', *Psychosomatic Medicine*, 27:3

Newton, K. M., Reed, S. S., Lacroix, A. Z., Grothaus, L. C., Ehrlich, K., and Guiltinan, J. (2006) 'Treatment of Vasomotor Symptoms of Menopause with Black Cohosh, Multibotanicals, Soy, Hormone Therapy, or Placebo', *Annals of Internal Medicine*, 145:12

North American Menopause Society (2011) 'The role of soy isoflavones in menopausal health: Report of the North American Menopause Society', *Menopause*, 18:7

Nuffield Health (2014) *One in four with menopause symptoms concerned about ability to cope with life*, 17 October, online

Olowali, Antje (2005) ' "Goldmother Created her Children on Earth" – The Kuna Culture', paper delivered at the Second World Congress of Matriarchal Studies

Osol, Arthur, Pratt, Robertson, and Altschule, Mark D. (1967) *US Dispensatory and Physicians Pharmacology* (Philadelphia, Lippincott)

Palma, F., Volpe, A., Villa, P., Cagnacci, A., et al., (2016) 'Vaginal atrophy of women in postmenopause. Results from a multicentric observational study', *Maturitas* 83 (online)

Parker, D. C., Rossman, L. G., and Vanderlaan, E. F. (1972) 'Persistence of rhythmic human growth hormone release during sleep in fasted and nonisocalorically fed normal subjects', *Metabolism*, 21:3

Parkes, A. S., Herbertson, M. A., and Cole, J. (1979) 'Fertility in Middle Age: Proceedings of the Eighth IPPF Biomedical Workshop', *Journal of Biosocial Science*, 11:Suppl. 6. London, Galton Foundation

Pastan, Linda (1978) *The Five Stages of Grief* (New York, W. W. Norton)

Pechey, J. (1699) *A Plain and Short treatise of an Apoplexy, Convulsions, Colick … and other Violent and Dangerous Diseases* (London)

Pettiti, D. B., Wingerd, J., Pellegrin, F., and Ramcharan, S. (1979) 'Risk of vascular disease in women: smoking, oral contraceptives, non-contraceptive estrogens, and other factors', *Journal of the American Medical Association*, 242:11

Pincus, G., Romanoff, L. P., and Carlo, J. (1954) 'The excretion of urinary steroids by men and women of various ages', *Journal of Gerontology*, 9:2

Ploss, H. H., and Bartels, M. and P. (1935) *Woman: an Historical, Gynaecological and Anthropological Compendium*, ed. and trans. E. Dingwall (London, William Heinemann)

Polit, D., and Larocco, S. (1980) 'Social and psychological correlates of menopausal symptoms', *Psychosomatic Medicine*, 42:3

Pollycove, Ricki, Naftolin, Frederick, and Simon, J. A. (2011) 'On the evolutionary origin and significance of menopause', *Menopause*, 18:3

Powell, M. (1972) *The Treasure Upstairs* (London, Pan Books)

Procope, B. (1968) 'Studies on the urinary excretion, biological effects and origin of oestrogens in post-menopausal women', *Acta Endocrinologica*, 60: Supplementum 135

Rees, M. C. P., and Barlow, D. H. (1991) 'Quantitation of hormone replacement induced withdrawal bleeds', *British Journal of Obstetrics and Gynaecology*, 98:1

Reinke, B. J., Ellicott, A. M., Harris, R. L., and Hancock E. (1985) 'The timing of women's psychosocial changes', *Human Development*, 28:5

Riphagen, F. E., Fortney, J. A., and Koelb, S. (1988) 'Contraception in women over forty', *Journal of Biosocial Science*, 20:2

Rosenthal, S. H. (1968) 'The involutional depressive syndrome', *American Journal of Psychiatry*, 124:11S

Ross, R. K., Paganini-Hili, A., Mack, T. M., Arthur, M., and Henderson, B. E. (1981) 'Menopause, oestrogen therapy and protection from death from Ischaemic Heart Disease', the *Lancet*, 18 April (2)

Rossetti, C. (1979–2000) *The Complete Poems: A Variorium Edition*, ed. R. W. Crump (Baton Rouge and London, Louisiana State University Press)

Roth, J. A., with the collaboration of Richard R. Hanson (1977) *Health Purifiers and Their Enemies: a Study of the Natural Health movement in the United States with a Comparison to its Counterpart in Germany* (New York, Prodist, London Croom Helm)

Rudolph-Touba, J. (1978) 'Marriage and the family in Iran', *The Family in Asia*, ed. M. S. Das and P. D. Bardis (New Delhi, Vikas)

Ruzicka, L. T., and Bhatia, S. (1982) 'Coital frequency and sexual abstinence in rural Bangladesh', *Journal of Biosocial Science*, 14:4

Sackville-West, V. (1931) *All Passion Spent* (London, L. & V. Woolf)

Sayers, D. L. (1939) *Strong Meat* (London, Hodder & Stoughton)

Schiff, I, Regenstein, Q., Tulchinsky, D., and Ryan, K. J. (1979) 'Effects of estrogens on sleep of hypogonadal women', *Journal of the American Medical Association*, 242:22

Scot, R. (1584) *A Discoverie of Witchcraft* (London, W. Brome)

Seaman, B. (1969) *The Doctor's Case Against the Pill* (New York, P. H. Wyman)

——, and Seaman, G., M.D. (1977) *Women and the Crisis in Sex Hormones* (New York, Rawson Associates)

Selye, H., Strebel, R., and Mikulaj, L. (1963) 'A Progeria-Like Syndrome produced by Dihydrotachysterol and its prevention by Methyltestosterone and Ferric Dextran', *Journal of the American Geriatric Society*, 11:1

Severne, L. (1979) 'Psychosocial aspects of the menopause', *Changing Perspectives on Menopause*, ed. A. Voda, M. Dinnerstein and S. O'Donnell (Austin, University of Texas Press)

Sévigné, Madame de (1927) *Letters of Madame de Sévigné to her Daughter and her Friends*, ed. Richard Aldington (London)

Sharma, V. K., and Saxena, M. S. L. (1981) 'Climacteric symptoms: a study in the Indian context', *Maturitas*, 3:1

Shatrugna, V., Kulkarni, B., Kumar P. A., et al. (2005) 'Bone status of Indian women from a low-income group and its relationship to the nutritional status', *Osteoporosis International*, 16:12

Sherman, B., Wallace, R. B., and Treloar, A. E. (1979) 'The menopausal transition: endocrinological and epidemiological considerations', in *Fertility in Middle Age: Proceedings of the Eighth IPPF Biomedical Workshop*, ed. A. S. Parkes, M. A. Herbertson, and J. Cole, published as Supplement 6 of the *Journal of Biosocial Science* (London, Galton Foundation)

Shock, N. W. (1986) 'Longitudinal Studies of Aging in Humans', *Handbook of the Biology of Aging*, 2nd edn, ed. C. E. Finch and E. L. Schneider (New York, Van Nostrand Reinhold), pp., 721–43

Shreeve, C. M. (1987) *Overcoming the Menopause Naturally: How to Cope – Without Artificial Hormones* (London, Arrow Books)

Sierra, B., Hidalgo, L. A., and Chedrau, P. A. (2005) 'Measuring climacteric symptoms in an Ecuadorian population with the Greene Climacteric Scale', *Maturitas*, 51:3

Simms, H. S., and Stolman, A. (1937) 'Changes in human tissue electrolytes in senescence', *Science*, No. 86, pp. 269–70; republished in *Aging*, ed. G. H. Emerson, Benchmark Papers in Human Physiology, 11 (Stroudsburg PA, Dourden, Hutchinson & Ross, 1977)

Smith, John (1723) *The curiosities of common water; or The advantages thereof in preventing and curing many distempers. Gather'd from the writings of several eminent physicians, and also from more than forty years experience* (London, J. Billingsley, J. Roberts, A. Dodd & J. Fox)

Smith, Stevie (1979) *The Holiday* (London, Virago)

—— (1985) *The Collected Poems of Stevie Smith* (Harmondsworth, Penguin)

Stamm, L. (1984) 'Differential power of women over the life course: a case study of age roles as an indicator of power', *Social Power and Influence of Women*, ed. L. Stamm and C. D. Ryff (Epping, Bowker)

Stevenson, G. S., trans. and ed. (1925) *The Letters of Madame: the Correspondence of Elizabeth Charlotte of Bavaria, Princess Palatine, Duchess of Orleans* (London, Chapman & Dodd)

Stone, S., Mickal, A., Rye, P., and Phillip, H. (1975) 'Postmenopausal symptomatology, maturation index, and plasma estrogen levels', *Obstetrics and Gynecology*, 45:6

Stroope, S., McFarland, M. J., and Uecker, J. E. (2015) 'Marital Characteristics and the Sexual Relationships of U.S. Older Adults: An Analysis of National Social Life, Health, and Aging Project Data', *Archives of Sexual Behavior*, 44:1

Stuart, M., (1979) *The Encyclopedia of Herbs and Herbalism* (London, Orbis)

Studd, J. W. W., ed. (2003) *Management of the Menopause* (Boca Raton, FL, Parthenon)

—— and Chakravarti, S., and Orain, D. (1977) 'The climacteric', *Clinics in Obstetrics and Gynaecology*, 4:1

—— and Thom, M. H., Paterson, M. E. L., and Wade-Evans, T. (1980) 'The prevention and treatment of endometrial pathology in post-menopausal women receiving exogenous oestrogens', *The Menopause and Post-menopause*, ed. N. and R. Paoletti and J. L. Ambrus (Lancaster, MTP Press)

—— and Thom, M. H. (1981) 'Oestrogens and endometrial cancer', *Progress in Obstetrics and Gynaecology*, ed. J. W. Studd (London, Churchill Livingstone)

Sturdee, D. W., and Brincat, M. (1988) 'The hot flush', *The Menopause*, ed. J. W. W. Studd and M. I. Whitehead, with a Foreword by R. M. Greenblatt (Oxford, Blackwell Scientific Publications)

—— and MacLennan, A. (2004) 'Evolution and Revolution at the Menopause', *Climacteric*, 7:4

—— and Wilson, K. A., Pipil, E., and Crocker, A. D. (1978) 'Physiologic aspects of the menopausal hot flush', *British Medical Journal*, 2:79

Summers, M., ed. (1967) *The Works of Aphra Behn* (New York, Phaeton)

Sutherland, E. (1985) 'New Life at Kyerefaso', *Unwinding Threads: Writing by Women in Africa*, ed. C. H. Bruner (London, Heinemann)

Sydenham, T. (1701) *The Whole Works of that Excellent Practical Physician*, trans. J. Pechey (London, R. Wellington)

Szasz, Thomas (1970) *The Manufacture of Madness: A Comparative Study of the Inquisition and the Mental Health Movement* (New York, Harper & Row)

Thompson, B., Hart, S., and Durno, D. (1973) 'Menopausal age and symptomatology in a general practice', *Journal of Biosocial Science*, 5, pp. 71–82

Thurman, J. (1982) *Isak Dinesen: The Life of a Storyteller* (New York, St Martin's Press)

Tiger, Virginia (1986) 'Woman of many summers: The Summer Before the Dark', *Critical Essays on Doris Lessing*, ed. V. Tiger and C. Sprague (Boston, G. K. Hall)

Tilt, E. J. (1857) *The Change of Life in Health and Disease* (London, John Churchill)

Tolstoy, Sophie Andreyevna (1929) *The Countess Tolstoy's Later Diary 1891–1897*, trans. Alexander Werth (New York, Paysan Clarke)

Travers, C., O'Neill, S. M., King, R., Battistutta, D., and Khoo, S. K. (2001) 'Greene Climacteric Scale: norms in an Australian population in relation to age and menopausal status', *Climacteric*, 8:1

Treloar, A., Boyton, R. D., Benn, B. G., and Brown, B. W. (1967) 'Variation of the human menstrual cycle through reproductive life', *International Journal of Fertility*, 12, pp. 77–126

Trye, M. (1675) *Medicatrix, or the Woman-Physician* (London, Henry Broome & John Leete)

Utian, W. (1978) *The Menopause Manual: A Woman's Guide to the Menopause* (Lancaster, MTP Press)

—— (1980) *The Menopause in Modern Perspective* (New York, Appleton, Century, Croffs)

—— (2012) 'A decade post-WHI, menopausal hormone therapy comes full circle – need for an independent commission', *Climacteric*, 15:320

Van Keep, P. A., and Kellerhals, J. (1974) 'The impact of socio-cultural factors on symptom formation: some results of a study on ageing women in Switzerland', *Psychotherapy and Psychosomatics*, 23:1–6

—— and Utian, W. H., and Vermeulen, A., eds (1982) *The Controversial Climacteric: The workshop moderators' reports presented at the Third International Congress on the Menopause held in Ostend, Belgium, in June, 1981, under the auspices of the International Menopause Society*

Van Look, P. F. A., Lothian, H., Hunter, W. M., et al. (1977) 'Hypothalamic– pituitary–ovarian function in perimenopausal women', *Clinics in Endocrinology*, 7:1

Vermeulen, A. (1983) 'Androgen secretion after age 50 in both sexes', *Hormone Research*, 18:1–3

Walker, B. G. (1985) *The Crone, Women of Age, Wisdom, and Power* (San Francisco, Harper & Row)

Wallace, R. B., Sherman, B. M., Bean J. A., Leeper, J. P., and Treloar, A. E. (1978), 'Menstrual cycle patterns and breast cancer risk factors', *Cancer Research*, 38:11 (Part 2)

Weber, M. T., Rubin, L. H., and Maki, P. M. (2013) 'Cognition in perimenopause: the effect of transition stage', *Menopause*, 20:5

Weissman, M. M. (1979), 'The myth of involutional melancholia', *Journal of the American Medical Association*, 242:8

[Wesley, John] 1747 *Primitive Physic, or an Easy and Natural Method of Curing Most Diseases*

Westcott, P. and Black, L. (1987) *Alternative Health Care for Women: A Compendium of Natural Approaches to Women's Health and Well-being* (Wellingborough, Thorsons)

Westkott, Marcia (1986) *The Feminist Legacy of Karen Horney* (New Haven and London, Yale University Press)

Whitehead, M. I., Campbell, S., Dyre, G., Collins, W. P., Pryse-Davies, J., Ryder, T. A., Rodney, M. I., McQueen, J., and King, R. (1978) 'Progestogen modification of endometrial histology in menopausal women', *British Medical Journal*, 2:6152

—— and McQueen, J., Minardi, J. and Campbell, S. (1978) 'Clinical considerations in the management of the menopausal endometrium', *Postgraduate Medical Journal*, 54 (2), pp. 59–64

Whiting, P. W., Clouston, A., and Kerlin, P. (2002) 'Black cohosh and other herbal remedies associated with acute hepatitis', *Medical Journal of Australia*, 177:8

Wier, J. (1568), *De Praestigiis Daemonum et incantationibus ac veneficiis libri sex* (Basel, Ex Officina Oporiniana)

Wilbush, J. (1988) 'Climacteric disorders – historical perspectives', *The Menopause*, ed. J. W. W. Studd and M. I. Whitehead (Oxford, Blackwell Scientific Publications)

Williams, R., Karacan, I., and Hursch, C. (1974) *Electroencephalography (EEG) of Human Sleep: Clinical Applications* (London, Wiley)

Wilson, G. I. (2000) *Understanding Old Age: Critical and Global Perspectives* (London, Sage Publications)

Wilson, R. A. (1966) *Feminine Forever* (London, W. H. Allen)

Winter, Susan (2000) *Older Women, Younger Men* (New York, Horizon Press)

Wiser, C. V. (1978) *Four Families of Karimpur* (Syracuse NY, Maxwell School of Citizenship and Public Affairs)

Witchel, Alex (1993) 'On Tour with Helen Gurley Brown; Go Ahead, Say it: Sex and the Senior Woman', *New York Times* (1 April)

Wollstonecraft, Mary (1792) *A Vindication of the Rights of Woman: with strictures on political and moral subjects* (London, J. Johnson)

Yeats, W. B. (1961) *Collected Poems* (London, Macmillan)

Index

A Note on the Type

The text of this book is set Adobe Garamond. It is one of several versions of Garamond based on the designs of Claude Garamond. It is thought that Garamond based his font on Bembo, cut in 1495 by Francesco Griffo in collaboration with the Italian printer Aldus Manutius. Garamond types were first used in books printed in Paris around 1532. Many of the present-day versions of this type are based on the *Typi Academiae* of Jean Jannon cut in Sedan in 1615.

Claude Garamond was born in Paris in 1480. He learned how to cut type from his father and by the age of fifteen he was able to fashion steel punches the size of a pica with great precision. At the age of sixty he was commissioned by King Francis I to design a Greek alphabet, and for this he was given the honourable title of royal type founder. He died in 1561.